Mosby's Fundame
ANIMAL HEALTH T[...]

SMALL ANIMAL ANESTHESIA

Mosby's Fundamentals of
ANIMAL HEALTH TECHNOLOGY

Series editor
Roger G. Warren, V.M.D.

SMALL ANIMAL ANESTHESIA
Roger G. Warren

SMALL ANIMAL SURGICAL NURSING
Diane L. Tracy, *Editor*

SMALL ANIMAL RADIOGRAPHY
Lawrence J. Kleine

PRINCIPLES OF PHARMACOLOGY
Richard Giovanoni

Mosby's Fundamentals of
ANIMAL HEALTH TECHNOLOGY

SMALL ANIMAL ANESTHESIA

Roger G. Warren, V.M.D.

The University of Florida,
School of Veterinary Medicine,
Gainesville, Florida

with 151 illustrations

The C. V. Mosby Company

ST. LOUIS • TORONTO • LONDON   1983

MOSBY

A TRADITION OF PUBLISHING EXCELLENCE

Editor: Eugenia A. Klein
Assistant editors: Kathryn H. Falk, Jean F. Carey
Manuscript editor: Sylvia B. Kluth
Book design: Jeanne Bush
Cover design: Diane Beasley
Production: Carolyn Biby

The C.V. Mosby Company
11830 Westline Industrial Drive, St. Louis, Missouri 63141

Library of Congress Cataloging in Publication Data

Warren, Roger G.
  Small animal anesthesia.

  (Mosby's fundamentals of animal health
technology)
  Bibliography: p.
  Includes index.
  1. Anesthesia in veterinary surgery.   I.   Title.
II.   Series.
SF914.W37   636.089′796   82-6421
ISBN 0-8016-5398-3   AACR2

C/VH/VH 9 8 7 6 5   05/C/642

Contributor

ALISTAIR I. WEBB
B.V.Sc., Ph.D., M.R.C.V.S., D.V.A., D.A.C.V.A.
Assistant Professor of Veterinary Anesthesiology,
Department of Medical Sciences,
University of Florida,
College of Veterinary Medicine,
Gainesville, Florida

Preface

Since the inception of the first formal college-level training program for animal health technicians (AHTs) in 1961, the demand for skilled veterinary paraprofessionals has grown appreciably. In 1975, the American Veterinary Medical Association (AVMA) assumed the responsibility for the accreditation of AHT programs and established the Committee on Animal Technician Activities and Training (CATAT). In the same year, the Association of Animal Technician Educators (AATE) was formed for the purpose of assuring quality instruction for students, providing guidance to graduate AHTs, and assisting educators and practitioners. Since then, many state veterinary licensing boards and practice acts have instituted examinations and certification requirements for AHTs.

In spite of a well-established and well-organized educational foundation, there has been no compilation of text material written expressly for the AHT. The Mosby series addresses this need by providing comprehensive information that will enable educators and practitioners to blend this material with both formal and in-service training programs. The text material is liberally illustrated and presented in a way that facilitates student and curriculum evaluation. Specific performance objectives are provided at the beginning of each chapter to aid the instructor in developing a curriculum or training program and to help the student in comprehending the focus of the material.

It is our hope that this series will expand and improve in concert with the burgeoning field of animal health technology.

Roger G. Warren

Contents

1

Preanesthetic considerations

PERFORMANCE OBJECTIVES

After completion of this chapter, the student will:

- Discuss those factors that affect the selection of a particular anesthetic method
- Describe the performances involved in a routine preanesthetic physical examination
- List the indications for use of preanesthetic medications in small animals
- Discuss the advantages and disadvantages of using a narcotic in preference to a tranquilizer for preanesthetic sedation
- Explain the term "neuroleptanalgesia"
- Know the commonly used drug combinations for the dog and cat
- List the general precautions associated with the use of preanesthetic sedative medications
- List the indications and contraindications for the use of muscle-paralyzing drugs during anesthesia
- Demonstrate the ability to solve routine drug dosage calculations, using common metric measurements and conversions

Before actually administering a general or local anesthetic to an animal, it is important to consider those factors that can influence the anesthetic state. The patient should be evaluated physically and physiologically before anesthesia is induced in order to avoid and/or predict possible complicating factors that may have a bearing on the success of the procedure. Drugs referred to as "preanesthetics" are given primarily to prepare the animal for the induction and maintenance of general anesthesia. Many of these have analgesic and sedative properties that allow chemical restraint of an animal for minor surgical procedures without the risk of a general anesthetic.

The use of preanesthetic drugs is still a matter of personal discretion among veterinarians. As medicine surely is not an exact science, so too must one realize that these drugs have both advantages and disadvantages. The veterinarian accustomed to using preanesthetic drugs rarely discontinues their use. However, it often becomes a dangerous habit to administer tranquilizers to every animal undergoing anesthesia, be it for a major or minor procedure. The use of preanesthetic drugs must vary according to the individual animal and the particular circumstances.

As the veterinary profession continues to grow and advance, so too will the role of the animal health technician (AHT) in both anesthesia and surgical services. As the AHT's responsibilities increase, it becomes imperative to gain an understanding of those concepts essential to the successful administration of anesthesia in small animal patients. The first chapter in this unit on small animal anesthesia is primarily concerned with proper patient evaluation before anesthesia and the use and disuse of preanesthetic drugs in dogs and cats. A short section on parenteral drug dosing has been included at the end of the chapter to introduce the student to basic concepts of drug calculations for parenteral administration of medications.

EVALUATING THE ANESTHETIC PROCEDURE

The major purpose for spending time and money evaluating all animals that are to receive anesthetic drugs is to determine those underlying factors that could lead to an "unexpected" anesthetic complication. In many instances, a particular anesthetic can be avoided if the animal has a superimposed disease or metabolic disorder that would be aggravated by a certain anesthetic drug or procedure. Avoiding a problem is always the most desirable course of action, especially when such a problem could result in the unnecessary loss of an animal's life.

Factors affecting selection of anesthetic method

Each of the following factors should be considered in selecting the most appropriate anesthetic method:

- Nature of the procedure
- Physical status of the animal
- Preanesthetic physical examination of the animal
- Availability of trained personnel
- Facilities and equipment for anesthesia
- Familiarity with anesthetic technique

Nature of the procedure

The term "procedure" refers to either a surgical operation or a diagnostic examination such as a radiograph, a myelogram, or a cerebrospinal fluid (CSF) tap. Several questions should be asked before beginning any procedure:

1. Is the procedure necessary to save the animal's life, or can it be postponed to a time when the animal can better withstand the stress of anesthesia and surgery? General anesthesia must be considered a major stress to an animal's physiologic state, especially when the animal must also cope with other stressful conditions such as metabolic disease, trauma, parasitism, dehydration, anemia, and fear.

2. What is the anticipated duration of the anesthesia needed to perform the procedure? Procedures in excess of 50 to 60 minutes require selection of the safest possible anesthetic drug and method.

3. Will the surgical operation result in possible anesthetic complications? Thoracic surgery, for example, lends itself to problems of patient ventilation once the negative pressure of the chest has been disrupted. The possibility of cardiac arrest is increased whenever the heart and/or vagus nerve are manipulated by the surgeon. Surgery on or around a major blood vessel could result in acute hypovolemic shock should the vessel be accidentally ruptured or lacerated by the surgeon or a surgical instrument.

4. Will the positioning required for the procedure interfere with the animal's normal respiratory or cardiovascular status under anesthesia? Every attempt should be made to maintain the animal in as normal a physiologic position as possible. Positions that overextend or hyperflex the limbs, neck, or head should be avoided. The animal's airway and endotracheal tube should be continually checked to ensure that they have not become kinked or obstructed in any way. Heavy drapes, towels, or instruments must not compress the chest of small dogs or cats. Care should be taken to avoid tilting the animal on the surgical table more than 10 to 15 degrees as this position may compress the diaphragm with abdominal viscera and impinge on the animal's ventilation and cardiovascular functions.

5. When the procedure is diagnostic (for example, a survey radiograph for hip dysplasia), is general anesthesia necessary, or can tranquilization or narcotic

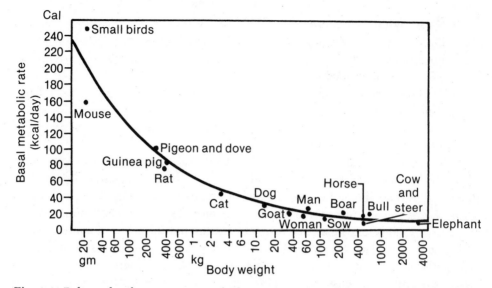

Fig. 1-1. Relationship between average body weight (horizontal axis) and basal metabolic rate per kilogram per day (vertical axis). Anesthesia lowers the metabolic rate and oxygen consumption. Shivering increases the metabolic rate in skeletal muscle tissue and hence increases oxygen demand.

sedation be used? Certain diagnostic procedures may result in serious complications such as seizures following a myelogram, anaphylactic shock resulting from an allergic reaction to the iodine injection during an intravenous pyelogram, abdominal hemorrhage following a liver punch biopsy, ruptured urinary bladder following a pneumocystogram, etc.

6. Can the surgical procedure be accomplished using local analgesia rather than general anesthesia? Local analgesia coupled with manual restraint may be less stressful than general anesthesia, especially to an older dog or cat. Many animals will tolerate short surgical procedures, such as suturing a minor laceration or removing a small skin tumor, with only a local analgesic injection and mild restraint. The concepts of "general" versus "local" anesthesia are discussed in Chapters 2 and 3.

Physical status of the animal

The rate at which anesthetic drugs are detoxified (metabolized) and eliminated from the body is directly related to the metabolic rate of the individual animal. The higher the basal metabolic rate, the faster the drug is metabolized and removed from circulation to the brain and other body compartments. Fig. 1-1 compares the basal metabolic rates for different species of animals according to weight and energy expenditure (measured in calories). Some of the physical factors to consider regarding the effect of an animal's metabolic rate on desirable drug dosage are considered here.

Species. Animals of a relatively large body mass and low metabolic rate (for example, dogs or sheep) require *less* of an anesthetic drug dosage per unit of body weight than smaller animal species that have a higher metabolic rate—for example, cats, rats, or birds (Fig. 1-1).

Size of breed. The smaller the breed of animal, the *greater* will be the relative dosage of anesthetic drug per unit of body weight required to produce and maintain anesthesia. A 45-kg German shepherd dog, for instance, requires less of a barbiturate dosage per kilogram than a 3-kg toy French poodle.

Breed and body type. Certain breeds of dogs and cats are particularly sensitive to the depressant action of barbiturate anesthetics. Animals that are naturally lean and muscular require *less* anesthetic drug than obese animals of a similar weight. Greyhounds, whippets, Afghans, and salukis are known for their tendency to become overly depressed from barbiturates because they have very small amounts of body fat for redistribution of the drug. These sighthound canines tend toward overdepression from barbiturates well into the recovery period and therefore require a substantially reduced dosage from that given other breeds. If the comparison is based on body type within one breed of dog or cat (for example, a fat beagle versus a lean, healthy beagle), the obese animal will have a lower metabolic rate and therefore require less of an anesthetic dosage per kilogram than the lean one. Lean animals also tend to recover from ultrashort-acting barbiturate anesthetics at a slower rate than their obese counterpart. In addition, brachycephalic breeds of dog or cat tend to have difficulty breathing under general anesthesia because of their relatively short nasal passages and large soft palates. Breeds such as pugs, Pekingese, Boston terriers, and Persian cats may require an anticholinergic drug to reduce salivary and tracheal secretions while they are under a general anesthetic. Further, it is wise to always intubate the trachea of a brachycephalic animal to ensure a patent airway during the anesthesia and recovery periods.

Condition of the animal. Animals that are dehydrated, anorexic, or in generally poor condition require less of an anesthetic dosage than healthy animals.

Age. Newborn animals begin life with a relatively low metabolic rate. At puberty, the metabolic rate reaches its maximum and gradually declines with increasing age. Neonatal and geriatric animals are more sensitive to the depressant action of anesthetic drugs because of their low metabolic rate and relatively inactive enzyme detoxification system. Anesthetics that require detoxification before they can be eliminated from the bloodstream must be used cautiously with such animals to avoid overly depressing them with a dosage normally administered to a healthy middle-aged animal. Animals between 3 and 12 months of age seem to require the largest relative dosage of anesthetic drug to produce and maintain the anesthetic state. Barbiturates should be avoided in animals younger than 3 months of age because of comparatively immature liver function.

Sex. Male animals have a slightly higher metabolic rate than females (see Fig.

1-1) and may therefore require more anesthetic drug per unit weight than their female counterpart. Sex hormones appear to have some influence over the response to a particular anesthetic drug, especially to the length of recovery from barbiturate anesthesia. Conflicting data, however, continue to make this issue controversial.

Disposition and activity level. Since the metabolic rate of an animal increases with activity or fear, very active or fearful animals require more of a sedative or anesthetic drug dosage than would a quiet, docile animal. Hypothyroidism causes a reduction in metabolic rate, and, consequently, an animal with this condition requires less of an anesthetic dosage than does a normal animal.

Trauma. Injured animals are often in a state of shock or weakened health. Caution must be exercised when administering general anesthesia to such animals, especially if internal injuries have caused liver, kidney, brain, respiratory, or cardiovascular impairment. Radiographs should be considered for any animal struck by a car to check for the possible sequelae of pneumothorax, collapsed lung, diaphragmatic hernia, ruptured urinary bladder, or abdominal hemorrhage.

Classification of physical status. The physical status of the animal should be determined by using the classification system adopted by the American Society of Anesthesiologists (ASA) (see Table 1-1). Following the preanesthetic physical examination, the appropriate classification numeral should be recorded in the animal's hospital record. Classification of risk may vary according to personal interpretation but will help in the selection of the safest anesthetic method for a variety of different situations.

Preanesthetic physical examination of the animal

All animals entering a hospital for elective surgery or diagnostic procedures that require anesthesia (anesthetic drugs) should routinely receive a *complete physical examination* before admission. Particular attention should be paid to the respiratory, cardiovascular, renal, and hepatic systems. The animal's owner should be made aware of the usual risk associated with anesthesia and surgery as well as any additional risk that may be discovered on physical examination. Some veterinary hospitals are requiring that, before the animal is admitted, the owner read and sign a hospital release form that carefuly states risks and liabilities.

Before beginning any medical/surgical procedure, a patient history must be taken. Particular questions should be asked regarding:
1. Previous illnesses, heat cycle, pregnancy, or surgeries
2. Existing diseases such as those affecting the heart, respiratory system, kidneys, or liver; any blood or neurologic disorders; and diabetes, cancer, heartworms, and parasitism
3. Exposure to drugs such as steroids, insulin, anticonvulsants, tranquilizers, anesthetics, organophosphates, insecticides, antibiotics (especially neomycin, polymyxin B, streptomycin, kanamycin, or gentamicin)

TABLE 1-1
Classification of patient's physical status*

Category	Physical condition	Examples of possible situations
Class I MINIMAL RISK	Normal healthy animal No underlying disease	Ovariohysterectomy; castration; declawing operation; hip dysplasia radiograph
Class II SLIGHT RISK	Animals with slight to mild systemic disturbances Animal able to compensate No clinical signs of disease	Neonate or geriatric animals; obesity; fracture without shock; mild diabetes; compensating heart or kidney disease; low-grade heartworm infestation
Class III MODERATE RISK	Animals with moderate systemic disease or disturbances Mild clinical signs	Anemia; anorexia; moderate dehydration; low-grade kidney disease; low-grade heart murmur or cardiac disease; moderate fever
Class IV HIGH RISK	Animals with preexisting systemic disease or disturbances of a severe nature	Severe dehydration; shock; anemia; uremia or toxemia; high fever; uncompensating heart disease, diabetes, or pulmonary disease
Class V GRAVE RISK	Surgery often performed in desperation on animals with life-threatening systemic disease or disturbances not often correctable by an operation. Includes all moribund animals not expected to survive 24 hours. Little need for general anesthesia as the moribund state renders the animal oblivious to pain	Advanced cases of heart, kidney, liver, lung, or endocrine disease; profound shock; major head injury; severe trauma; pulmonary embolus

*An "E" is added to the classification if the procedure is of an emergency nature.

4. Tendency of the animal toward drug reactions or allergies
5. Previous blood transfusions
6. Recent feedings

A complete physical examination should be conducted by the veterinarian with technical assistance provided by the AHT. (AHTS are presently certified in many states to assist or perform basic physical examinations in the animal owner's presence provided they are acting under the direct supervision of a licensed veterinarian.) The examination should include:

1. Determination of body temperature
2. Auscultation of heart and lung sounds
3. Determination of pulse status
4. Examination of eyes, conjunctiva, mouth, pharynx, tongue, teeth, nose, gingiva, and lips
5. Examination of mucous membranes of the eyes, mouth, and genitalia for color and capillary refill time
6. Examination of skin and hair coat for degree of hydration, signs of allergy, dermatitis, or parasitism
7. Palpation of superficial lymph nodes
8. Palpation of abdominal organs
9. Determination of common reflexes used to monitor the patient during general anesthesia (refer to Chapter 2)
10. Evaluation of central nervous system (CNS), especially when epidural anesthesia or myelograms are anticipated
11. Determination of the animal's temperament, activity level, and gait
12. Determination of the animal's packed cell volume (PCV), hemoglobin (Hb), and total protein (TP)

In addition, the following procedures, where they are indicated, should be completed before administering anesthetic drugs:

1. Electrocardiogram (ECG) in animals with either high risk cardiac disease or abnormal pulse
2. Laboratory tests on all animals in ASA Class II or above or on animals over 6 years of age. These should include CBC, BUN, SGPT, creatinine, urinalysis, or any other appropriate clinical laboratory test.
3. Thoracic and/or abdominal radiographs in all major trauma cases or in aged animals when trauma or disease may be suspected
4. Correction or stabilization of patient with acidosis, dehydration, electrolyte imbalance, anemia, infection, parasitism, malnutrition, or renal, hepatic, or cardiovascular imbalance
5. Administration of appropriate intravenous fluids to high risk patients: for example, animals over 6 years of age, patients with renal or hepatic disease, and those undergoing procedures lasting more than 45 to 60 minutes and/or involving significant blood loss. Examples of commonly used fluids are:
   a. *Ringer's lactate*—a balanced electrolyte solution for most operative procedures
   b. *Normal saline*—fluid of choice in animals with metabolic alkalosis due to vomiting and/or excessive diarrhea
   c. *Dextrose*—useful for supplying calories to animals under 4 to 6 months of age or those with diabetes. The fluid should contain at least 5.0% dextrose.

d. *Dextrose 2.5% in* $^1/_2$*-strength saline:*—suitable for general operative procedures or if animal has been slightly anorexic or dehydrated before anesthesia

e. *Plasma*—useful in cases of burns, anticipated blood loss when whole cross-matched blood is unavailable, and total plasma protein levels below 5.0 gm/dl

6. Witholding of food from the animal for 8 to 12 hours before anesthesia—24 to 36 hours if intestinal surgery is to be performed. Water is allowed up to 4 hours before anesthesia unless the procedure involves the stomach or digestive tract, when water should be withheld for 8 to 12 hours. Animals with known kidney disease and most geriatric animals should never be deprived of water for longer than 2 hours.

It is sometimes impossible to perform all these procedures in addition to a complete physical examination in high risk emergency patients where time is often a major factor in the survival of the animal. There may not be time to wait for laboratory test results, for instance, in a nonelective operation such as repairing a ruptured urinary bladder or a traumatic perforation in the abdomen of a dog. Discretion combined with decisive action must be shown in emergency situations. Elective procedures allow for a greater degree of flexibility in choosing anesthetic drugs or systems best suited for the animal. Safe anesthesia and successful surgery are both dependent on a systematic preanesthetic routine for evaluating the patient to detect those factors that could influence an individual animal's response to anesthetic drugs. The importance of a well-organized and thorough approach cannot be overemphasized, as more and more the duties of history taking and patient evaluation are becoming the responsibility of the trained AHT. Nowhere is this organized and systematic approach more valuable in the avoidance of "unexpected" events than in the busy, high surgical volume small animal practice.

Availability of trained personnel

The ultimate responsibility for the safety of patients in an animal hospital resides with the attending veterinarian, who may find well-trained and experienced AHTs a practical investment. They are invaluable for restraining and calming excitable animals. More than this, they can be important members of a team approach to safe and successful anesthesia and surgery. The duties of preanesthetic medication, anesthetic induction, and patient monitoring are only a few of the responsibilities within the capabilities of a conscientious and properly educated AHT.

Facilities and equipment for anesthesia

It is best if the area for inducing general anesthesia and preparing the animal for surgery is close to but separate from the room where sterile surgery is performed. Such a room is commonly termed the "prep" room. It should be well lighted, quiet, and designed for easy cleaning of table and floor surfaces. It should also be well organized and uncluttered with all equipment and supplies required for anesthesia maintained in adequate supply and ready for use (see Fig. 1-2). If inhalation anesthesia is used extensively, the "prep" room should be included in the centralized piping of compressed oxygen and nitrous oxide. Since flammable anesthetic gases are rarely, if ever, used today, it is safe to use electrical clippers and vacuum cleaners in the preparation room.

An anesthetic emergency box should be within easy reach and continually checked to ensure that all items are in good supply and not beyond expiration date. A small- to medium-sized fishing tackle box is often used for an emergency box, as it is portable and contains folding drawers to store drugs separately. As an aid to reducing a panic response to emergency situations, it is wise to post one or several protocol flow charts designed to facilitate the selection of drugs in the treatment of shock and cardiac arrest. The chart(s) should be placed on a wall within easy view in the surgery and recovery room areas, secured to the emergency box or attached to the ECG machine (see Table 1-2).

Equipment and supplies useful in the preparation room, operating room, and recovery room for the anesthesia of small animal patients include:

General items
Stainless steel "prep" table
Animal positioner
Movable cart
Urine collection pan
Accurate stand-on weight scale (metric reading)
Infant scale (metric) for weighing small animals such as birds, kittens, and puppies
Cloth towels or blankets
Cotton, gauze, adhesive tape, sterile sponges
"Prep" tray
Alcohol dispenser
Sterile lubricant
Ophthalmic ointment
Clippers with surgical blades (no. 40)
Bandage scissors
Intravenous catheters, jugular catheters
Sterile instruments for cut-down use
Sterile gloves of assorted sizes
Caps and masks
Intravenous fluid selection in 250, 500, and 1,000 ml containers
Fluid administration sets
IV infusion stands
Blood administration and collection sets
3-way stopcocks
Rectal thermometer
Stethoscopes (regular and esophageal)
Antiseptic for use on endotracheal tubes, rubber breathing tubes, etc.

Tourniquet
Small tool kit
Narcotics safe and log book
Sterile syringes and hypodermic needles of assorted sizes
Suction apparatus with sterile tubing
Stainless steel waste bucket
Ceiling- or wall-mounted examination lamps
Blood gas analyzer
Emergency drug box (see Appendix G for contents)
Restraining rope or gauze ties
Insulating table pad or warming blanket
Cardiac defibrillator
Monitoring equipment (should include ECG monitor)
Ambu resuscitator bag
Ventilator to assist or control breathing
Oxygen therapy cage
Anesthesia forms
Euthanasia solution
Death reports

Related items

Compressed oxygen and nitrous oxide supply
Anesthesia machine (more than one preferred)
Inhalation masks of various sizes
Nonrebreathing system for animals under 8 kg
Corrugated rubber breathing tubes
Reservoir bags: 1-, 3-, and 5-L capacity
Carbon dioxide absorbing granules
Tracheostomy tubes
Endotracheal tubes of assorted sizes
Endotracheal tube adapters
Endotracheal tube cuff inflator (for example, 5 ml syringe)
Stylet for use on small endotracheal tubes
Hemostatic forceps
Laryngoscope with assorted blade sizes
Flashlight or penlight
Spare batteries and bulbs for laryngoscope and flashlight
Preanesthetic medications
Injectable general anesthetic drug(s)
Topical anesthetic jelly or spray for desensitizing cat larynx
Inhalation anesthetic drug(s)
Local analgesic solution(s)
Epidural anesthesia kit
Movable stool for anesthetist
Scavenging system for waste anesthetic gases

Most movable items used for anesthesia or surgical purposes should be stored outside the sterile operating room. If, due to the small size of the facility, these items must be stored in the sterile surgery room, they should be enclosed in cabinets that are free of surfaces for dust collection.

TABLE 1-2

Flowchart for the prevention and treatment of cardiopulmonary arrest (CPA)

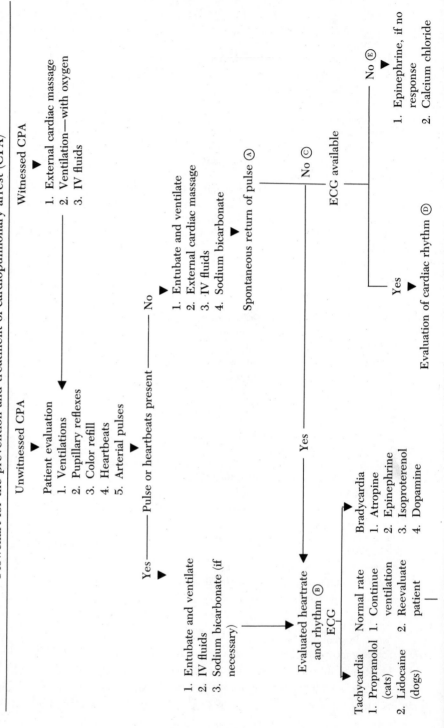

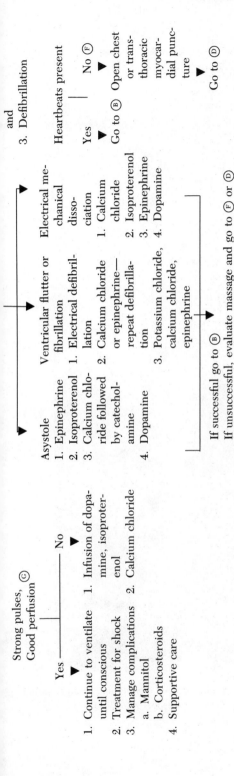

Strong pulses, Ⓒ
Good perfusion

Yes ——————— No

1. Continue to ventilate
   until conscious
2. Treatment for shock
3. Manage complications
   a. Mannitol
   b. Corticosteroids
4. Supportive care

1. Infusion of dopa-
   mine, isoproter-
   enol
2. Calcium chloride

Asystole
1. Epinephrine
2. Isoproterenol
3. Calcium chlo-
   ride followed
   by catechol-
   amine
4. Dopamine

Ventricular flutter or
fibrillation
1. Electrical defibril-
   lation
2. Calcium chloride
   or epinephrine—
   repeat defibrilla-
   tion
3. Potassium chloride,
   calcium chloride,
   epinephrine

Electrical me-
chanical
disso-
ciation
1. Calcium
   chloride
2. Isoproterenol
3. Epinephrine
4. Dopamine

If successful go to Ⓑ
If unsuccessful, evaluate massage and go to Ⓕ or Ⓓ

and
3. Defibrillation

Heartbeats present

Yes   No Ⓕ

Go to Ⓑ   Open chest
             or trans-
             thoracic
             myocar-
             dial punc-
             ture

             Go to Ⓓ

From Muir, W.M., and others: An outline of veterinary anesthesia. In Fenner, W.R., editor: Quick reference to veterinary medicine, New York, 1982, Harper & Row, Publishers, Inc.

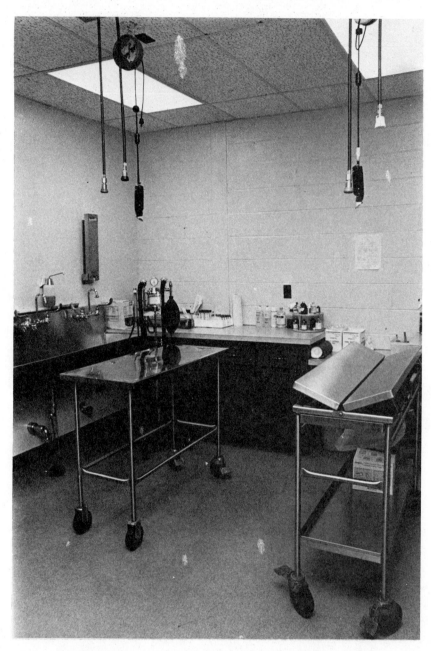

Fig. 1-2. Surgical "prep" room. Note ceiling drops for compressed oxygen and nitrous oxide and electric clippers. Movable "prep" carts allow for patient transport into the surgery room.

While the list on pp. 10 and 11 may be extravagant for the small, one-veterinarian practice, it may, in some ways, be incomplete for the large volume, multiveterinarian practice. Additions or deletions are a matter of personal preference. To some, a more than adequate inventory of anesthetic equipment and supplies is one reflection of preparedness. Even though a drug or piece of equipment may be used only on rare occasions, its availability in an emergency situation can sometimes save an animal's life.

Familiarity with anesthetic technique

A general rule of thumb in veterinary anesthesia is that procedures of very short duration are performed under ultrashort-acting barbiturates, such as thiamylal or thiopental, whereas procedures of a long duration (>30 minutes) require a longer-acting barbiturate (for example, pentobarbital) or inhalation anesthesia. Veterinarians who perform surgery unassisted by technicians may elect to use pentobarbital for long procedures or a combination of pentobarbital and an ultrashort-acting barbiturate. The amount of trained help available to the veterinarian greatly influences the choice of anesthetic. Inhalation anesthesia usually requires at least one individual trained in the safe use and care of the anesthesia machine, endotracheal intubation, and patient monitoring. In the 1930s, it was an accepted concept that once a doctor had mastered a particular anesthetic technique it was not advantageous to change to an unfamiliar one. Although it is true that the greatest success usually comes with that technique or anesthetic drug most frequently used, new anesthetic drugs and techniques are being introduced at a rate that has doubled and tripled since ether anesthesia, introduced in 1842, was used for all anesthesia cases. Veterinarians graduating in the 1980s must choose from a multitude of drugs and techniques.

The AHT must be as concerned as the veterinarian about selection of and familiarity with anesthesia technique. The veterinarian's success rate will in part rest with the proper training and education of technicians, especially concerning indications and contraindications of various anesthetic drugs.

RATIONALE FOR PREANESTHETIC MEDICATION

Any drug administered to a patient within 1 hour of general (or local) anesthesia is referred to as a "preanesthetic" or a "preoperative" medication or simply a "preop." The majority of preanesthetic drugs are given by injection, usually intramuscularly or subcutaneously and, on occasion, intravenously.

Indications

Preanesthetic drugs are administered to veterinary patients for a variety of reasons:

- To aid in the restraint of the animal by quieting the patient, reducing anxiety, and decreasing hyperactivity
- To reduce or minimize pain, especially if the animal has suffered a fractured limb and must be moved or manipulated before anesthetic induction
- To facilitate the induction phase of general anesthesia by eliminating or reducing the excitatory stage. These drugs also help to reduce delirium and excitement during the recovery from general anesthesia.
- To minimize the vagal-mediated reflexes associated with the depressant action of general anesthetics and intubation of the trachea. Many anesthetic drugs can cause bradycardia; some also cause excessive secretion from salivary and tracheal glands. Intubation of the trachea can cause a strong vagal stimulus resulting in bradycardia and/or laryngospasm. Excessive salivation in the anesthetized animal could result in aspiration pneumonitis after surgery, while the animal is unconscious and unable to swallow.
- To augment the general anesthetic drug in order to decrease the total amount of anesthetic drug needed to produce and maintain anesthesia. The chances of overdosing the animals with anesthetic drug are less if the animal first receives a sedative drug.
- To aid in the performance of local analgesia techniques by providing sedation and reducing anxiety

Contraindications

All premedication drugs, except the anticholinergics, are considered central nervous system (CNS) depressants. It must be remembered that these drugs will cause a certain degree of respiratory and cardiovascular depression, especially if used in high doses. Thus caution must be exercised when dealing with animals in respiratory or cardiac failure. The administration of sedatives or narcotics is often eliminated or used in greatly reduced dosages with high risk patients. Animals in hypotensive shock should not receive tranquilizers or narcotics unless careful monitoring is combined with the use of intravenous fluids.

The use of atropine and other related preanesthetic medication can interfere with interpretation of the patient's pupil size and response to light by causing dilation of the pupil. Excessive administration of atropine, especially via the intravenous route, can lead to atropine poisoning, which can sometimes be fatal.

Some professionals believe that anticholinergic drugs, like atropine, are contraindicated as routine preanesthetics because they cause a sustained paralysis of the ciliated epithelium in the trachea and bronchi. Their use results, on occasion, in overly thick mucous production after anesthesia and an inability to clear secretions from the tracheobronchial tree. Some veterinarians therefore do not use atropine as a preanesthetic medication.

CLASSIFICATION AND USE OF PREANESTHETIC MEDICATIONS

Table 1-3 summarizes the classification of preanesthetic drugs according to their general sedative action and provides some commonly used examples. Since every drug has both a generic (chemical) name and one or more trade names, the student should be concerned at first with learning only the generic name. (Appendix E gives the generic and trade names for all anesthetic drugs mentioned in this text.)

The student is, of course, not expected to memorize drug dosages. It is foolhardy to believe that one set dosage can be used under all circumstances. Many variables relative to the specific animal and situation alter drug dosage. In the following discussion of individual preanesthetic medications, drug dosages have deliberately been omitted in order to emphasize drug action. (Drug dosages for the commonly used preanesthetics are given in Table 1-4.) It is, however, important that the AHT become familiar with drug calculations before handling or administering anesthetic drugs.

Under no circumstances is the AHT permitted to prescribe *any* drug for an animal. Only under the direct and immediate supervision of a licensed veterinarian can a technician administer anesthetic or preanesthetic drugs to an animal.

Preanesthetic drugs will be discussed according to the following five categories:
- Anticholinergics
- Tranquilizers
- Narcotics
- Neuroleptanalgesics
- Dissociative agents

Anticholinergics (sympathomimetics)

Drugs in this category are given primarily to counteract certain actions of tranquilizers, narcotics, and general anesthetics—that is, bradycardia, excessive salivation, and increased vagal tone caused by anesthetics, tracheal intubation, or surgical manipulations.

Atropine sulfate is a commonly used anticholinergic drug. It and similar drugs have additional uses for small animals unassociated with their preanesthetic properties:
- As an antidote or organophosphate intoxication
- As an antispasmodic to control diarrhea and/or vomiting
- As a mydriatic applied as an ophthalmic solution to examine the retina of the eye

Anticholinergic drugs, when given at preanesthetic dosages, do not provide analgesia. They act by competing with acetylcholine (a neurotransmitter) at various effector sites in the nervous system, namely the exocrine glands, iris, and heart. When they are used for preanesthetic medication in small animals, anticholinergics have certain advantages and disadvantages.

TABLE 1-3

Classification of preanesthetic drugs with examples

Preanesthetic drugs				
Nonsedative		*Sedative*		
Anticholinergics	*Muscle paralyzers**	*Tranquilizers*	*Narcotics*	*Dissociative agents*
Atropine	Curare	Promazine	Morphine	Phencyclidine
Scopolamine	Succinylcholine	Acetylpromazine	Apomorphine	Ketamine
Aminopentamide	Pancuronium	Chlorpromazine	Meperidine	Tiletamine
Glycopyrrolate	Gallamine	Triflupromazine	Fentanyl	
		Droperidol	Oxymorphone	
		Diazepam	Etorphine	
		Xylazine	Nalorphine	
		Lorazepam		

Neuroleptanalgesics

Fentanyl citrate (Innovar Vet)

Acepromazine-oxymorphone

*Muscle-paralyzing drugs should never be administered until an adequate state of general anesthesia has been induced. Use of muscle-paralyzing drugs alone is considered inhumane.

Advantages*
- Stabilization of heart rate by counteracting vagal tone, thereby increasing heart rate
- Prevention of excessive secretions from the salivary and tracheal glands, which results in drying of the mouth and upper respiratory tract

Disadvantages
- The production of excessively thick mucus from the trachea and bronchi
- Increased anatomic dead space caused by a dilation of bronchial airways, which could be of importance in brachycephalic animals or those with chronic respiratory disease. (Intubation of the trachea in these animals is, therefore, extremely important.) Anticholinergics are contraindicated in certain cases of heart disease.

In addition, anticholinergic drugs also cause dilation of pupils and decreased intestinal peristalsis.

Overdosage signs

Increasing dosages of anticholinergic drugs can lead to CNS excitability, delirium, coma, and death. Dogs seem to be more sensitive to atropine poisoning than cats, probably because cats (as well as rabbits) have larger amounts of the enzyme atropine esterase in their liver for removing atropine from the bloodstream. The intravenous dose that causes CNS excitement in dogs is about half what it is in cats. Signs of atropine poisoning can occur in either species when the total dosage given exceeds 2.0 to 5.0 mg/kg. In most clinical situations it is rare to see atropine poisoning as a result of a single dose.

Precautions

Atropine and related drugs should be used with caution:
- In animals with cardiac disease associated with arrhythmias and/or tachycardia
- In animals with uncompensating respiratory disease or distress
- In constipated animals because of the drug's antiperistaltic action
- In animals with severe renal dysfunction

Specific examples of anticholinergic drugs

Atropine sulfate. Obtained from the leaves of the deadly nightshade plant, atropine is the most commonly used anticholinergic preanesthetic for small animals. Atropine is often referred to as a "belladonna (the word "belladonna" means "beautiful lady") alkaloid" and is related to the mydriatic action of atropine on the pupils of the eye. In ancient times, dilated pupils in women was considered a sign of beauty.

*The lists throughout this chapter are not presented in order of increasing or decreasing importance.

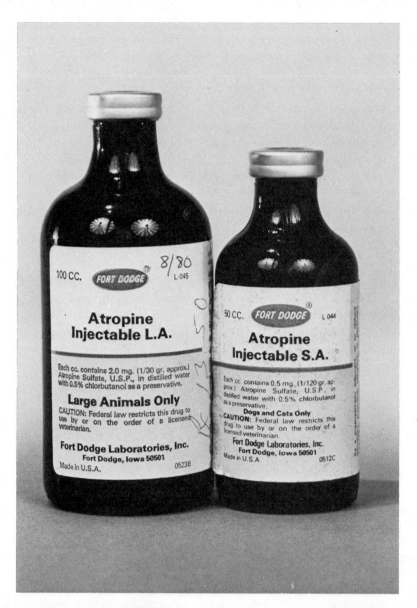

Fig. 1-3. Atropine multidose vials. The two bottles appear similar except for size and label-ing. Thus careful inspection can prevent cases of inadvertent drug overdosage.

Availability. Atropine is supplied as a sterile solution containing $^1/_{120}$ grain/ml (0.5 mg/ml) for parenteral injection. Some drug companies supply two different strength solutions of atropine (see Fig. 1-3). One must *always* read and inspect the drug container before removing and administering medication.

Route of administration. Atropine is usually given by intramuscular or subcutaneous injection 20 to 30 minutes before anesthetic induction. It can be mixed and given in combination with most tranquilizers and phencyclidine drugs. When used to prevent narcotic-induced bradycardia, it is best given 15 to 30 minutes before the narcotic drug.

Intravenous administration requires caution, but atropine can be given via this route when an immediate action is desired, as in sudden bradycardia or organophosphate poisoning. Since atropine has clinical uses other than as a preanesthetic, it should be aspirated into the syringe *first* if it is being administered in combination with a tranquilizer or dissociate anesthetic drug. Dosage is quite variable depending on the species. When given subcutaneously, its duration of action is 60 to 90 minutes.

Other anticholinergic drugs

- Scopolamine hydrobromide (hyoscine). Nicknamed "scope," it has a sedative action on some species.
- Methylatropine nitrate
- Aminopentamide
- Glycopyrrolate. Duration of action is almost twice that of atropine. It does not readily cross the blood-brain barrier and is therefore less of a depressant.

Tranquilizers (ataractics, neuroleptics)

A tranquilizer drug, by definition, acts to quiet or calm the animal. In human medicine, tranquilizers are widely used to treat emotional and psychoneurotic states as well as for relief of anxiety and stress. There have been attempts recently to treat aggressive behavior and/or neurotic pets with low dosages of tranquilizing drugs; however, the results are often difficult to assess objectively in veterinary patients. The majority of tranquilizer drugs used for preanesthetic purposes in small animals are derived from the compound phenothiazine. Tranquilizers other than these are referred to as nonphenothiazine tranquilizers and are classified separately.

No fewer than 10 different phenothiazine-derived drugs are currently available for use as preanesthetic medications. Their use as such is related to their general actions as sedative, antihistaminic, antiemetic, and antiarrhythmic drugs. In addition, they have a synergistic or additive effect when used in combination with general anesthetic drugs. There are presently in excess of 20 phenothiazine-derived drugs employed for the treatment of psychiatric patients, chlorpromazine being the prototype. Within the veterinary profession only about five to six of these are used for preanesthetic purposes.

The general discussion of tranquilizers that follows concerns primarily the phenothiazine-derived drugs. *Acepromazine* will be used as a common example for veterinary patients. It is not the intent of this text to recommend one tranquilizer over another, since variations in response always have to be taken into account, as will the particular circumstance in which a tranquilizer drug is being employed. In cases where nonphenothiazine tranquilizers differ significantly from the general mode of action, notation will be made; otherwise all tranquilizer drugs can be considered similar in action.

Advantages
- They produce a calming effect and permit easier restraint and handling of anxious animals.*
- They reduce the amount of general anesthetic drug required for a surgical level of anesthesia.
- They provide an antiarrhythmic action on the heart. Low dosages of a phenothiazine tranquilizer help protect the heart against cardiac arrhythmias associated with anesthetic induction and sympathetic stimulation due to high levels of circulating epinephrine.
- They decrease the possibility for excitement or hysteria during anesthetic induction and/or recovery.
- They provide a profound degree of sedation and analgesia when combined with a narcotic.
- They do not produce physical dependence (addiction) as do most narcotic sedatives. The vast majority of tranquilizer drugs are not subject to Schedule II federal regulations (see p. 35). Special records of their use and distribution are not required, nor must they be kept in a special narcotics safe. The main exception to this ruling is the drug diazepam, which is presently being reclassified as a Schedule II substance.

Tranquilizers also have the following actions considered advantageous under certain circumstances:
- They produce an antiemetic effect by directly suppressing the vomiting center in the brain and are therefore used to prevent vomiting due to carsickness.
- They provide an antipruritic effect from their antihistamine action and are used to prevent licking of wounds or chewing of feet, bandages, or splints.
- Diazepam has a therapeutic action against myelogram-induced seizures or seizures resulting from an overdose of a local analgesic drug. In addition, diazepam is the only tranquilizer indicated for use in epileptic patients or patients with seizure disorders.

---

*Tranquilizers are sedative in nature, but they *do not* provide any significant degree of analgesia. Animals tend to appear calm and asleep when tranquilized; however, if provoked or manipulated in such a way as to elicit pain, they are quite capable of responding. The use of muzzle restraint should be considered if the animal has suffered a fractured limb or other painful injury and must be manipulated before induction of anesthesia. Tranquilizer drugs do not produce unconsciousness or anesthesia.

Disadvantages

- Tranquilizers produce varying degrees of respiratory depression.
- They produce varying degrees of hypotension. *All* tranquilizers cause a decrease in blood pressure and should be either avoided or used judiciously in animals with cardiovascular disease, hypovolemic shock, or serious dehydration.
- They produce hypothermia and involuntary muscle shivering.
- They produce ataxia and incoordination.
- They produce prolapse of the nictitating membranes in the eye (see Fig. 1-4), making ocular examination difficult.
- They cause a loss of conditioned responses and behavioral training, and they delay reaction time.
- Phenothiazine tranquilizers appear to lower the seizure threshold in epileptic animals and may actually precipitate a convulsive episode. These tranquilizers are therefore contraindicated for use in animals with epilepsy or any other convulsive disorder such as strychnine poisoning, organophosphate poisoning, and hypocalcemic tetany.
- Phenothiazine tranquilizers, on rare occasions, may produce an allergic photosensitive skin reaction in susceptible individuals. Signs are often triggered by sunlight and take the form of a skin rash or sunburn.
- Phenothiazine tranquilizers should not be given to animals with blood clotting disorders or blood dyscrasias—for example, von Willebrand's disease in dogs.
- Federal regulations prohibit the use of tranquilizing drugs in animals being slaughtered for human consumption.
- They cross the placental barrier and may adversely affect the newborn if used during parturition or cesarean section.
- They are nonreversible and without antidote.

Overdosage and toxicity

Increasing dosages of a tranquilizer can result in progressive restlessness, disorientation, and eventually CNS convulsions, coma, and death. In actuality, it would require a gross error in dosage to kill a healthy dog or cat with a single dose of tranquilizer. However, serious *hypotension* can result from the administration of routine dosages, especially in animals with preexisting cardiovascular disease. Further, there are *no* antidotes or reversal drugs to counteract the hypotension, respiratory depression, and/or CNS excitability that can result from tranquilizer overdosage. If severe hypotension does occur, intravenous fluids should be administered to counteract the circulatory depression. If needed, a barbiturate can be administered to depress the CNS and quiet any seizures induced by the tranquilizer. Occasionally, a normal dose of a potent tranquilizer, such as acepromazine or chlorpromazine, may result in excitement rather than sedation in certain animals. Incon-

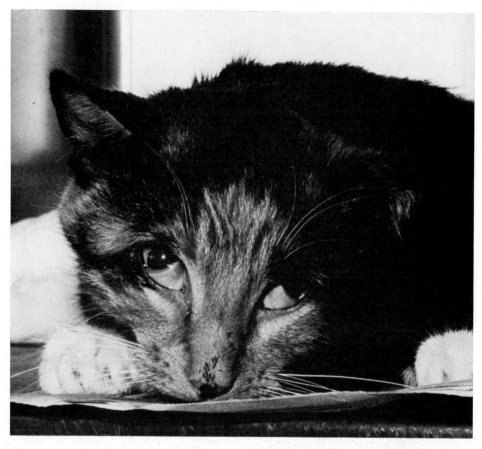

Fig. 1-4. Prolapsed third eyelid following subcutaneous administration of acepromazine (1 mg) to a 4-kg cat.

sistencies of this nature are not uncommon in veterinary patients. Nor are they limited only to tranquilizers. If an animal exhibits excitement or restlessness following a normal dose of tranquilizer it is best to be gentle and work quietly to induce general anesthesia. Noise, rough handling, or administration of additional tranquilizer may aggravate the situation and excite the animal even more. Some veterinarians prefer to combine a tranquilizer with a narcotic for greater preanesthetic sedation. Adverse reactions to tranquilizing drugs should always be noted clearly on the animal's permanent record.

In summary, the common signs of toxicity and/or overdosage for all tranquilizer drugs are:
- Cardiovascular hypotension
- CNS excitability leading to convulsions, coma, and death if a sufficiently large dose is administered

- Hypersensitive skin reactions triggered by exposure to sunlight (phenothiazines)
- Possible jaundice and/or blood dyscrasias with chronic use (phenothiazines)
- Hyperactive limb movements and body positions associated with high dosages
- Severe respiratory depression when combined with the central respiratory depressant action of a narcotic and/or general anesthetic.
- Interaction with and/or potentiation of other drug actions. For example, tranquilizers can increase barbiturate sleeping time.
- Unusual personality changes. Cases have been reported where a normally friendly dog has become vicious and aggressive, even toward its owner, following a standard dose of a drug like chlorpromazine or droperidol. Typically, such behavior alterations appear 12 to 24 hours following the administration of the tranquilizer and persist for about 24 hours, although longer periods have been noted by some owners. Similar occurrences have also been reported in humans.

In general, most tranquilizer drugs in use today are relatively safe and effective when administered at the recommended dosages.

General precautions

Tranquilizing drugs should be used with discretion or eliminated as a preanesthetic medication in cases where:
- The animal is in a state of shock, whatever the cause
- The animal is weak, dehydrated, or severely debilitated
- The animal has a known sensitivity to tranquilizing drugs
- The animal is already receiving depressant medication
- The animal is in a state of advanced kidney, liver, or cardiovascular disease
- The animal has suffered severe trauma, especially to the head or chest
- The animal has a history of epilepsy or is actively displaying signs of a seizure disorder (phenothiazines). In addition, the phenothiazine tranquilizers should be avoided as preanesthetics in animals undergoing diagnostic myelograms or cerebrospinal fluid (CSF) taps.

Specific examples of tranquilizers

Those tranquilizers most often used in dogs and cats for preanesthetic sedation are:

- Acepromazine
- Promazine
- Chlorpromazine
- Triflupromazine
- Ethyl isobutrazine
- Promethazine
- Triflumeprazine
- Diazepam
- Droperidol
- Xylazine

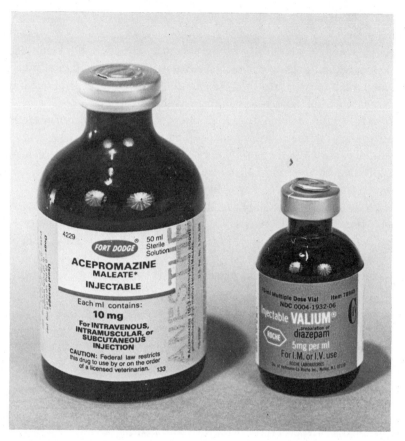

Fig. 1-5. Acepromazine maleate and diazepam vials. Note protective cap on each bottle and controlled substance symbol on the diazepam label.

Phenothiazine derivatives

Acepromazine maleate (acetylpromazine). This drug is commonly referred to as "ace." At the present time it is one of the most widely used tranquilizing drugs for small animals and is considered a potent neuroleptic for all species, including wildlife.

AVAILABILITY. Acepromazine is supplied as a sterile 1.0% yellow solution containing 10 mg/ml for parenteral injection. It is also available for oral use as 10 or 25 mg tablets. Acepromazine is marketed for veterinary use only (Fig 1-5).

ROUTE OF ADMINISTRATION. When used as a preanesthetic, acepromazine is most often given by the subcutaneous or intramuscular route. When given subcutaneously, 15 to 30 minutes should be allowed to pass before inducing general anesthesia. If given intramuscularly, a wait of 5 to 10 minutes is sufficient to allow for maximum sedative effects before induction. Acepromazine may also be given intravenously; however, this route is not recommended due to the potent hypotensive effect of acepromazine. If an immediate sedative effect is desired, the veterinarian may administer the drug intraveneously followed by induction of general anesthesia with a barbiturate or inhalation anesthetic drug. Intravenous injection of this or any other preanesthetic drug must always be done with caution at a lowered dosage and under the *direct* supervision of the attending veterinarian.

ADVANTAGES. The advantages of using acepromazine over other drugs as a preanesthetic sedative in dogs and cats are that:

- It has a potent sedative action.
- It has a wide margin of safety and can therefore be administered over a wide dosage range in healthy animals.
- It has a low toxicity.
- It produces predictable sedation in a wide variety of domestic and wildlife species.
- It produces good muscle relaxation and can be used in combination with dissociative anesthetics to decrease muscle rigidity.
- It does not precipitate with atropine and can therefore be mixed with atropine and administered from one syringe as a single preanesthetic injection.
- It has an additive effect when combined with a narcotic.

In addition, acepromazine also has all the advantages of tranquilizers previously listed.

DISADVANTAGES. The specific disadvantages of acepromazine are related to its potent hypotensive, hypothermic, and phenothiazine properties. The general disadvantages of all tranquilizers apply also to acepromazine.

PRECAUTIONS OR COMPLICATIONS. See general precautions of tranquilizer drugs discussed earlier. The LD_{50}* dosages for acepromazine in mice have been determined for oral, subcutaneous, and intravenous routes of administration†:

Oral LD_{50} = 256 mg/kg

Subcutaneous LD_{50} = 130 mg/kg

Intravenous LD_{50} = 61 mg/kg

On close inspection of these LD_{50} figures in mice, the deaths occurring from the intravenous route are considerably greater than for the subcutaneous or oral

---

*LD_{50} represents the lethal dose (LD) of a substance that when administered to a significantly large number of animals (usually mice) will kill 50% of them. In the example used for acepromazine, if 100 mice were given the drug by intravenous injection at a dosage of 61 mg/kg, approximately 50 would die and 50 would survive. In research on drug toxicity, the LD_{50} dosage is considered the end point for studying the lethal nature of any substance. LD_{100} values are rarely, if ever, investigated when determining the lethal toxicity of a drug.

†Lumb, W.V., and Jones, E.W.: Veterinary anesthesia, Philadelphia, 1973, Lea & Febiger, p. 187.

routes of administration. Thus the precaution against administering acepromazine by intravenous injection except by the most experienced of personnel is essential.

Promazine hydrochloride

AVAILABILITY. Promazine is supplied as a sterile solution containing 25 mg/ml (2.5%) or 50 mg/ml (5.0%) for parenteral injection. It is also supplied in tablets of 10, 25, 50, 100, and 200 mg and as a syrup containing 2 mg/ml. Promazine is cleared for use in both human and veterinary patients.

ROUTE OF ADMINISTRATION. As a preanesthetic, promazine is generally administered subcutaneously or intramuscularly. If administered intravenously, it must be given slowly to effect and with extreme caution. Perivascular irritation and/or thrombophlebitis are possible consequences of intravenous use.

ADVANTAGES. Promazine is similar in action to acepromazine although somewhat less hypotensive and less sedating. Before the manufacture of acepromazine, promazine was the most widely used tranquilizer for both large and small animals. Considered safe for use with dogs and cats, it can be mixed with atropine.

DISADVANTAGES. See disadvantages of tranquilizer drugs discussed earlier.

PRECAUTIONS OR COMPLICATIONS. See general precautions concerning tranquilizer drugs discussed earlier.

Chlorpromazine hydrochloride. Chlorpromazine was one of the first phenothiazine derivatives to be used as a preanesthetic sedative. Synthesized in 1950, chlorpromazine is considered the prototype of phenothiazine-derived tranquilizers. It possesses profound sedation and a prolonged duration of action (usually greater than 8 hours).

AVAILABILITY. Chlorpromazine is supplied as a sterile solution containing 25 mg/ml for parenteral injection. It is also available for both oral and rectal administration. For oral use, chlorpromazine is supplied in tablets containing 10, 25, 100, or 200 mg; in time-released capsules ("spansule") containing 30, 75, 150, 200, or 300 mg; and as a flavored syrup containing 10 mg per teaspoon (5 ml). Rectal suppositories are available in 25 and 100 mg sizes. In addition, chlorpromazine is available in gallon bottles containing a concentration of 30 mg/ml for human use. The reason for such a large variety of available forms of chlorpromazine is its extensive use with humans as an antiemetic, as a treatment for mental and emotional disorders, and for alleviation of uncontrollable hiccups.

ROUTE OF ADMINISTRATION. When used for preanesthetic sedation, chlorpromazine is usually given by intramuscular or subcutaneous injection. The intravenous route is not recommended except at a greatly lowered dosage and under extreme caution, as chlorpromazine, even more than acepromazine, can cause severe hypotension. The profound hypotensive action of chlorpromazine, like other potent phenothiazine-derived tranquilizers, can produce shock. The hypotension is a result of both central CNS depression and alpha blockade of peripheral blood vessels, causing widespread vasodilation. Intravenous administration of a potent tranquilizer such as chlorpromazine can cause a condition referred to as orthostatic hypotension:

severe hypotension as a result of positioning the patient in a standing posture when the head is rapidly elevated above the heart. The word "orthostatic," borrowed from human medicine, refers to anything that is caused by standing erect. In dogs and cats care should always be taken when the animal is heavily sedated with a phenothiazine-derived tranquilizer or is under general anesthesia not to make *sudden* position or posture changes that affect the flow of blood to or from the head. This may be a potential problem during radiography positioning, cerebrospinal fluid (CSF) taps, tilting of the patient on the surgery table, and transporting of a tranquilized or anesthetized animal back to its recovery cage. Thus the animal should be maintained in as near a horizontal position as possible at all times. Cases of orthostatic hypotension have been know to occur in heavily sedated human patients while they are transported by elevator from one floor to another.

ADVANTAGES. Chlorpromazine as a preanesthetic medication has certain advantages over other tranquilizers:
- Prevention of vomiting during anesthetic induction and recovery
- Potent sedation allowing for easier restraint during induction of anesthesia and greater reduction in the volume of general anesthetic drugs
- Good muscle relaxant capability

In addition, see advantages of tranquilizer drugs discussed earlier.

DISADVANTAGES. In addition to those factors previously listed, chlorpromazine has become less popular as a preanesthetic for small animals due mainly to its:
- Prolonged sedation (>8 hours)
- Inconsistent or unpredictable sedative action, especially in the cat and horse
- Potent hypotensive actions
- Potential to produce a greater photosensitivity reaction in susceptible animals than other commonly used phenothiazine-derived tranquilizers
- Tendency to cause local irritation and pain when given intramuscularly
- The possibility of incorrect intravenous technique, resulting in accidental perivascular injection, which can cause localized cellulitis, pain and necroses of skin
- Tendency of solution to discolor if kept in bright light

PRECAUTIONS OR COMPLICATIONS. In addition to those discussed earlier, the use of chlorpromazine in dogs and cats can lead to:
- Orthostatic hypotension due to sudden positional changes
- Perivascular irritation
- Prolonged recovery from sedative and ataxic actions
- CNS excitement rather than sedation in some cats

Triflupromazine hydrochloride

AVAILABILITY. Triflupromazine is supplied as a sterile solution containing 3, 10, or 20 mg/ml for parenteral injection. The 20-mg/ml concentration is generally used by veterinarians and the 3-mg/ml concentration reserved for intravenous use. Triflupromazine is also available for oral use in 10, 25, or 50 mg tablets and as a liquid containing 10 or 50 mg/ml. Rectal suppositories are available containing 35 or 70 mg. Triflupromazine is marketed as both a human and a veterinary drug.

ROUTE OF ADMINISTRATION. Triflupromazine may be given by subcutaneous, intramuscular, or intravenous routes for preanesthetic sedation. If given intravenously, the dose must be reduced and caution exercised. When administered intravenously, the precautions and side effects are similar to chlorpromazine. Intravenous use in cats and small dogs is discouraged.

ADVANTAGES. As a preanesthetic, triflupromazine has specific advantages over other tranquilizing drugs:

- Greater antiemetic effect
- Less hypotensive effect than acepromazine or chlorpromazine, while similar to promazine in clinical effects
- Usefulness in combination with oxymorphone as a preanesthetic neuroleptanalgesic for both cats and dogs

DISADVANTAGES. In addition to those factors previously listed, triflupromazine has side effects similar to chlorpromazine and may cause a higher incidence of hyperexcitability or spastic reactions than is normally seen with other tranquilizing drugs.

PRECAUTIONS OR COMPLICATIONS. See "General precautions concerning tranquilizer drugs."

OTHER PHENOTHIAZINE TRANQUILIZERS. Additional phenothiazine-derived tranquilizing drugs available for veterinary use are ethyl isobutrazine, triflumeprazine, promethazine, and propiopromazine.

Nonphenothiazine derivatives

Diazepam. A benzodiazepine compound with mild sedative properies, diazepam is similar in action to chlordiazepoxide (see Fig. 1-5).

AVAILABILITY. Diazepam is supplied as a sterile oil solution containing 5.0 mg/ml for parenteral injection. Propylene glycol, sodium benzoate, and benzoic acid are included to solubilize the diazepam. Diazepam is not water soluble. Thus it cannot be given as a mixture with any other water soluble drug such as atropine because an insoluble precipitate will form. Diazepam is also supplied in 2, 5, and 10 mg tablets for oral administration, and it is available as a powder for mixing with food or a pellet for subcutaneous implantation in feedlot animals. Its use for these domestic animals is primarily its mild tranquilization and its antistress and growth-enhancing effects.

ROUTE OF ADMINISTRATION. When used as a preanesthetic drug, diazepam should be given *intravenously*. It should be administered just before induction of anesthesia with a thiobarbiturate or inhalation agent. When given intramuscularly or subcutaneously, diazepam is poorly absorbed. When administered intravenously, care must be taken to assure a slow injection as propylene glycol, the carrier vehicle, is a cardiovascular depressant.

ADVANTAGES. Since diazepam is not considered a potent sedative, it is rarely used as a preanesthetic sedative except:

- In animals with a known history of epilepsy
- In animals with an active seizure disorder
- In animals undergoing CSF taps or myelogram studies
- In animals with neurologic disorders requiring surgery
- In animals with head injuries such as skull fracture and concussion
- In animals with cardiovascular disease, since diazepam is less depressant on the heart and peripheral blood vessels than most other tranquilizers
- In geriatric or obese animals
- When local analgesics are to be given for spinal or epidural blocks
- When muscle relaxation is desired without profound sedation, as in muscle strain of limb or spine
- To alleviate seizures due to local analgesic drug toxicity

DISADVANTAGES. Diazepam has certain disadvantages in common with most tranquilizers. It is not, however, contraindicated in seizure disorders, nor is it associated with hypersensitive skin reactions as are the phenothiazine tranquilizers. Its use in veterinary anesthesia has been limited primarily because:

- It must be administered intravenously. Diazepam is not soluble in water. When given intramuscularly, it is quite painful and irritates local tissue. It may also cause a perivascular irritation if deposited around a vein rather than into it.
- Diazepam cannot be mixed with atropine in the same syringe because precipitation will occur.
- Diazepam has no antiemetic action.
- Diazepam may cause excitement rather than sedation in some animals, often producing an exaggerated sniffing response in dogs.
- It should be administered through an intravenous catheter by *slow* injection to lessen the chance for cardiovascular depression and/or venous irritation.

PRECAUTIONS OR COMPLICATIONS. Less information is available about diazepam's toxic effects and possible complications than the somewhat older phenothiazine-derived tranquilizers. The first six "General precautions of tranquilizer drugs" apply also to diazepam (see p. 25). In addition, care should be taken that the diazepam is administered slowly and intravenously. (Propylene glycol can cause bradycardia, hypotension, and apnea if injected too rapidly by the intravenous route.) If hyperexcitement occurs, the veterinarian should be prepared to control the animal and administer a thiobarbiturate immediately. Perivascular irritation will occur if diazepam is accidentally injected outside the vein.

Droperidol. A butyrophenone derivative, droperidol is considered a more potent tranquilizer than promazine and chlorpromazine; however, it is shorter-acting (8 to 12 hours) and is rarely used alone as a preanesthetic sedative, although it is capable of producing sedation equal to the phenothiazine tranquilizers. It is most often used in combination with the narcotic, fentanyl, for preanesthetic sedation and analgesia. Droperidol is rarely administered to cats.

AVAILABILITY. Droperidol is supplied as a sterile solution containing 2.5 mg/ml for parenteral injections. It is available in 10 ml vials or 2.0 and 5.0 ml ampules. Innovar Vet, a commercially available preparation, has a concentration of 20 mg/ml (2.0%) combined with fentanyl.

ROUTE OF ADMINISTRATION. Droperidol is water soluble; therefore, it can be mixed with atropine. It can be given by subcutaneous, intramuscular, or intravenous injection. The intramuscular or intravenous route is preferred.

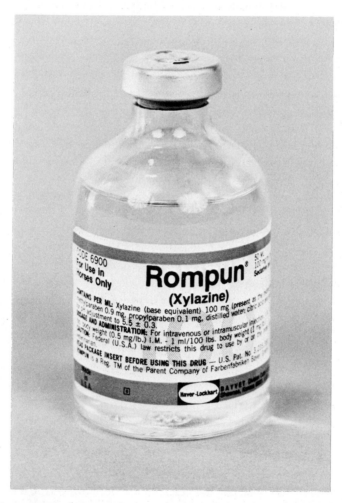

Fig. 1-6. Xylazine bottle (100 mg/ml). Note that the label contains both the trade name and generic name of the drug.

ADVANTAGES. Droperidol has the following advantages in that:

- It does not by itself produce any clinical signs of respiratory depression when used at recommended dosages
- It has a relatively short duration of action (6 to 12 hours)
- It provides good antiemetic action
- It has a protective action, similar to the phenothiazine tranquilizers, against epinephrine-induced arrhythmias
- It has a wide margin of safety

DISADVANTAGES. Droperidol is relatively expensive and may cause muscle tremors, hyperexcitability, and/or behavioral changes in some animals, especially during the recovery period.

PRECAUTIONS OR COMPLICATIONS. These are essentially the same as for all tranquilizer drugs.

Xylazine. A nonphenothiazine, nonnarcotic sedative derived from thiazine, xylazine possesses both analgesic and muscle-relaxing properties. Although not a true tranquilizer because of its analgesic property, it is presented here because it is used as a preanesthetic sedative.

AVAILABILITY. Xylazine is supplied as a sterile 2.0% solution containing 20 mg/ml for parenteral injection in dogs and cats. Xylazine is also available for use in the equine as a sterile 10.0% solution containing 100 mg/ml. Often this form is diluted and administered to dogs or cats (see Fig. 1-6).

ROUTE OF ADMINISTRATION. When used for preanesthetic sedation alone or in combination with other tranquilizers or anesthetics, xylazine is usually given by intramuscular injection. Cautious administration of a reduced dosage via the intravenous route may be employed for a more rapid onset of action. Administration by the subcutaneous route generally does not produce the desired degree of sedation and analgesia.

ADVANTAGES. In comparison to other sedative tranquilizers, xylazine has the advantages of:

- Providing good analgesia and muscle relaxation when used alone
- Providing sufficient analgesia and sedation when combined with another tranquilizer, nitrous oxide, or a local analgesic to perform minor surgical or diagnostic procedures. Sedation lasts 1 to 2 hours. Xylazine combined with ketamine is often administered to cats for short surgical procedures lasting under 20 to 30 minutes.
- Significantly reducing the total dosage of barbiturate anesthetics required to produce a surgical level of general anesthesia. When xylazine is given as a preanesthetic, the total calculated dosage of ultrashort-acting barbiturate required for anesthetic induction can be reduced by 25% to 75%
- Permitting combination with other tranquilizers, ketamine, ultrashort-acting barbiturates, halothane, or methoxyflurane

- Being one of the few drugs capable of inducing vomiting in cats. Xylazine will cause emesis in about 90% of cats and 50% of dogs when administered by the intramuscular route unless, of course, the animal received a phenothiazine tranquilizer either before the xylazine or combined with xylazine. In most instances a preanesthetic drug that induces vomiting would be an undesirable attribute. It is listed here as an advantage only because it is so difficult to induce vomiting in a cat, and there are occasions when evacuation of stomach contents may be desirable before the induction of general anesthesia—for example, if a cat were to have been fed or watered a short time before it was to be anesthetized. It is far better to have the cat vomit while it is conscious than to deal with emesis or regurgitation during anesthetic induction. Many general anesthetic drugs will cause a reflex emptying of the stomach as the animal loses consciousness. An unconscious animal is no longer able to swallow or cough up material from its trachea. If stomach contents were to enter an anesthetized animal's trachea and/or lungs, the chances for serious complications would be magnified (see Chapter 2).

DISADVANTAGES. In addition to the general problems with tranquilizer drugs, xylazine has the following specific disadvantages:

- It has an unpredictable analgesic effect when used alone or with another tranquilizer.
- It can cause severe bradycardia, hypotension, hypoventilation, and second degree heart block when administered intravenously, especially in debilitated animals.
- It can result in profound sleep in some dogs and cats. This may be partially reversed using doxapram, a respiratory stimulant.

PRECAUTIONS OR COMPLICATIONS. In addition to those discussed earlier, xylazine must be used with extreme caution in dogs or cats having:

- Any cardiovascular disease, especially if it is associated with disturbances in atrial or ventricular rhythm
- Concurrent therapy with digitalis or any other cardiorhythmic drug
- Artificial pacemaking devices to control heart rate and myocardial contractions
- Any degree of respiratory dysfunction, whether due to disease or injury

Narcotics (hypnotic, opiate)

Narcotic drugs, one of the oldest and most important classes of anesthetic drugs, usually produce a greater degree of CNS depression than do tranquilizers. The source of narcotics ranges from the juice of the unripened opium seed to present day nonopium, synthetic narcotics. Opium's analgesic and euphoric properties have been known since ancient times. The word "opium" is taken from the Greek word, "opion," which means juice—the drug, opium, being a crude extract obtained from the juice of unripened poppy seed capsules. The first semipure natural derivative of opium was isolated in 1803 and named "morphine" after the Greek god of dreams, Morpheus. Morphine is that portion of the opium poppy that gives the drug its analgesic property and is still the standard against which all newer analgesic drugs are compared. Few narcotic drugs, be they natural or synthetically derived, are superior to morphine in analgesia. The word "narcotic" denotes a state of sleep with analgesia. The sleep state produced by a narcotic is considered incomplete and arousable, whereas the sleep associated with general anesthesia is one of non-arousal, even with a painful stimulus. When used as preanesthetic or postanesthetic drugs, narcotics provide analgesia at low dosages and sedation with analgesia at higher dosages.

The early Greek physicians were aware of opium's tendencies to produce both physical and psychologic dependence (addiction). All narcotics capable of producing analgesia are considered addicting. In addition, they all produce respiratory, cardiovascular, and CNS depression as well as other undesirable side effects separate from their analgesic nature. Narcotics such as morphine and heroin produce varying degrees of euphoria (a feeling of well-being), which makes humans prone to psychologic dependence on the drug. The chemical nature of these drugs leads both humans and experimental animals to a physical dependence on the drug. Since animals have no access to drugs and do not develop psychologic dependence on them, addiction to drugs like morphine, heroin, or alcohol is not a complication as it is in human anesthesia. The respiratory and cardiovascular effects of narcotics, however, must be considered as dangerous to animals as they are to humans.

The Controlled Substances Act of 1970

Narcotics are considered Schedule II drugs according to The Controlled Substances Act passed by Congress in the fall of 1970. The Act is designed to strengthen existing state and federal law enforcement authority in the area of drug abuse and help prevent illegal drug dealing in the United States. The Act also establishes a system to regulate the legitimate use and handling of controlled drugs by qualified individuals, drug manufacturers, and drug ordering companies. The Controlled Substances Act requires qualified individual users of controlled drugs to register with the Drug Enforcement Administration (DEA) and maintain proper records and inventories for all controlled drug stocks. The DEA, a branch of the U.S. Department of Justice, assigns each qualified person or institution a registration number that must be used in ordering or prescribing a controlled drug. Special order forms are required when purchasing any Schedule II drugs.

The Act classifies all drugs subject to control into five classes or schedules. Each schedule has specific criteria for inclusion of a drug and allows flexibility to review and revise drugs according to their potential for abuse. As new drugs come into the market, they may be brought under this control as information becomes available relative to their potential for abuse. Drugs already under control may be reclassified or removed from the schedules entirely. Not every drug on the market is subject to the Controlled Substance Act. Individual states also have statutes for controlling dangerous and narcotic drugs.

The degree to which a particular drug is controlled and the conditions of its record keeping, inventory requirements, and requirement of specific order forms for its purchase are dependent on which schedule it falls into. Schedule I drugs are those with the greatest potential for abuse and therefore come under maximum control. In addition, Schedule I drugs have no currently accepted medical use in the United States. Some examples of specific drugs and their schedule classification according to the Controlled Substance Act of 1970 are:

Schedule I: LSD, marijuana, mescaline, peyote, and certain narcotics such as heroin
Schedule II: Pentobarbital, morphine, meperidine, fentanyl, apomorphine, amphetamine
Schedule III: Thiamylal, thiopental, codeine, nalorphine, levallorphan
Schedule IV: Phenobarbital, chloral hydrate, diazepam, promazine, acepromazine, methohexital
Schedule V: Terpin hydrate with codeine

Schedule V drugs have the lowest potential for abuse. Federal law allows these drugs to be sold on a restricted over-the-counter basis while some states require that such drugs be sold only on a prescription basis.

Controlled substances for parenteral injection must be manufactured under federal guidelines. Multidose vials are packaged with a special protective cap to discourage tampering during shipping. Any bottles received without a protective seal should be reported immediately to the proper authorities. Controlled drugs have the capital letter "C" printed on their labels. The Roman numeral representing the drug's schedule number is printed within the "C" (see Fig. 1-7).

Technicians, by law, cannot dispense Schedule II substances from their respective containers except under the direct supervision of an individual licensed by the DEA to handle and prescribe such drugs. It is important to realize the controls and restrictions placed upon Schedule II drugs as it may be the AHT's responsibility to maintain the inventory and record books for these drugs. The responsibility for maintaining accurate records and safekeeping of any controlled drug ultimately resides with the veterinarian.

Preanesthetic use of narcotic drugs in dogs and cats

The majority of narcotic analgesics have traditionally been used only for dogs since their tendency to produce an excitatory rather than a sedative action is greater in cats, especially with morphine. Excitement can also occur in dogs, particularly if the narcotic is given too rapidly by the intravenous route. Administering a tranquilizer before or in combination with the narcotic reduces the excitatory side effects. Premedication with atropine is a common procedure to counteract the bra-

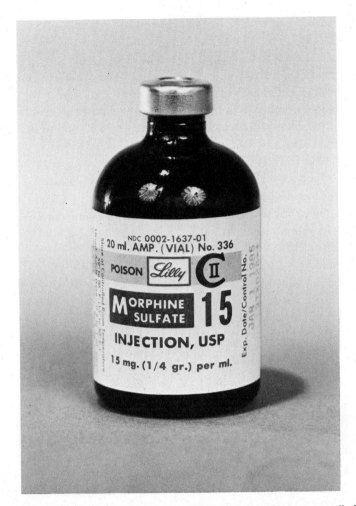

Fig. 1-7. Controlled substance label to show the label for a Schedule II controlled substance. Note also that a drug label must contain the expiration date—in this case, Jan. 1, 1985.

dycardia associated with narcotics. Administration is usually via the intramuscular or subcutaneous route 10 to 30 minutes before induction with a general anesthetic drug. Some narcotics may be given slowly by intravenous injection and at a reduced dosage. Yet caution must be observed, as the intravenous route may result in CNS excitement and/or serious cardiovascular and respiratory depression.

Advantages
Narcotics are often preferred to tranquilizers for preanesthetic medication because:

- They provide good to excellent analgesia when administered at a low dosage. Analgesia may be desired before general anesthesia as well as postoperatively to comfort the animal and help prevent neurogenic shock.
- They provide good sedation and calming at higher dosages. They are capable also of producing light sleep. They do not, however, render the animal totally unconscious or oblivious to the deep pain that accompanies surgical manipulations of the abdomen, thorax, spinal cord, or fractured bones.
- Their depressant actions (for example, sedation, bradycardia, and respiratory depression) are reversible with drugs called narcotic antagonists (see pp. 49-52). Overdosage with a narcotic, therefore, can be minimized if it is detected before the depressant effects become irreversible. Narcotic drugs should *never* be used unless a narcotic antagonist drug is immediately available. In addition, atropine should be available for treating bradycardia that often accompanies narcotic overdosage.
- They stimulate evacuation of both the upper and lower gastrointestinal tract. Some, but not all, narcotics act directly on the CNS of dogs to cause an initial vomiting and defecation before the animal is sedated. For instance, morphine classically produces vomiting and defecation within 5 to 10 minutes after it is injected intramuscularly or subcutaneously in dogs. When a drug like morphine is used as a sole preanesthetic sedative, it is a wise practice to place the dog in a run following the injection so it is less likely to vomit or defecate on itself. If surgery must be performed on a dog that has recently ingested food or water, premedication with morphine is desirable for evacuation of stomach contents, thereby decreasing the likelihood of reflex vomiting under general anesthesia. Use of a tranquilizer before or in combination with the narcotic may cancel the emetic action of the narcotic.
- They can be used in *low* dosages for analgesia and sedation in cats (see Table 1-4). Combining the narcotic with a tranquilizer or administering the tranquilizer 5 to 10 minutes before injecting the narcotic eliminates a great deal of the excitatory side effects of the narcotic drug. When used in cats, the subcutaneous route is preferred.
- They are of particular benefit as a preanesthetic medication for dogs with heart conditions such as congestive heart failure, mitral valve insufficiency, and heartworm disease. Low dosages of narcotic drugs have minimal depressant effects on the myocardium. Morphine, for instance, is sometimes used in low dosages to treat dogs suffering from acute congestive heart failure more because of its beneficial actions on the heart than for its sedative or analgesic properties.
- They allow for a significant reduction (50% to 75%) in the amount of general anesthetic drug required to perform surgery or diagnostic procedures. Narcotics may also be used during general anesthesia to enhance analgesia.

Due to their potent analgesic and sedative action, narcotics are often used for minor surgical procedures in dogs where the index for pain is considered low—for example, suture repair of superficial skin lacerations, removal of a crushed toenail, or extraction of a fishhook from the lip of a fractious dog. Narcotics may also be used for procedures requiring analgesia rather than deep surgical anesthesia—for example, diagnostic radiographs for visualization of a fractured bone where manipulation of the affected limb would otherwise elicit considerable pain, dentistry involving teeth scaling and extraction of loose incisor teeth, or the placement of a urinary catheter. When used for minor procedures, the narcotic sedation can be potentiated by a tranquilizer. This combination lessens the possibility of narcotic excitement and decreases the total amount of narcotic required to perform the procedure.

Disadvantages

Obviously no CNS depressant drug is without undesirable side effects.

- Narcotics depress respiration and blood pressure to a greater degree than tranquilizers and often cause panting along with decreased ventilation.
- They decrease heart rate, cardiac output, and oxygen consumption.
- They require a special narcotics license for their purchase and use. Federal law requires that strict records of narcotic use be maintained within the hospital. A daily inventory of individual usage must be kept and made available for inspection by state and federal agents without notice. Narcotics invite theft; therefore, all narcotics must be kept in a nonmovable safe at all times. Narcotic drugs must never be left on counter tops or in areas where the public can view them. After withdrawing a narcotic dose from the bottle, the vial should be returned immediately to locked storage.
- Narcotics are not always predictable as they can produce excitement or sedation depending on the species as well as the individual animal. Cats are notoriously sensitive to morphine. If given a dosage greater than 1.0 mg/kg, cats may experience varying degrees of morphine mania, characterized by widely dilated pupils, salivation, and anxiety. Higher dosages may lead to extreme CNS excitation and spinal convulsions that can persist for hours or terminate in coma and death. Although dogs can tolerate higher dosages than cats, fatal doses of narcotics in the dog may also be preceded by CNS excitement and convulsions. Death is more often a result of respiratory and cardiovascular depression.
- Narcotics tend to make the animal hyperreactive to sound. An animal under the effect of narcotic sedation should be treated and allowed to recover in a quiet room. If the telephone were to suddenly ring or an instrument were to hit the floor, an animal that has received a narcotic or narcotic-tranquilizer mixture may jump suddenly or even fall from the table. This exaggerated

auditory response is due to the stimulatory effect of certain narcotics on spinal cord reflexes.

• Narcotics stimulate defecation and/or vomiting that create unpleasant working conditions. In addition, the stimulatory effect of some narcotics on vomiting and defecation are contraindicated in such cases as gastrointestinal obstruction, diaphragmatic hernia, punctured lung, ruptured spleen, etc.

• They may lead to postoperative vomiting and/or constipation.

• Narcotics can cross the placenta and depress the newborn's ability to initiate breathing at the time of delivery. Narcotic drugs are often used as part of a balanced anesthesia technique for bitches in need of an emergency cesarean section. Although the risk to the bitch is minimized by such a technique, the chance for respiratory depression in the newborn puppy is a distinct disadvantage of the narcotic. It is important not to administer the narcotic to the bitch until everything is in readiness and surgery can proceed as quickly as possible following the administration of the narcotic.

• When narcotics are combined with a tranquilizer, the degree of respiratory and cardiovascular depression is greater than when either drug is used alone for sedation. Although the depressant actions of the narcotic can be reversed with a narcotic antagonist, such is not the case with the tranquilizer. Depression resulting from the tranquilizer portion of the mixture must be supported until the tranquilizer has been metabolized by the liver and excreted in the urine (a period usually requiring 6 to 24 hours).

• Narcotics decrease body temperature by 1° to 2° C or more, especially when used in combination with general anesthetic drugs for abdominal or thoracic surgery. Tranquilizer drugs also cause some degree of hypothermia.

• They may cause apnea at high dosages.

Signs of narcotic overdosage
Any of the following signs may indicate an overdosage of narcotic drugs:

• Excessive salivation associated with anxious behavior

• Extreme excitement often precipitated by restraint or noise

• Shallow respirations, low respiratory rate, and cyanosis. If the animal is breathing 100% oxygen, the cyanosis may not be manifested until the pure oxygen is discontinued and the animal begins to breathe room air. (See Chapter 6 for a more detailed discussion of cyanosis and pulmonary function.)

• Bradycardia resulting in a heart rate of less than 70 to 75 beats per minute, which is associated with extreme sedation and/or disturbance of cardiac rhythm

• Hypotension resulting in a prolonged capillary refill time or a blood pressure reading of less than 70 to 80 mm/Hg systolic pressure

• Tonic convulsions

• Pinpoint pupil constriction

General precautions

Narcotics should be used with extreme caution or eliminated altogether as pre-anesthetic medication in the following situations:

- Circulatory shock from any cause
- Trauma to the head, thorax, or spinal cord
- Severe limb trauma
- Any type of respiratory or cardiovascular disease
- Debilitating liver or kidney disease
- With untamed animals such as the raccoon, skunk, or ferret
- With cats or dogs with a known sensitivity to one or more narcotic drugs
- With animals that may have received another CNS depressant drug at a referring animal hospital or that have accidentally ingested such intoxicants as alcohol, marijuana, cocaine, or sleeping pills

Specific examples of narcotic drugs

The following list of narcotic drugs is generally used for preanesthetic analgesia and/or sedation. In addition, these drugs may be employed during the anesthetic period as well as postoperatively to provide additional analgesia and prevent excitement or pain during the recovery period. Following the list is a brief discussion of those narcotic drugs most often used in dogs and cats (refer to Table 1-4 for specific drug dosages):

- Morphine
- Meperidine
- Oxymorphone
- Fentanyl
- Apomorphine

Morphine sulfate. Used primarily for its analgesic action, morphine is derived from opium, which is extracted from the unripened seed capsules of the poppy plant.

Availability. Morphine is supplied as a sterile solution containing 10 15, 20, or 30 mg/ml, or as a solution combined with atropine sulfate for parenteral injection. It is also available in 5, 8, 10, 15, and 30 mg tablets.

Route of administration. Subcutaneous or intramuscular injection (intravenous route to be avoided)

Advantages. As a preanesthetic medication, morphine:

- Is inexpensive
- Mixes with atropine
- Provides excellent analgesia
- Stimulates vomiting (and defecation)
- Significantly reduces the amount of general anesthetic needed to induce and maintain surgical anesthesia

- Calms the animal and allows for easier restraint
- Provides analgesia and sedation postoperatively
- Is useful in cardiac disease
- Is reversible

Disadvantages. In addition to the disadvantages of narcotic drugs discussed earlier, morphine has the specific disadvantages of:

- Being contraindicated in cats unless given at a greatly reduced dose and in combination with a tranquilizer
- Causing unpredictable CNS excitement in some dogs, thereby defeating its action as a sedative. Administration of intravenous barbiturate to treat morphine excitement or additional amounts of general anesthetic to induce the anesthetic state may be required in an excited animal.
- Causing postoperative vomiting and/or constipation
- Being a potent respiratory depressant
- Being contraindicated in cases of intestinal obstruction or diaphragmatic hernia due to its stimulation of vomiting and defecation
- Causing hyperreactivity to auditory stimuli

Precautions. See the general precautions associated with the use of narcotic drugs discussed earlier.

Meperidine hydrochloride. A synthetic analgesic drug similar in action to morphine but with fewer side effects, meperidine's analgesic and sedative actions are less than morphine.

Availability. Meperidine is supplied as a sterile 5% or 10% solution containing either 50 or 100 mg/ml for parenteral injection. The lower concentration is generally used for small animals. It is also available for oral use in 50 or 100 mg tablets.

Route of administration. For preanesthetic analgesia and mild sedation, it is administered by intramuscular or subcutaneous injection. When given subcutaneously, 20 to 30 minutes should be allowed for complete action. On occasion, it may be given intravenously, usually to dogs. Rapid intravenous injection may overstimulate the CNS, causing convulsions and a precipitous fall in blood pressure. Meperidine is the narcotic most often used when a dog or cat requires postoperative analgesia and sedation.

Advantages. As a preanesthetic medication, meperidine:

- Provides good analgesia. It is approximately one tenth as potent as morphine and has a wide margin of safety.
- Can be used for intraoperative analgesia
- Reduces the likelihood of postanesthetic excitement during the recovery period
- Does not usually stimulate vomiting or defecation
- Can be used in cats
- Can be used alone or combined with a low dose of tranquilizer for additional

sedation and for decreasing the dosage of general anesthetic drug by 50% to 60%

• Is reversible

Disadvantages. In addition to the disadvantages of narcotic drugs discussed earlier, meperidine has the specific disadvantages of:

• Being more expensive than morphine
• Being less predictable in its sedative action, especially in cats
• Having a shorter duration of action than morphine
• Being less suitable for use in animals with heart disease because of its hypotensive action

Precautions. Refer to the general precautions associated with the use of narcotic drugs discussed earlier.

Oxymorphone hydrochloride. A synthetic narcotic analgesic drug similar in action to morphine but with less respiratory depression at clinical dosages, oxymorphone has analgesic and sedative actions that are considered to be 10 times as potent as morphine on a milogram per kilogram basis.

Availability. Oxymorphone is supplied as a sterile solution containing either 1.0 mg/ml (0.1%) or 1.5 mg/ml (0.15%) for parenteral injection. It is unavailable for oral use.

Route of administration. For preanesthetic analgesia and sedation it is usually given by intramuscular or subcutaneous injection. It may be given to dogs by intravenous injection if analgesia is immediately required. However, caution must be applied as with any narcotic given via this route, and the dosage should be reduced. Intravenous injection is not recommended in cats because of (1) their sensitivity to narcotics and (2) oxymorphone's potent action.

Advantages. As a preanesthetic medication oxymorphone:

• Provides good to excellent pre- and postanesthetic sedation and analgesia
• Can be used in both dogs and cats
• Has minimal depressant action on respiration or cardiovascular function when used at clinical dosages
• Does not usually stimulate vomiting or defecation
• Can be used alone or in combination with a tranquilizer to enhance the sedative action and decrease by 50% to 75% the total amount of general anesthetic required
• Has a specific reversal drug, naloxone, or it can be reversed by other narcotic anatagonists

Disadvantages. There are no specific disadvantages to oxymorphone although it is subject to the general disadvantages of all narcotic drugs.

Precautions. Refer to the general precautions associated with the use of narcotic drugs discussed earlier.

Fentanyl citrate. A potent narcotic analgesic similar in action to morphine, fentanyl is considered to be *100* times more potent than morphine as an analgesic. Fentanyl is used primarily in dogs and most often in combination with the tranquilizer, droperidol.

Availability. Fentanyl is supplied as a sterile solution containing 0.05 mg/ml (0.005%) in 2.0 and 5.0 ml vials for parenteral injection. It is not often used alone as a preanesthetic sedative or analgesic, although it may be given in conjunction with general anesthesia to enhance analgesia. When combined with droperidol in the commercial product, Innovar Vet, fentanyl is supplied at a concentration of 0.4 mg/ml (0.04%). Fentanyl is unavailable for oral use.

Route of administration. As a preanesthetic medication in combination with droperidol, it is usually administered by intramuscular injection. It may also be given intravenously at a reduced dosage for analgesia during a surgical procedure.

Advantages. As a preanesthetic medication fentanyl:
- Provides excellent analgesia at very low dosages
- Combines well with a tranquilizer to provide sedation and analgesia suitable for performing minor surgery, dentistry, or diagnostic procedures. The combination available commercially as Innovar Vet is often used as part of a balanced technique for cesarean section anesthesia in dogs.
- Does not cause vomiting; however, defecation may still occur
- Has a relatively short and mild depressant activity on respiration and cardiovascular function, making it well suited for outpatient use, for use in debilitated dogs during emergency surgery, or for cardiac procedures. Onset of action is rapid by intramuscular or intravenous injection.
- Decreases the total amount of general anesthetic required for a surgical level of anesthesia by 50% to 80%
- Can be reversed by narcotic antagonists

Disadvantages. In addition to the disadvantages of narcotic drugs discussed earlier, fentanyl:
- Is more expensive than other narcotics
- Is contraindicated in cats
- Causes defecation and/or transient diarrhea in some dogs, especially when given by intramuscular or subcutaneous injection
- May result in severe respiratory depression and/or a rigid chest wall, necessitating controlled ventilation
- Often causes panting and/or increased salivation
- Causes a significant bradycardia, especially when given intravenously. Atropine given before the fentanyl by subcutaneous or intramuscular injection will usually prevent salivation and bradycardia. Atropine should always be available when using fentanyl or any other narcotic. Should severe bradycardia occur, atropine may be administered intravenously to restore a normal heart rate.

Precautions. Refer to the general precautions associated with the use of narcotic drugs discussed earlier.

Apomorphine hydrochloride. A direct product of morphine with strong emetic action, apomorphine has mild sedative and analgesic action and is used primarily to induce vomiting in dogs. Apomorphine is not used as a preanesthetic sedative or analgesic even though it possesses these properties to a mild degree.

Availability. It is supplied in tablet form containing 6.5 mg of apomorphine.

Route of administration. If crushed and mixed with sterile saline, the solution may be injected subcutaneously or intramuscularly. Vomiting usually occurs in 5 to 10 minutes. Another method of administration is to crush one-half of a 6.5 mg tablet into a fine powder and place it into the dog's lower conjunctival sac; vomiting usually occurs within 3 to 5 minutes.

Advantage. It directly stimulates the vomiting center of the brain to cause emesis and thus is useful in some cases of poisoning to empty the stomach (the usual dose is $1/2$ to 1 tablet).

Disadvantages. In addition to the general disadvantages of narcotic drugs, apomorphine:

- Is used with dogs only (does not stimulate vomiting in cats)
- Can result in respiratory depression if given repeatedly or in high dosages
- May result in aspiration pneumonitis
- Can cause serious problems if given to animals with problems such as a bowel obstruction resulting from a sharp foreign body in the small intestine, a diaphragmatic hernia, or dilated esophagus
- Will not induce vomiting if the dog was previously given a tranquilizer or narcotic drug
- Causes an initial stimulation of the vomiting center followed by a depression (as with morphine). If the initial dose of apomorphine does not cause emesis, subsequent doses are of little use.
- Will potentiate other CNS depressants
- Should not be administered by ocular route in dogs with conjunctivitis, glaucoma, or other ophthalmalogic disorders

Neuroleptanalgesics

Neuroleptanalgesia is a state of CNS depression and analgesia produced by the combined actions of a narcotic analgesic and a tranquilizer (neuroleptic). Total unconsciousness does not occur and arousal of the sedative state is possible with a painful or auditory stimulus. Several narcotic-tranquilizer combinations are employed. Innovar Vet is the only commercially available combination and is presently the most widely used neuroleptanalgesic for dogs.

When administered at clinically recommended dosages, there is little cardiovascular depression and minimal toxic side effects associated with neuroleptanalgesia.

Severe respiratory depression or apnea, however, is possible, and particular attention must be paid to the animal's respiratory rate, tidal volume, and mucous membrane color.

Because neuroleptanalgesia combinations employ the use of a narcotic drug, they are considered Schedule II controlled substances. Strict records must be maintained of their inventory and hospital usage. The narcotic must be kept in a special locked safe along with any other Schedule II drugs. A special DEA license and order form are also required for purchase.

The contraindications and precautions associated with the use of neuroleptanalgesia are related to the individual narcotic and tranquilizer drugs as well as those general disadvantages and precautions listed for each category of preanesthetic medication.

Primary use in dogs and cats

Neuroleptanalgesic combinations are generally used in dogs, although some combinations can be used in cats for pre- and postanesthetic sedation and analgesia. Atropine may be used to prevent or counteract the salivation or bradycardia sometimes associated with the use of a narcotic. The narcotic and tranquilizer are usually mixed together in the same syringe and administered by intramuscular injection 10 to 15 minutes before inducing general anesthesia. Intravenous administration is possible in medium to large dogs but discouraged in cats. The duration of narcotic analgesia is 20 to 40 minutes, depending on the particular drugs used and whether they are given by the intravenous or intramuscular route. Caution must be shown when administering CNS depressant drugs by the intravenous route. Narcotic antagonist drugs should be available should serious respiratory depression occur. Ventilation may require support in cases of apnea.

Advantages

Combinations of a narcotic and a tranquilizer for use as a preanesthetic medication have the general advantages associated with the use of either drug alone. In addition, neuroleptanalgesic combinations can be useful for:
- Preanesthetic and postoperative analgesia with sedation
- Reducing the total dosage of general anesthetic by 50% to 90%
- Balanced anesthesia in conjunction with a local analgesic or as part of a technique using nitrous oxide and oxygen, a muscle paralyzer, and/or a local analgesic for purposes of major surgery, for example, cesarean section
- Minor surgical procedures of short duration (less than 30 minutes)
- Diagnostic radiographs or other manipulative procedures such as vaginal examinations and skin biopsy
- Dental procedures such as teeth scaling or minor tooth extraction when general anesthesia may effect a greater risk

- Performing certain treatments in aggressive or anxious animals, such as anal gland packing and irrigation and cleaning of ears
- Geriatric animals or animals unable to withstand general anesthesia
- Grooming purposes

Disadvantages

In addition to the disadvantages previously attributed to each individual drug, the combination of a narcotic with a tranquilizer:

- Causes moderate to severe respiratory depression and can produce apnea
- Causes a hypersensitivity to auditory stimuli and therefore requires a quiet work and recovery area
- Is not totally reversible in that the tranquilizer portion of the combination has no antagonist. Depression resulting from the narcotic drug may be reversed with a narcotic antagonist. Unfortunately, the animal may still require attention and support if an overdose of tranquilizer were given. Even after administration of a narcotic antagonist, the animal may continue to show signs of ataxia, sedation, hypothermia, and hypotension until the effects of the tranquilizer drug have worn off.
- Often causes defecation or transient diarrhea
- Often stimulates panting and can cause stiff chest wall, making artificial ventilation difficult unless a muscle-paralyzing drug is given
- Often causes bradycardia
- Can result in spontaneous limb movements or extensor rigidity
- May result in clonic convulsions with overdosages
- Occasionally causes restlessness and delirium vocalization during the recovery period, especially if the recovery area is noisy or heavily trafficked
- In some instances may result in aggressiveness and/or personality changes during the recovery period. The degree of variability in the analgesic and calming effect of neuroleptanalgesia can be disturbing. There have been a few reports of disposition changes lasting up to several days after the use of a neuroleptanalgesic combination. Usually such prolonged effects are related to an overdose of the drug combination.
- Does not produce as predictable analgesia and sedation in the cat as in the dog
- Requires a narcotics license to order and administer. The usual restrictions and record keeping are required because of the narcotic drug's classification as a Schedule II substance.
- Potentiates the depressant action of barbiturates and inhalation anesthetics. The possibility for overdosage of either is greater when neuroleptanalgesics are used for preanesthetic medication. Dosages of barbiturates should be reduced accordingly.

It is important to realize that when narcotics or narcotic combinations are employed for the relief of acute physical pain, there always exists the chance for overdosing the animal once the painful stimulus has been removed. An animal with severe pain will tolerate considerably large doses of narcotics, sometimes even with no obvious signs of relief. Should the pain suddenly subside, as in the passage of a kidney stone from the ureter into the urinary bladder, the animal may rebound into a serious state of respiratory depression if large doses of narcotic were used for analgesia. Reversal of a large overdosage may not be satisfactory in all cases. It is extremely important that the animal be watched closely for signs of respiratory depression, bradycardia, and prolonged capillary refill time during its recovery from a narcotic overdosage. Intubation of the trachea with ventilatory support should be performed when severe respiratory depression occurs.

Specific examples of neuroleptanalgesic combinations

The following examples of commonly used neuroleptanalgesic drug combinations will be discussed only in regard to their generally accepted use in the dog or cat.

Fentanyl + droperidol (Innovar Vet)

Accepted use. Dog only. Not approved for use in cats

Availability. Innovar Vet is supplied as a premixed sterile solution for injection in 20 ml multidose vials, with a concentration of 0.4 mg/ml of fentanyl (narcotic) and 20.0 mg/ml of droperidol (tranquilizer).

One important disadvantage of Innovar Vet is that it allows no flexibility of dosage between narcotic and tranquilizer since it is a premixed solution (see Table 1-4). The human product, Innovar, contains lower concentrations of each drug and is more expensive than Innovar Vet.

Route of administration. Intramuscular or intravenous. Subcutaneous administration usually requires a greater dosage and therefore presents an increased chance for overdosage.

Oxymorphone + triflupromazine

Accepted use. Dog and cat

Availability. It is supplied individually, according to each injectable drug: oxymorphone (1.0 mg/ml or 1.5 mg/ml) and triflupromazine (20 mg/ml). Oxymorphone may also be used in combination with other tranquilizers such as acepromazine to produce varying states of sedation.

Route of administration. Dogs—intramuscular, subcutaneous, or intravenous injection; cats—intramuscular or subcutaneous injection

Meperidine + acepromazine

Accepted use. Dog and cat

Availability. It is supplied individually according to each injectable drug: meperidine (50 mg/ml) and acepromazine (10 mg/ml). Generally, the acepromazine is given at a much lower dosage than when it is being used alone for tranquilization. The purpose of the acepromazine is to augment the narcotic and provide mild sedation. Large doses of acepromazine are to be avoided since it is not reversible, has a long duration of action, and is hypotensive.

Route of administration. Dogs—intramuscular, subcutaneous, or intravenous injection; cats—intramuscular or subcutaneous injection

Narcotic antagonists

Narcotic antagonist drugs are synthetically produced and similar in structure to morphine. There are three antagonist drugs commonly used to abolish the depressant effects of narcotics:

- Nalorphine
- Naloxone
- Levallorphan

Primary use in the dog and cat

The primary use of narcotic antagonists is to reverse the severe respiratory depression characteristic of an overdosage of any narcotic or narcotic/tranquilizer combination. Narcotic antagonists also reverse the analgesia, bradycardia, vomiting, defecation, sedation, hypothermia, miosis, panting, and euphoria associated with the use of narcotic drugs. They will not reverse the milder degrees of respiratory depression associated with low doses of narcotics. Antagonist drugs can also be used to reverse the respiratory depression in puppies or kittens delivered by cesarean section under a narcotic analgesic for balanced anesthesia. Approximately one-tenth to one-twentieth of the adult dose of antagonist can be injected into the umbilical vein of the newborn or applied as a drop underneath the neonate's tongue.

Antagonists do not reverse the depressant effects of tranquilizers, barbiturates, or other general anesthetics. They should not be used to treat respiratory depression caused by any drug(s) other than narcotics. Since antagonists are actually synthetic narcotics, they impart a mild CNS depressant effect of their own, similar to morphine. It is important to realize that if any of these drugs are given to an animal that has not received a previous dose of narcotic, they can produce CNS depression due to their mild narcotic action. If used indiscriminantly to treat depression from drugs other than narcotics, they may add to the depressed state and cause an even greater degree of respiratory depression. It is possible to overdose an animal with a narcotic antagonist, producing signs similar to overdosage with a narcotic drug— for example, respiratory depression, hypothermia, bradycardia, or even seizures. If the first dose of a narcotic antagonist does not reverse the depressant effects of a narcotic, it is unwise to give additional doses since they will do little to improve the depression and may lead to an overdosage of the antagonist. Naloxone has the least depressant activity of the three commonly used narcotic antagonists and may be given as a repeated dose provided the total dosage requirement is not exceeded.

Route of administration

A narcotic antagonist drug should always be available when narcotics are being used. The antagonist acts fastest when administered by the intravenous route but may also be given intramuscularly or subcutaneously when immediate narcotic reversal is not required. The initial effects of an intravenous injection are seen within 15 to 30 seconds. The panting respiration created by the narcotic is altered to a more normal tidal volume and rate of breathing. (If respiratory depression occurs during the period of general anesthesia due to a previously administered narcotic or a supplemental dose of narcotic, a small dose of antagonist can be given intravenously to effect, thereby restoring a more adequate ventilation without interfering with the level of general anesthesia.) Within 1 to 2 minutes after administering the antagonist, 80% to 90% of the narcotic-induced respiratory depression and 50% to 75% of narcotic sedation are reversed. Reversal of the respiratory depression lasts from 1 to 4 hours depending on the amount of narcotic given and the dose of antagonist used. A relatively small dosage of antagonist is capable of reversing a large dose of narcotic.

Specific examples of narcotic antagonists

The three most commonly used narcotic antagonist drugs for dogs and cats are nalorphine, levallorphan, and naloxone. Since these drugs are synthetically related to morphine, they are considered narcotics in themselves and therefore subject to the federal controls concerning all Schedule II substances. Fig. 1-8 shows two commonly used antagonist drugs with some of the narcotics they can reverse.

Nalorphine hydrochloride. Synthetically derived from morphine, nalorphine is used extensively in dogs to antagonize morphine, meperidine, or fentanyl (Innovar Vet). It also antagonizes respiratory depression caused by overdoses of heroin, codeine, oxymorphone, methadone, and most other natural or synthetic narcotics. In addition, it has been used as an antidote to intoxication from the commonly available commercial products, propoxyphene (Darvon) and pentazocine (Talwin).

Route of administration. Most often given intravenously. May be given by subcutaneous or intramuscular injection although the therapeutic effect is less and the onset of action is slower.

Availability. Nalorphine is supplied as a sterile solution containing 0.2 mg/ml (ampules) or 5.0 mg/ml (multidose vials) for parenteral injection.

Levallorphan tartrate. Similar to nalorphine, levallorphan antagonizes the same narcotics as nalorphine. However, it is approximately 5 to 10 times more potent than nalorphine in reversing respiratory depression.

Route of administration. Intravenous injection is preferred.

Availability. Levallorphan is supplied as a sterile solution containing 0.05 mg/ml (ampules) or 1.0 mg/ml (multidose vials) for parenteral injection.

Naloxone hydrochloride. Synthetically derived from the narcotic analgesic, ox-

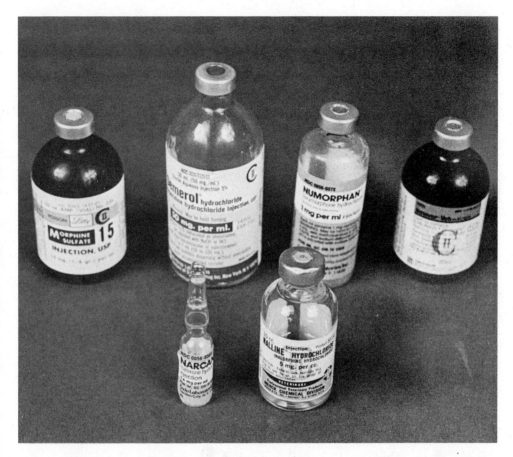

Fig. 1-8. The top row shows four narcotic drugs commonly used with animals: from left to right, morphine, meperidine, oxymorphone, and Innovar Vet. The bottom row shows two antagonist drugs that can be used to reverse the depressant effects of a narcotic: from left to right, naloxone and nalorphine.

ymorphone, naloxone specifically reverses the depressant effects of oxymorphone. It also antagonizes other narcotic analgesics such as morphine, meperidine, and fentanyl. Although naloxone is more expensive than other antagonists, it presently enjoys the advantage of causing little, if any, respiratory depressant activity. It is approximately 10 times as potent as nalorphine and 3 times as potent as levallorphan in reversing respiratory depression due to narcotic overdose. When naloxone is used to reverse the respiratory depression caused by its parent compound, oxymorphone, analgesia remains even after the respiratory depression has been abolished. Naloxone also antagonizes the commercial analgesic product, Talwin, and can be used to treat dogs or cats accidentally intoxicated with this product.

Route of administration. Intravenous injection preferred. For every 1.5 mg of oxymorphone, 0.02 mg (0.05 ml) of naloxone should be administered for reversal. The maximum 4 hour dose should not exceed 0.4 mg.

Availability. Naloxone is supplied as a sterile solution containing 0.4 mg/ml for parenteral injection. Multidose vials are unavailable.

Other preanesthetic medications

A number of other anesthetic drugs can be used as preanesthetic medications. Some of these include such injectable drugs as short-acting barbiturates for preoperative sedation and low doses of dissociative anesthetic drugs, such as ketamine, for preanesthetic immobilization and sedation of cats (see Chapter 3). These drugs however, are not often used as preanesthetics by small animal practitioners. (Although ketamine may be used as a preanesthetic in cats, it will not be discussed in this chapter; however, its dosage for this purpose is included in Table 1-4.)

Muscle paralyzers

A brief account of muscle-paralyzing drugs is given here in order to introduce the student to their general use and indications and contraindications. Further reading on individual muscle-paralyzing drugs is recommended whenever these drugs are used on a routine basis in conjunction with a general anesthetic. These drugs, in practice, are never administered until a state of unconsciousness has been obtained in the patient.

Muscle-paralyzing drugs are also referred to as *muscle relaxants.* These drugs act by interrupting normal impulse transmission at the nerve-to-muscle synapse (neuromuscular junction). They act primarily on voluntary (skeletal) muscles to cause a flaccid paralysis. Since these drugs almost always result in paralysis of the intercostal and diaphragmatic muscles, they must be used with extreme caution. The term "muscle paralyzer" is preferred to "muscle relaxant" because of the potential to paralyze ventilation. THEY POSSESS NO SEDATIVE OR ANALGESIC PROPERTIES AND SHOULD NEVER BE USED AS THE SOLE ANESTHETIC DRUG. Their use during anesthesia is only as an adjuvant to other general anesthetic drugs to produce a more complete relaxation of skeletal muscles.

Muscle-paralyzing drugs produce a progressive paralysis of skeletal muscles, beginning with the muscles of the face, neck, tail, and limbs. The abdominal muscles, intercostals, and diaphragm are then paralyzed in subsequent order. Death can easily result from clinical doses if the animal is not artificially ventilated, death being directly attributable to respiratory paralysis. It is considered inhumane to use these drugs without some means for artificially ventilating the animal and without general anesthesia. Tracheal intubation must always precede the administration of these drugs when they are used for complete muscle relaxation. It is also strongly advised that a source of 100% oxygen be available.

Many of the currently used muscle-paralyzing drugs can be partially or totally

TABLE 1-4

Suggested dosage ranges of some common preanesthetic medications for use in healthy dogs and cats*

Drug name	Canine dosage (mg/kg)†	Feline dosage (mg/kg)†
Atropine	0.02-0.10	Same
Scopolamine	0.01-0.02	Same
Glycopyrrolate	0.01-0.02	Same
Succinylcholine	0.2-0.4 (IV)	0.5-1.0 (IV) (very short duration)
Pancuronium	0.05-0.1 (IV)	Same
Neostigmine	0.02-0.05 (IV) preceded by atropine (.04 mg/kg) (do not repeat more than 3 times)	Same
Acetylproma-zine	0.05-0.20 (not to exceed 4.0 mg)	Same
Chlorpromazine	1.0-5.0	1.0-2.0
Promazine	2.0-6.0	4.0-6.0
Triflupromazine	2.0-4.0	4.0-8.0
Xylazine	1.0-2.0	0.5-1.0
Diazepam	0.2-1.0 (IV) (not to exceed 10.0 mg)	Same (not to exceed 5.0 mg)
Morphine	0.1-2.0	0.05-0.10
Meperidine	1.0-5.0	0.5-2.0
Oxymorphone	0.1-0.2 (up to 5.0 mg)	Total dose = 0.5-1.0 mg
Fentanyl	0.01-0.05 (IV)	Not recommended
Innovar Vet®	1 ml/5-10 kg (IM) or 1 ml/10-30 kg (IV)	Not recommended
Naloxone (0.4 mg/ml)	0.05-0.5 ml (IV) (not to exceed 1.0 ml over 4 hours)	0.05-0.25 ml (IV) (not to exceed 0.5 ml over 4 hours)
Nalorphine (5.0 mg/ml)	0.5-1.0 ml (IV, IM, or SQ)	0.2-0.5 ml (IV)
Ketamine	Not recommended	5-10 (IM)

*Dosage is given as a range rather than a single value to emphasize the variability seen within a single species. Animals that are sick or depressed require significant reduction in dosage. Route of administration is assumed to be subcutaneous unless specified within parentheses.
†To convert dosage figures to mg/lb, divide by 2.2.

reversed with the antagonist drug, neostigmine. Those muscle-paralyzing drugs that act as depolarizing agents on the neuromuscular junction are not reversible, for example, succinylcholine. Artificial ventilation may also be needed during the recovery period even when a reversal drug is used. Hypoventilation is a serious complication in the use of any muscle-paralyzing drug and incomplete reversal of the paralyzer is not uncommon. Artificial ventilation should be maintained until the animal has recovered its *full* ability to move air into and out of its lungs and is able to hold its head upright. A nerve stimulator is helpful in determining when to safely extubate a paralyzed patient.

The muscle-paralyzing drugs most often used for dogs and cats act locally at the neuromuscular junction to decrease nerve impulse conduction through skeletal muscle tissue, thereby producing a localized relaxation (paralysis) of muscle. General anesthetics, on the other hand, cause muscle relaxation by depressing the CNS, resulting in a decrease in skeletal muscle tone due to a centralized action. Unfortunately, profound muscle relaxation from general anesthetic drugs is difficult to obtain without also causing serious depression of respiration and blood pressure.

Common muscle-paralyzing drugs are generally classified as either *depolarizing* or *nondepolarizing*.
- Depolarizing muscle-paralyzing drug: succinylcholine
- Nondepolarizing muscle-paralyzing drugs:
   a. Curare
   b. Gallamine
   c. Pancuronium

Nondepolarizing muscle-paralyzing drugs are reversible with neostigmine, provided the neuromuscular junction has not been overly suppressed. Reliance on neostigmine to totally restore a paralyzed animal's normal ventilation is unwise since neostigmine is an antcholinesterase drug and not without its own side effects—namely, bradycardia and increased bronchial and salivary secretions. Administration of atropine (0.04 mg/kg) should always precede neostigmine to counteract these muscarinic side effects. To avoid a cumulative muscarinic effect, neostigmine should not be repeated more than two or three times (see Fig. 1-9).

Indications
- To produce better skeletal muscle relaxation during surgical procedures such as orthopedics or deep abdominal surgery in large dogs
- To facilitate controlled ventilation as in thoracic surgery
- To facilitate a difficult tracheal intubation or break a laryngospasm in cats (usually given shortly after an ultrashort-acting barbiturate)
- To aid in the reduction of dislocated joints, especially in large dogs
- To decrease the amount of general anesthetic drug in debilitated animals (as part of a balanced anesthetic technique)

Contraindications
- With animals with moderate to severe respiratory, liver, or kidney disease
- With animals suffering from glaucoma or undergoing surgery of the eye (succinylcholine raises intraocular pressure)
- With animals being concurrently treated with any of the following antibiotics: neomycin, streptomycin, polymyxin, gentamicin, or any other "mycin" antibiotic. These antibiotics tend to potentiate the paralytic action and increase the duration of paralysis from muscle relaxants.

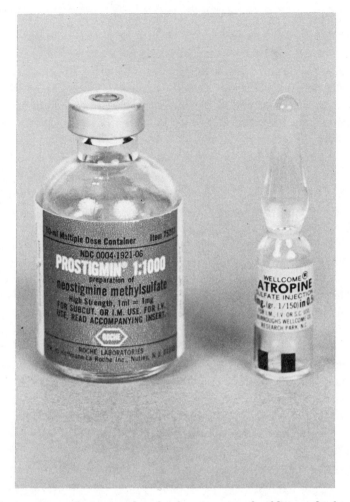

Fig. 1-9. Neostigmine and atropine drug bottles. Atropine should precede the neostigmine to lessen the chance for muscarinic side effects.

- With animals that have been recently treated with organophosphate insecticides or other anticholinesterase medications—for example, flea and tick dips, flea collars, or flea sprays. These medications tend to increase the intensity of paralysis and prolong the recovery period.
- With animals with electrolyte imbalance, especially involving potassium and/or calcium ions. (Prolonged respiratory paralysis or cardiac arrest could result from indiscriminant use of muscle-paralyzing drugs in such animals.)
- With animals with known or suspected histories of susceptibility to malignant hyperthermia
- With animals that are not first put under general anesthesia (use of muscle-paralyzing drugs before general anesthesia is considered inhumane)

PARENTERAL DRUG DOSING

Drug dosages for animals are usually given a range to compensate for such variables as age, breed, personality, and physical status of the species as well as the route by which the drug is administered. For the most part anesthetic drugs are dosed in milligrams per kilogram of body weight. It is important that the AHT become familiar with the metric system, especially as it pertains to conversions between pounds and kilograms and to working with percentage solutions (see Appendix B).

When asked to administer a drug to an animal, the AHT should be able to calculate with minimal delay the dosage according to the veterinarian's preference. It is good practice to check and *double check* all calculations of anesthetic drugs before their administration. The AHT should never administer a potent drug to an animal without the assurance that the dose is accurate and appropriate for the situation. Once injected there may be no means of retrieving an overdose. A watchful technician can often discover an error in dosage before it is administered and therefore serves an invaluable role as part of a necessary guardian system concerning the animal's welfare. If an error in dosage is suspected, the technician must never adjust it without first consulting the veterinarian.

Preanesthetic tranquilizer calculation

Calculating anesthetic drug dosages is a relatively simple procedure. Before proceeding with the calculation, the following information is essential:
1. The weight of the animal in kilograms (kg)
2. The concentration of the drug being administered (mg/ml)
3. The recommended dosage of the drug (usually given in milligrams per kilogram [mg/kg]).

In most cases the only variable is the animal's weight. The recommended dosage will vary somewhat among species and according to the situation, but the drug's concentration should not vary.

Below is an example of calculating the dosage for a preanesthetic injection of acepromazine to be administered subcutaneously to a 20 kg dog:
- Weight of dog = 20.0 kg
- Concentration of acepromazine = 10.0 mg/ml
- Recommended dosage of acepromazine = 0.2 mg/kg by subcutaneous injection

To find the dosage in this case multiply the dog's weight by the dosage:

$$20.0 \text{ kg} \times 0.2 \text{ mg/kg} = 4.0 \text{ mg}$$

The final step is to calculate the volume of acepromazine required since it is supplied as a 1.0% solution containing 10.0 mg/ml. This is done by setting up a simple algebraic equation to solve for X, (X representing the unknown volume of acepromazine to be injected):

(a) $\dfrac{10.0 \text{ mg}}{1.0 \text{ ml}} = \dfrac{4.0 \text{ mg}}{X \text{ ml}}$

(b) $\dfrac{10.0 \text{ mg} \cdot X \text{ ml}}{1.0 \text{ ml}} = 4.0 \text{ mg}$

(c) $10.0 \text{ mg} \cdot X \text{ ml} = 4.0 \text{ mg} \cdot 1.0 \text{ ml}$

(d) $X \text{ ml} = \dfrac{4.0 \text{ mg}}{10.0 \text{ mg}} \cdot 1.0 \text{ ml}$

(e) $X = 0.4 \text{ ml}$

In this example the dog would be given 0.4 ml of acepromazine by subcutaneous injection. A 1.0 ml tuberculin syringe should be used to accurately measure and administer the 0.4 ml volume (see Fig. 1-10).

When calculating drug dosages, one should always follow a step-by-step procedure until completely familiar with the drug and its concentration. The following steps are recommended when administering drugs by parenteral injection:

1. Record animal's weight in kilograms.
2. Multiply animal's weight (in kg) by the recommended drug dosage (in mg/ kg) to get the total mass (mg) of drug needed for the animal.

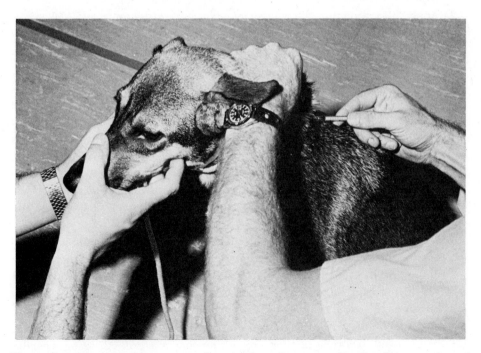

Fig. 1-10. Subcutaneous injection in dog. A tuberculin syringe (1 ml) is being used to administer 0.4 ml of acepromazine while the AHT gently restrains the dog's head.

3. Set up a proportional equation between the concentration of the drug as it is supplied (in mg/ml) and the total mass needed for the particular animal to get the final volume for administration.

4. Verify correct dosage, route of administration, and animal's identity before administering the drug(s).

5. Select the appropriate size syringe and hypodermic needle for injection of the drug. A 22 gauge needle (or smaller) should be used for the subcutaneous injection to minimize discomfort. If the solution being injected is viscous, a larger hypodermic needle is necessary to deliver a smooth and rapid injection.

6. Aseptically remove (aspirate) the desired volume of drug from its container.

When aspirating a drug from a multidose vial, it is essential to maintain the sterility of the drug by practicing strict asepsis. Contamination of a multidose vial with bacteria and/or chemical residues may inactivate the drug and/or lead to infection of the animal in the form of a local abscess or generalized septicemia.

The following procedure is recommended when aspirating and administering an injectable drug from a multidose vial:

1. Select the appropriate sized sterile syringe and hypodermic needle. Attach needle to syringe without contaminating the syringe tip or any portion of the hypodermic needle. Leave needle capped until ready for use.

2. Apply 70% alcohol to the rubber injection cap on the multidose vial. Allow enough time for the alcohol to disinfect the surface (1 to 5 minutes), and scrub surface lightly. Remove any residual alcohol with sterile gauze or cotton before aspirating the drug.

3. Invert multidose vial and introduce hypodermic needle through the vial stopper at a slight angle (see Fig. 1-11). This causes minimal damage to the rubber stopper by creating a resealable entry hole through the stopper, preventing subsequent leakage of the drug or contamination of the vial contents with small pieces of rubber. Avoid inserting the needle through the stopper at a perpendicular angle, as this creates a larger entry hole and induces contamination. Alternate sites on the rubber stopper through which the needle is introduced, and use as small a gauge needle as practical to pierce the stopper.

4. Aspirate the desired volume of drug into the syringe. If a vacuum has developed within the multidose vial, aspiration will be difficult. Hold the plunger of the syringe to prevent any of its contents from entering the multidose vial should a vacuum be present. On the other hand, if the vial contains excessive pressure, the plunger of the syringe may be forced out of the barrel unless it is held firmly. Excessive pressure or vacuum within the multidose vial can be relieved before aspirating by introducing a sterile 22 gauge needle through the stopper while holding the vial upright. This allows the air space

Preanesthetic considerations

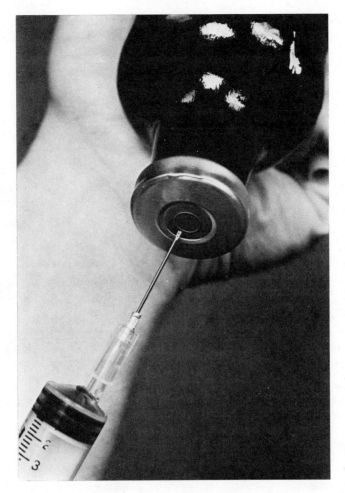

Fig. 1-11. Correct needle entry into multidose vial. The bevel of the needle enters the multidose vial at an angle of about 30 degrees.

    within the vial to equilibrate with atmospheric pressure. Injecting air into a multidose vial before aspirating may be contraindicated with certain drugs, as the air may decrease the potency and/or cause precipitation of the drug.

5. Remove the needle from the vial and replace the sterile protective cap. (During aspiration the needle cap should be held in the fingers or placed on a surface so as not to contaminate the inner protective surface.) Apply alcohol to the vial stopper before returning it to its proper location.

6. Hold syringe so needle is up and gently tap the syringe by flicking the barrel with a finger to displace any large air bubbles to the top. Expel air bubbles through the needle. Replace protective needle cap.

7. Administer the injection in an aseptic manner (Fig 1-12).
8. Dispose of needle and syringe in appropriate manner. Do not discard un-
   capped needles or reusable syringes into regular wastebasket. Once used,
   the needle should be destroyed and placed in a special container for eventual
   incineration. Unless the syringe is to be reautoclaved, it should also be destroyed following use and held for incineration.

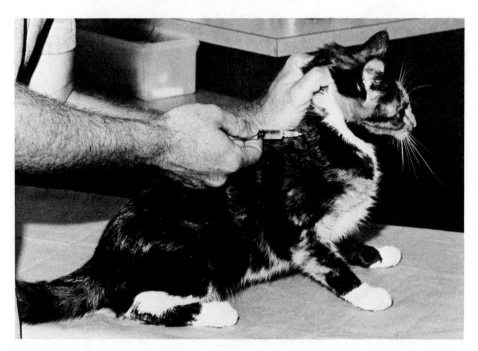

Fig. 1-12. Subcutaneous injection in cat—without assistance. The left hand restrains the
cat's head while pulling up slightly on the skin over the dorsum of the neck. The injection
is made into the subcutaneous space beneath the raised skin. If the cat becomes unruly,
upward tension on the neck raises the front feet off the table surface, thereby permitting
more control.

2

Assessing the depth of general anesthesia

PERFORMANCE OBJECTIVES

After completion of this chapter, the student will:

- List the common vital signs and reflexes used when evaluating an animal's physical status while under general anesthesia

- Discuss the three criteria of general anesthesia

- List the classic stages of general anesthesia and differentiate each stage according to changes in vital signs and reflex activity

- Discuss the purposes of patient monitoring

- Describe routine methods for monitoring important parameters during the anesthetic period

- List the general signs associated with an animal's recovery from general anesthesia

- Discuss the potential problems that may occur during the animal's recovery period

- List the common emergency situations associated with the routine administration of general anesthesia to small animal patients

- Discuss the etiology, signs, and preventive measures associated with aspiration pneumonitis in the dog or cat

VITAL SIGNS

The following common vital signs can be used in conjunction with reflexes to evaluate the animal's physical status while under the effects of an anesthetic drug:
1. Heart rate and rhythm
2. Respiratory rate, rhythm, and depth
3. Arterial pulse
4. Body temperature
5. Mucous membrane color
6. Capillary refill
7. Pupil size and response to light
8. Intraocular pressure

It is important to evaluate as many of these vital signs as possible before administering any drugs that depress the CNS. A written anesthesia form should be used to record preanesthetic vital signs, especially in high risk patients (see "Monitoring the anesthetized patient"). This information can then be used as a baseline for comparing the effects of all subsequent drugs on the animal's normal vital signs.

Heart rate and rhythm

Normal awake value: Dog = 70-110 beats/minute
Cat = 90-140 beats/minute

Most general anesthetic drugs cause the heart rate to decrease—usually only about 10%—once a surgical plane has been obtained. Animals that normally have a slow heart rate (that is, 80 beats per minute) may show no significant decrease under anesthesia. Anesthetic drugs tend to decrease body temperature and metabolism, which in turn tend to lower the heart rate depending on the degree of hypothermia. On the other hand, the heart rate is likely to increase during the induction of general anesthesia because of a transitory excitation of the CNS. A heart rate of less than 70 beats per minute in dogs or 80 beats per minute in cats is considered bradycardiac. The characteristic rhythm of the heart sounds may also be altered by anesthetic drugs, some having a more pronounced effect than others (see Table 2-1).

Many anesthetic drugs directly irritate the heart muscle (myocardium) and predispose the heart to dysrhythmias. The early signs of cardiac irritability can often be detected by the use of an electrocardiogram, cardiac monitor, or Doppler apparatus. A noticeable change in the rhythm of the heart may be a sign of impending cardiac arrest even when there is no anesthetic overdosage. The heart rate and rhythm can be determined by using a stethoscope to auscultate both left and right chest walls in the area of the third to sixth ribs. Under anesthesia an esophageal stethoscope provides a better means for listening to heart and lung sounds while an electrocardiographic monitor should be used on all high risk patients to observe electric conduction through the atria and ventricles of the heart. Monitoring equip-

TABLE 2-1

Generalized classification of anesthetic drugs and techniques with examples

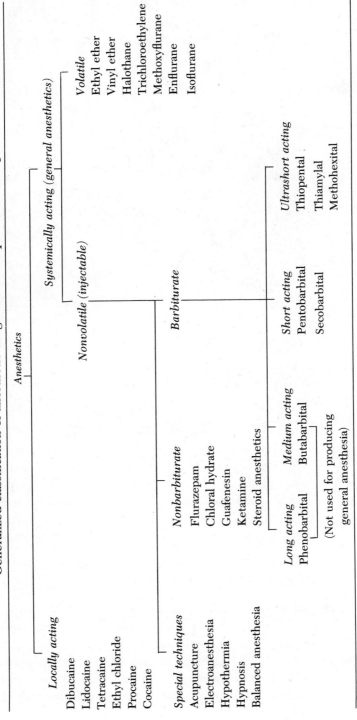

Anesthetics

Locally acting
Dibucaine
Lidocaine
Tetracaine
Ethyl chloride
Procaine
Cocaine

Special techniques
Acupuncture
Electroanesthesia
Hypothermia
Hypnosis
Balanced anesthesia

Systemically acting (general anesthetics)

Nonvolatile (injectable)

Barbiturate

Long acting
Phenobarbital

(Not used for producing general anesthesia)

Medium acting
Butabarbital

Short acting
Pentobarbital
Secobarbital

Ultrashort acting
Thiopental
Thiamylal
Methohexital

Nonbarbiturate
Flurazepam
Chloral hydrate
Guafenesin
Ketamine
Steroid anesthetics

Volatile
Ethyl ether
Vinyl ether
Halothane
Trichloroethylene
Methoxyflurane
Enflurane
Isoflurane

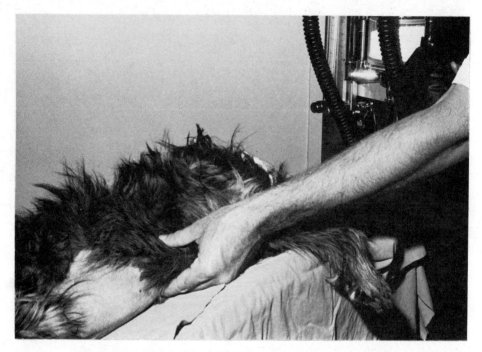

Fig. 2-1. Direct palpation of heartbeat. Dog's head is to the right.

ment is discussed later in this chapter. In small dogs and cats heart rate may also be determined by direct palpation of the animal's ventral chest wall to detect the apex beat (see Fig. 2-1).

When auscultating heart sounds, one should simultaneously palpate the pulse rate to determine if there is a significant discrepancy between the two. This can be done by palpating the femoral artery pulse while listening to the heart sounds with a stethoscope. When the heart rate is significantly higher than the pulse rate, the resulting *pulse deficit* may be indicative of a failing or inefficient heart. Determination of an existing pulse deficit should be part of the routine preanesthetic physical examination.

Respiratory rate, rhythm, and depth

Normal awake value in dog and cat = 20-30 breaths/minute

The term "respiration" is often used interchangeably with the term "ventilation," which is synonymous with "breathing." The most accurate term to describe the movement of air or gas into and out of the lungs, the normal exchange of oxygen from the lung alveoli into the pulmonary blood, and the normal elimination of carbon dioxide from the pulmonary blood into the lungs is "ventilation." The student should be aware of the distinctions many physiologists make between respiration and ventilation. From a purist's point of view "respiration" should be reserved for those biophysic and biochemic processes that have to do with the binding of oxygen to hemoglobin, the release of oxygen into the tissues for cellular metabolism, and the production and elimination of carbon dioxide at a cellular level. In this text, respiration refers to the mechanical aspects of ventilation and diffusion of gases between lung alveoli and pulmonary blood flow—namely the intake of oxygen (O_2) and elimination of carbon dioxide (CO_2).

Every time an animal breathes, it takes into its lungs approximately the same volume of air as it exhales. This volume of air (or gas) is referred to as the *tidal volume* (V_T). The tidal volume of an animal under general anesthesia can be estimated by multiplying the animal's weight (kg) by 10 to 15 ml (see Fig. 6-3). (The normal resting tidal volume is approximately 10 ml/kg.) The number of times an animal breathes in a minute is referred to as the *respiratory rate*. The tidal volume multiplied by the breathing rate gives the minute volume ($\dot{V}_E$) of respiration, which is often a more meaningful value than the tidal volume or rate of breathing alone. The student should become familiar with the terms used to describe the various volumes in the lungs and the concepts of anatomic versus mechanical dead space (see Chapter 6).

Depth of respiration refers to the size of the tidal volume. A shallow depth of respiration indicates a less than normal tidal volume. A sigh is a greater than normal tidal volume and is a normal physiologic response in the awake animal, designed to expand partially collapsed lung alveoli, thus preventing *atelectasis*.

The rhythm of respiration involves the time relationship between the inspiratory and expiratory phases of breathing. A normal at-rest rhythm consists of an inspiratory phase lasting about 1 to $1^{1}/_{2}$ seconds followed by a longer expiratory phase lasting 3 to 4 seconds. Normal inhalation involves an active expansion of the thorax followed by an elastic recoil to expel lung gases out of the trachea and into the atmosphere. When thoracic expansion is impaired or the normal airway is obstructed, the rhythm of respiration is altered. Abdominal breathing produces a less than normal tidal volume with a short, jerky rhythm sometimes referred to as "rocking boat" breathing. Adequate tidal volume should be evaluated by closely observing bilateral expansion of the chest walls (or lungs if the chest is open) and/or determination of arterial blood gas values.

All general anesthetic drugs and most preanesthetic sedatives decrease tidal volume by reducing the ability of the intercostal muscles to adequately expand the thorax. Most also decrease the rate of breathing and thus the minute ventilation. Tidal volume is decreased by 25% to 30% under general anesthesia while the rate of breathing generally drops to about 10 to 16 breaths per minute. The induction period generally causes an increased rate of breathing and/or breath holding. For example, halothane anesthesia may cause an increased respiratory rate coupled with a decreased tidal volume.

The term "hypoventilation" is often taken to mean a less than normal rate of breathing. Hyperventilation refers to a higher than normal respiratory rate and tidal volume. However, hyperventilation and panting are not to be confused since they have different underlying causes. Panting (tachypnea) is characterized by rapid yet shallow breathing and an open mouth. Panting is the normal response to an increase in body temperature and is a dog's or cat's major means for eliminating excess body heat. In the dog narcotics often produce a panting respiratory pattern resulting from their effect on the portion of the brain controlling body temperature and respiration. Hyperventilation is most often a response to a greater than normal arterial carbon dioxide (CO_2) tension. Hypoventilation is a decreased response to normal arterial CO_2 tension and is characterized by a decreased rate and tidal volume. The majority of general anesthetic drugs produce a hypoventilation that results in an increased arterial CO_2 tension (hypercapnia) (see Chapter 6 for explanation of arterial gas tensions). Rapid and shallow respirations in an anesthetized animal are often due to a buildup of CO_2 in the arterial blood, causing a respiratory acidosis. They may also be the result of hypoxia or hyperthermia due to fever or a rare condition known as *malignant hyperthermia*. Increased respiratory rate could also indicate a lightening of the anesthetic depth, especially during the administration of inhalation anesthesia. The anesthetist must be aware of all these possibilities in order to properly assess the cause for ventilatory changes and take appropriate action, if necessary.

Arterial pulse

The pulse should be palpated in one or more major arteries and the rate as well as the character of the pulse wave noted. A weak pulse wave may indicate hypotension. The pulse rate and heart rate should always be equal. In cats, palpation of a peripheral artery is more difficult than in dogs (unless the dog weighs less than 4 to 5 kg). If the femoral or lingual artery pulse is unpalpable, the systolic blood pressure may be critically low. Arteries that can be used for palpating the pulse, depending on accessibility, are:
- Femoral artery (medial aspect of upper thigh)
- Carotid artery (either side of trachea on neck)
- Lingual artery (ventral midline of tongue)
- Volar metacarpal artery (palmar aspect of paw distal to accessory carpal pad)
- Dorsal tarsal artery (dorsal aspect of hock joint)

Body temperature

Normal awake body temperature in dogs and cats = 38°-39° C

All tranquilizers, narcotics, and especially general anesthetics cause a decrease in normal body temperature (hypothermia). For anesthetic procedures of longer than 30 minutes' duration, a means of preventing heat loss from the animal's skin should be a routine procedure. One of the major causes of patient heat loss is the animal's placement on a cold stainless steel operating table. At the very least, a layer of newspaper, towels, or an insulated pad should be laid between the animal and the operating table. Cool air from air-conditioning units must never flow over the animal or the anesthetic vaporizer.

Prolonged general anesthesia (in excess of 60 minutes) can drop the normal body temperature 2° to 3° C. This degree of hypothermia, combined with a surgical procedure in which there is additional heat loss from a large abdominal or thoracic incision, can produce a body temperature of 35° C or below after 60 to 90 minutes of surgical anesthesia. In cases where extensive heat loss is anticipated, a circulating warm water pad is recommended to prevent serious hypothermia. Careless use of electric heating pads can be dangerous. Unless the lowest temperature setting is used, the heating pad can cause second or third degree burns where it contacts the animal's skin.

Body temperature during anesthesia is best monitored with a direct reading thermometer since use of a glass rectal thermometer to monitor body temperature may give a false reading. In addition, repeated readings of a rectal thermometer becomes time-consuming and, at times, impossible if the surgical procedure does not permit easy access to the animal's rectum. Direct reading thermometers can be placed in the rectum or esophagus of the animal and provide a constant readout of changes in body temperature. Hypothermia slows the rate at which the liver metabolizes anesthetic drugs, thereby prolonging anesthetic recovery. Severe hypothermia can also result in cardiac instability and shivering during recovery. Thus there is concern if the body temperature drops below 35° to 36° C.

Color of mucous membranes

Mucous membranes are normally medium pink, and some of the areas for observing their color are:
- Conjunctiva (always observing both eyes)
- Gingiva
- Tongue
- Lips and cheek (see Fig. 2-2)
- Prepuce or penis in males
- Vulva membranes in females (see Fig. 2-3)
- Inner margin of rectum
- Surgical incision

The color of the skin, wound edges, and internal organs may also be used to evaluate the animal's state of circulation and oxygenation. Periodically, the AHT should request an inspection of these areas by the surgeon. Mucous membranes of the mouth and tongue may be pigmented in dogs like the Chow and Labrador retriever. Therefore these areas should not be used to interpret color.

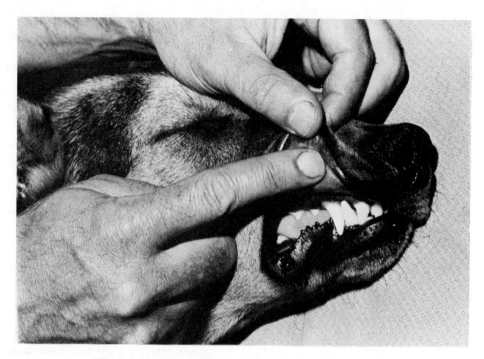

Fig. 2-2. Capillary refill test on buccal mucous membrane.

When administering 100% oxygen mixed with a volatile anesthetic, it is difficult to assess the true state of oxygenation to tissues like the mucous membranes. Awareness of this masking potential is important when administering high concentrations of oxygen to animals that may be in a condition of impaired respiratory and/or cardiovascular stability. Often such an animal will appear pinker under inhalation anesthesia than before, which should not be confused with improved health.

Capillary refill

Normal capillary refill time: Dog and cat = 1-2 seconds
Normal systolic blood pressure: Dog and cat = 110-180 mm/Hg
Normal diastolic blood pressure: Dog and cat = 70-90 mm/Hg

It is uncommon in general practice to directly monitor an animal's arterial blood pressure. To do so would involve additional time, expense, and insult to the animal since it involves cannulation of a major artery (for example, the femoral artery) under strict asepsis. Currently an ultrasonic Doppler and blood pressure cuff (sphygmomanometer) are being used to indirectly measure systolic blood pressure from the distal extremities of dogs (see Fig. 2-18).

A crude yet valuable means for monitoring an animal's tissue perfusion is the

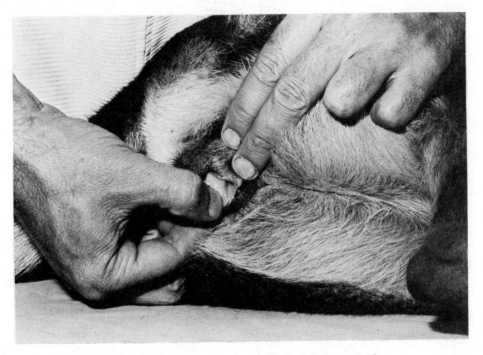

Fig. 2-3. Examination of vulvar mucous membrane in dog.

capillary refill test. Gentle but firm pressure is applied to the gingiva or inner surface of the lip (see Fig. 2-4). The pressure is then quickly released and the time required for the return of normal color to the area is noted. Applying finger pressure on the mucous membrane of the gums compresses the small capillaries, temporarily blocking blood perfusion to the area. Releasing the pressure allows the capillaries to fill with blood. The blanched white color seen when the pressure is initially released represents a section of capillary bed void of blood, and therefore void of hemoglobin and oxygen. As long as the heart is pumping with sufficient pressure, blood will reexpand the compressed capillaries, and flow will return to the area, bringing with it hemoglobin and oxygen. Oxygenated hemoglobin provides the normal pink color of mucous membranes. When hemoglobin is not combined with oxygen, it casts a bluish hue to mucous membranes (cyanosis). Cyanosis is difficult to diagnose from mucous membrane color unless the hemoglobin concentration is less than 5 gm/100 ml (see Table A-2 in Appendix A for normal hemoglobin [Hb] values).

When systolic pressure drops below 70 to 80 mm/Hg, the time for capillary refill will be noticeably longer and sluggish. When blood pressure drops below 50 to 60 mm/Hg, the capillaries may not refill at all. A severely hypotensive or hypothermic animal will show no discernible capillary refill since peripheral circula-

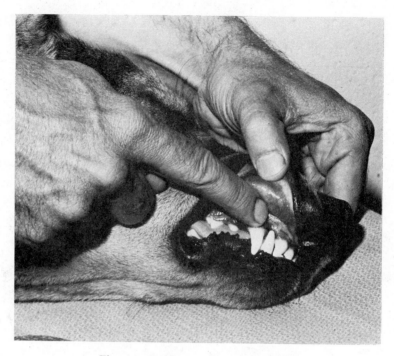

Fig. 2-4. Capillary refill test on gingiva.

tion will have shut down and the entire mouth will appear cold and colorless.

The majority of general anesthetic drugs have a depressant effect on the myocardium, causing it to contract with less than normal force. Consequently, blood pressure is reduced at surgical planes of anesthesia with almost all general anesthetic drugs. As anesthetic depth increases, blood pressure decreases until eventually an overdosage situation will occur. Tranquilizer and narcotic drugs also lower blood pressure. Systolic and diastolic blood pressures decrease slightly or remain normal in most healthy animals during general anesthesia. It is the dehydrated, weakened, or diseased animal that is most likely to have serious hypotension under general anesthesia.

Pupil size and response to light

When a bright light is directed into the pupil of a normal awake animal, the pupil will respond by constricting to a smaller diameter (miosis means constricted pupils). If the animal is placed in a dark area, the pupil will dilate to a larger than normal diameter (mydriasis means dilated pupils). Two involuntary responses (direct and indirect) occur when a bright light is directed into the pupil. An animal's left pupil will constrict if light is directed at it (direct response). The right pupil will also constrict (indirect response). The same responses will occur, only in reverse, if the light is directed at the right eye (see Fig. 2-5).

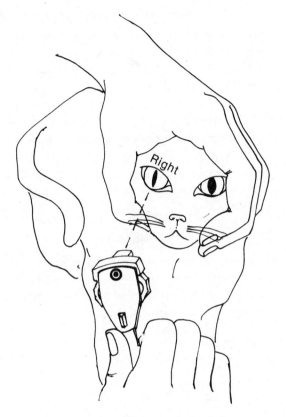

Fig. 2-5. Pupillary response to light.

If the brain goes without circulation or loses its oxygen supply for longer than a few minutes, permanent brain damage may result. One of the first areas to be affected is the portion of the brain that perceives vision and controls this pupillary response to light. The last areas of the brain to be affected are the vital centers controlling respiration and heart rate. It is possible under certain conditions for the brain to be without oxygen for a short period (as might occur in a temporary obstruction to the animal's airway or suffocation due to strangulation on a leash) and the animal to survive. Once a brain center has been damaged it generally cannot repair the loss; consequently, an animal could be blind and without locomotion yet continue to breathe and have a heartbeat (very few people would, of course, want such an animal for a pet). Pneumonia, secondary to the animal's inability to change its position to prevent fluid accumulation in the lungs and to protect its airway against aspiration, is often the cause of death in brain-damaged animals as well as in humans. An animal that has suffered severe brain damage due to anoxia or is clinically dead will have widely dilated pupils and lack pupillary responses to light.

Intraocular pressure

In the normal awake animal, the maintenance of pressure within the aqueous and vitreous humors of the eye is related to blood pressure. This intraocular pressure prevents the eyeball from collapsing on itself. If blood pressure is critically low, the intraocular pressure also will drop. *Caution* must be used when pressure is applied to the globe of the eye, especially in animals that have either poor cardiovascular stability or bradycardia. Excessive pressure may cause a reflex slowing of the heart due to stimulation of vagal nerves supplying the eye. A weak or unstable heart may be incapable of compensating, resulting in serious bradycardia and/or cardiac arrest. Thus intraocular pressure is rarely applied except as an aid to verify death following euthanasia or other causes. It is *not* recommended for monitoring anesthetized animals.

REFLEXES

Involuntary reflexes are used primarily as a means for determining the depth of general anesthesia. Combined with an evaluation of vital signs, they are a means for assessing the animal's relative health status under anesthesia. Following is a list and discussion of reflexes commonly used during anesthesia:
- Palpebral reflex
- Corneal reflex
- Oral-pharyngeal reflex
- Laryngeal reflex
- Ear pinna reflex
- Pedal reflex
- Patellar reflex

Palpebral reflex (blink reflex)

When the hairs along the lateral aspect of the upper eyelid are lightly touched, the conscious animal will respond by blinking. This is a protective reflex designed to prevent injury to the globe of the eye from foreign material in the air. This reflex is easily demonstrated on the awake or lightly anesthetized animal (see Fig. 2-6).

Corneal reflex

Gently touching the cornea of the eye with a soft clean object will elicit a protective reflex blinking of the eye. This technique should *not* be attempted on an awake animal as a sudden movement of the animal's head could result in injury to the cornea. In addition, it is not recommended for routine use as excessive pressure and/or chemical irritation might cause trauma to the cornea.

Oral-pharyngeal reflex

Trying to open or place an object into an awake animal's mouth results in an attempt on the part of the animal to close its jaws, especially if the pharyngeal area

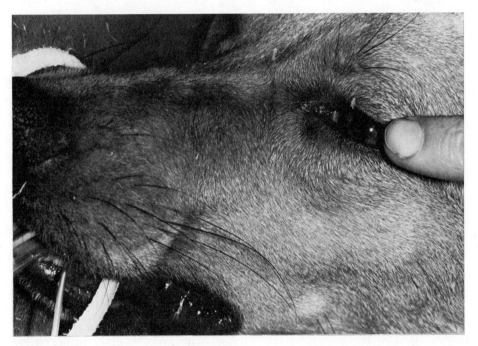

Fig. 2-6. Palpebral reflex in a dog. The dog has been anesthetized with thiamylal and is in stage III, plane 2, of general anesthesia. The eyeball is centrally fixed, and the pupil is neither overly constricted nor dilated.

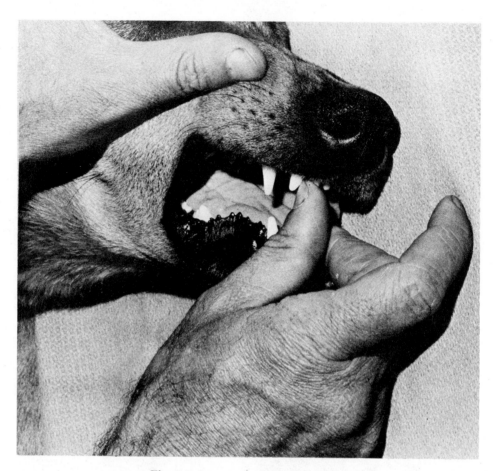

Fig. 2-7. Jaw muscle tone test on dog.

is touched. This is a protective reflex designed to prevent injury to the delicate structures of the mouth and pharynx and to prevent foreign objects from entering the trachea. This reflex is best tested in the lightly anesthetized animal by placing the thumb and middle finger into the front of the animal's mouth and attempting to open it by spreading the two fingers apart (see Fig. 2-7). The animal, although lightly anesthetized, will resist by increasing its jaw muscle tone. This reflex should be avoided in the animal that is awake and not conditioned to having its mouth opened. When testing this reflex on lightly anesthetized animals, care should be exercised to avoid being accidentally bitten. This reflex should not be used to gauge the depth of anesthesia in animals that have fractures of the maxilla or mandible.

Laryngeal reflex

Touching the larynx in the awake animal with any object will evoke a forceful cough and immediate closing of the epiglottis and vocal cords. This is a protective reflex to prevent aspiration of solid or liquid material into the trachea. Obviously, this reflex should never be attempted in an awake animal. The vocal cords can enter into spasm and prevent adequate ventilation should stimulation of this reflex be attempted in an animal not properly anesthetized. This reflex should not be tested for periodic evaluation of anesthetic depth. Loss of this reflex is necessary for tracheal intubation and requires general anesthesia with or without the combined use of a muscle-paralyzing drug.

Ear pinna reflex

Lightly touching the hairs along the lateral aspect of the upper ear canal causes a flicking movement of the pinna, a protective reflex to prevent foreign material from entering the ear canal. Some veterinarians test this reflex to help determine the depth of general anesthesia. When this and other reflexes are absent, it can be assumed that the animal is sufficiently anesthetized to perform surgery. Others, however, believe that the depth of anesthesia necessary to abolish this reflex is too variable to be reliable. (Oftentimes the animal does not lose this reflex until an overdosage depth is reached.) The return of this reflex in the dog can be used as one sign of recovery from anesthesia.

Pedal reflex (toe pinch)

Extending the rear limb while simultaneously pinching the middle toe of the same limb will stimulate a reflex withdrawing (flexion) of the limb (see Fig. 2-8). This is a spinal response to a noxious stimulus, that is, deep pain. This reflex may also be abolished if a local analgesic drug such as lidocaine or procaine is used to regionally anesthetize the caudal portion of the spinal cord. Since this reflex requires the maintenance of nervous pathways within the caudal portion of the spinal cord, anything that blocks this portion of the spinal cord will abolish the reflex, that is, epidural block will result. Animals in a coma due to head injuries or those under a surgical plane of general anesthesia will exhibit no reflexes that require brain activity. Comatose animals therefore would be unlikely to show any of the reflexes mentioned, or they would exhibit greatly diminished responses compared to the normal awake animal.

When testing the pedal reflex on the awake animal, it is not necessary to pinch the toe hard to elicit a withdrawal response (if too much pressure is applied to the toe, one may elicit a "bite" response as well!). Yet it is important to pinch the toe bone of the anesthetized animal with sufficient strength to produce a stimulus strong enough to be perceived by the brain as pain. Some people have used a hemostat to pinch the toe, others stab the toe with a hypodermic needle, but neither of these traumatic methods is necessary if the toe is adequately pinched. Using a hemostat or a needle could result in crush marks or infected needle holes on the toe, all of which are embarrassing and difficult to explain to the animal's owners should they notice. And they will!

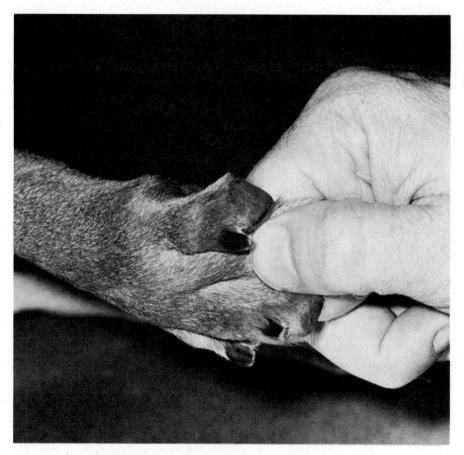

Fig. 2-8. Pedal reflex in a dog. The fourth toe on the uppermost rear limb is compressed between thumb and forefinger. If the animal is at a proper surgical stage of general anesthesia, reflex withdrawal of the limb should be either very slight or absent.

Patellar reflex

The patellar reflex is also know as the knee jerk reflex. When the rear limb is supported on its medial surface in a slightly flexed position and the patellar ligament is precisely struck with a solid object, the limb distal to the knee quickly extends or jerks (see Fig. 2-9). This is probably a protective reflex designed to remove, or be removed from, the irritating source of stimulation by fully extending the limb in a kicking movement. It does *not* require a complete spinal cord pathway to the brain and therefore could be present even when the spinal cord is severed or the animal is in a mild coma. In order to abolish this reflex, the caudal portion of the lumbar spine would have to be transected, crushed, or regionally anesthetized or the nerves that carry the stimulus to the spinal cord and/or back to the extensor muscles of the knee would have to be impaired. Since this reflex does not require the brain or major portion of the spinal cord, it may be present in paralyzed animals as long as the blood supply to the hind limb is present and the nerve pathways involved are intact. In order for this reflex to be abolished by general anesthetics, the depth of anesthesia would have to be extreme unless the anesthetic drug being used also produces profound muscle relaxation.

Since all seven reflexes mentioned in this section (except pupil response) require skeletal muscle contraction, they cannot be used to judge the depth of anesthesia if a muscle-paralyzing drug is used in combination with the anesthetic, nor can they be used to properly assess the depth of ketamine anesthesia since ketamine does not conform to the classic signs of general anesthesia (see Chapter 3).

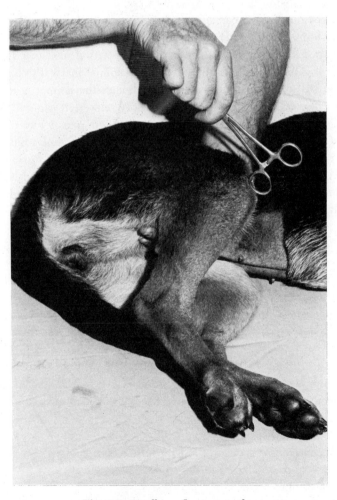

Fig. 2-9. Patellar reflex test in dog.

The student must constantly bear in mind that, although vital signs and reflexes have been discussed individually, one must never rely on only one or two signs to determine an animal's depth of anesthetic depression. All signs and reflexes must be continuously evaluated when monitoring the patient's state of health under anesthesia, be it generally or locally produced.

GENERAL ANESTHESIA
Criteria for the state of general anesthesia

The state referred to as *general anesthesia* is characterized by three basic criteria in animals, all of which are under CNS control:
- Relaxation of skeletal muscles
- Reduction of protective reflexes
- Unarousable sleep (that is, unconsciousness)

The main reason why local analgesic drugs are not used as extensively in animals as they are in humans is due primarily to the fact that animals are more difficult to restrain. It is possible to anesthetize a local region with drugs such as lidocaine or procaine, but it is nearly impossible to expect an animal that is the least bit apprehensive to lie still on a surgical table. Even though the animal is unable to feel local pain because of the drug's action on sensory nerves, it can still move voluntarily, especially when surprised by a sudden noise or a person entering the room. A human patient can be given a preanesthetic injection of meperidine, blocked by injection of a local analgesic drug, and *told* to remain motionless during the surgical procedure. Although general anesthesia is considered a greater risk to the patient than local anesthesia, this risk is necessary with animals in order to provide the surgeon with a surgical field that will not move away or bite.

The three criteria for general anesthesia in animals are obtainable by the sole use of anesthetic drugs such as barbiturates, halothane, methoxyflurane, enflurane, or ether. They may also be obtained by combining two or more weaker agents in a balanced approach. For instance, when a narcotic, barbiturate, muscle paralyzer, and nitrous oxide can be administered to an animal, it is possible to produce analgesia, unconsciousness, depression of reflexes, and skeletal muscle relaxation without risking the deeper planes of anesthesia produced by the barbiturate alone.

Characteristics of a general anesthetic drug

When a general anesthetic drug is administered to an animal in gradually increasing concentrations, the following sequence of events occurs as a result of progressive CNS depression:
1. Analgesia and amnesia
2. Loss of consciousness (sleep); loss of muscle coordination
3. Reduction of protective reflexes
4. Blockade of afferent stimuli

5. Skeletal muscle relaxation
6. Mild respiratory depression; mild cardiovascular depression
7. Severe respiratory and cardiovascular depression
8. Apnea
9. Cardiac standstill

The anesthetic drug being administered will determine the relative degree of depression for each level. Methoxyflurane, for instance, produces a greater degree of analgesia and muscle relaxation than halothane. Halothane, on the other hand, produces a relatively greater degree of analgesia than the barbiturate anesthetics. Yet halothane results in more cardiovascular depression than does ether.

The above sequence is also influenced by the use of other depressant drugs combined with or given before general anesthetic drugs. Barbiturates are not good analgesics at concentrations necessary for surgical anesthesia. It is possible to increase the degree of analgesia from barbiturates by increasing their concentration in the bloodstream. However, the depressant action of the barbiturate on respiration and cardiovascular function is also increased, thereby increasing the possibility of an overdosage. The potential for overdosage can be lessened by combining the analgesic action of a narcotic preanesthetic with the general anesthetic actions of the barbiturate. Interestingly enough, barbiturates at low dosages are good amnesics and are often used in humans as "truth serum."

For surgical purposes, it is important to reach and maintain the depth of anesthesia somewhere between level 5 and level 6 in the sequence of CNS depression. Unfortunately, almost every general anesthetic drug will produce some degree of respiratory and cardiovascular depression. Overdosage from a general anesthetic begins with level 7 and progresses to level 9. Level 10, although not listed, would be death, or permanent brain damage—a level obviously to be avoided.

One of the major criteria for evaluating the state of general anesthesia is blockage of pain sensation (level 4). Good sedation, muscle relaxation, and analgesia are of course paramount. If the patient is not properly anesthetized, pain will be perceived and often remembered. Even though the animal may be unconscious and unable to move, it responds to pain by exhibiting one or more of the following signs:

- Increase in heart rate
- Increase in respiratory rate
- Rise in blood pressure
- Pupil dilation
- Sweating (observe footpads)
- Salivation
- Movement of limbs, head, or tongue
- Oscillation of eyeball (nystagmus)

Classic stages of general anesthesia

Classically, there are four stages of general anesthesia. The original classification was based on the actions of diethyl ether but has been modified to accommodate the modern anesthetics, halothane and methoxyflurane. In practice, however, general anesthesia cannot be so conveniently divided into these four stages since the transition from one stage into another is never as clear-cut and observable as this clinical discussion. Many factors interplay to alter signs and reflexes. Preanesthetic drugs, including atropine, influence the animal's progression into and out of each stage. These general descriptions aid only in the total assessment of anesthetic depth. Just as there are many different dog and cat personality types, there are equally as many different ways in which a single species may react to a single anesthetic drug.

Following is a general description of the classic four stages of general anesthesia as they are experienced with halothane (see Fig. 2-10). The student should realize that these classic stages may also be applied to the barbiturate anesthetic drugs, although some of the signs and reflexes would differ slightly from those seen with halothane, ether, and methoxyflurane.

Stage I

This subjective stage is of little importance in animals. It begins with the moment the anesthetic drug is introduced into the body and ends with the loss of consciousness. Coordinated movements are lost. Hallucinations and vocalization may occur. Analgesia is absent in this stage, yet amnesia may occur. In humans, stage I is representative of the "truth serum" stage observed when subanesthetic dosages of a barbiturate are administered. Humans respond verbally during this stage yet are unable to remember any conversation. The pupils are responsive to light and are normal in size (unless dilated by atropine or constricted by a narcotic). All protective reflexes persist. Respiration and heart rate are basically normal.

Stage II (excitatory stage)

Stage II is characterized by exaggerated responses to all sensory stimuli. Animals may be delirious, howl or cry, or struggle involuntarily, limbs may paddle uncontrollably, and vomiting may occur, especially if the stomach contains food, water, or air. In general, the CNS is hyperreactive, and this stage is very dangerous. It is paradoxic that most general anesthetics appear to stimulate the CNS before (and after) depressing it. In actuality, the anesthetic drug causes a selective depression of higher inhibitory centers within the brain, thereby allowing excessive stimulation to proceed unchecked. Although preanesthetic sedation diminishes or eliminates this stage during the induction of anesthesia, there is always the possibility the animal may show a degree of excitement or delirium as it recovers from surgical anesthesia. Anesthetics are capable of producing a state of unarousable

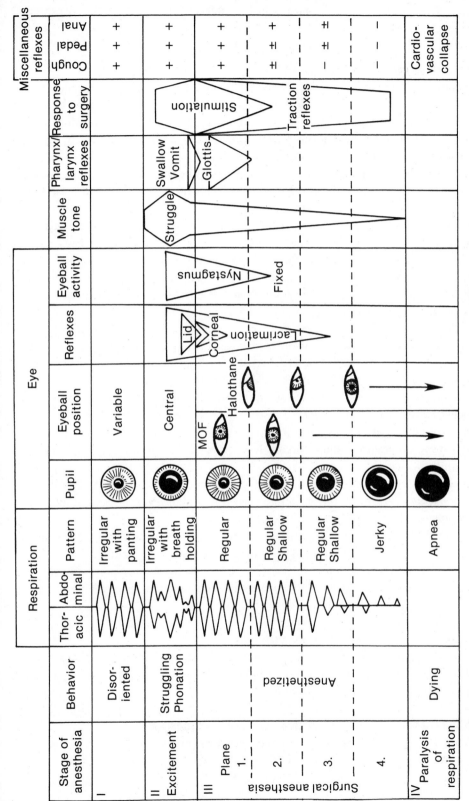

Fig. 2-10. The signs and stages of general anesthesia (as modified from Guedel's stages for diethyl ether in 1920 [assumes no premedication]). *I*, Initial administration to loss of consciousness; *II*, loss of consciousness to onset of regular respiratory pattern; *III* (2), eyeball centrally fixed (ether and methoxyflurane [Mof]); *III* (4), diaphragmatic breathing to apnea; *IV*, respiratory arrest.

sleep, yet they also produce varying degrees of CNS excitement as the animal enters and emerges from this state.

Some anesthetic drugs produce a greater degree of excitement than others, especially if their induction time and recovery time are prolonged. Some animals respond to general anesthesia with great resistance, unconsciously reacting with extreme excitement to light levels of the drug. The manner and method by which the anesthetic is administered may also determine the degree to which the animal passes through this excitatory stage. Inexperience on the part of the anesthetist often results in the slow administration of subanesthetic concentrations, thereby increasing the time it takes to bring the animal through stage II and increasing the possibility and severity of excitement. Pentobarbital and ether are notorious for producing an exaggerated stage II on both induction of and recovery from anesthesia, especially if they are administered without preanesthetic sedation. The degree to which this excitatory stage manifests itself also varies according to species: dogs tend to vocalize and struggle more than cats. If not properly restrained, animals could easily injure themselves. Involuntary movements could cause the animal to fall from the table and sustain a fracture or compound any previous fractures(s) or injuries that have occurred before anesthesia. Sometimes animals may unconsciously injure the restrainer or anesthetist by biting or scratching. If vomiting occurs, aspiration of stomach contents into the lungs is possible, resulting in serious complications or even the death of the animal (see "Aspiration emergencies").

Characteristic signs of stage II. These include changes in:
- Respiration: pattern becomes irregular and may result in panting, hyperventilating, or breath holding (breath holding at this stage is not a true form of apnea)
- Cardiovascular activity: rapid pulse and increase in blood pressure. Possibility of *cardiac arrest* due to exaggerated stress and high levels of circulating catecholamines
- Pupillary activity: eyeball centrally fixed with dilated pupil (nystagmus may occur)
- Corneal reflexes: present
- Oral reflexes: present with noticeable chewing, yawning, or swallowing
- Laryngeal reflex: present
- Pedal reflex: present and exaggerated
- Patellar reflex: present and exaggerated

Stage II ends when the animal is no longer excited, respiration becomes more regular as the animal loses voluntary control of breathing, and reflexes begin to become abolished or obtunded (dulled).

Stage III (sleep stage or surgical stage of anesthesia)

Stage III is characterized by a progressive depression of respiration, circulation, muscle tone, and protective reflexes. This is also referred to as the *working stage:*

one in which a surgical level of anesthesia occurs and is maintained by the anesthetist. Stage III is further divided into *four planes* as a means for more precise evaluation of the patient's vital signs and reflexes. Sometimes the line between life and death under anesthesia is all too thin. The anesthetist's major responsibility is the safety of the patient. Overdosage and subsequent death can usually be avoided by paying strict attention to the animal's vital signs and reflexes during this important stage of anesthesia. The focus of attention must be on the life of the patient to the point where surgery or diagnostic procedures may have to be delayed or cancelled should the animal experience an adverse reaction to an anesthetic drug.

Following is a list and discussion of the four planes within stage III. Some variation in vital signs and reflexes will occur depending on the particular anesthetic drug(s) being administered (see Fig. 2-10):

Plane 1. Considered a *light* plane of anesthesia

Plane 2. Considered a *medium* plane of anesthesia and may be thought of as the normal plane of surgical anesthesia

Plane 3. Considered a *deep* plane of anesthesia and is *undesirable* for all but a few highly painful surgical procedures

Plane 4. Considered an *overdosage* plane of anesthesia—respiration becoming totally paralyzed and the cardiovascular system collapsing

The following discussion of each plane in stage III assumes no preanesthetic medication with atropine or sedative drugs since use of these drugs will interefere to some degree with the assessment of anesthetic depth.

*Stage III, plane 1.*Characteristics of this stage are:

• Respiration: rate of 12 to 20 breaths per minute. Regular and smooth rhythm. Rate will increase if the animal is given a painful stimulus, for example, a firm toe pinch or scalpel incision.

• Heart rate: 90 to 120 beats per minute (slightly higher in cats)

• Pulse: regular and strong

• Eye position: rotates medially; slight nystagmus may be present; nictitating membrane prolapsed (see Fig. 2-11)

• Pupil: constricted and responsive to light. Barbiturate and narcotic drugs result in marked pupillary constriction (atropine tends to dilate the pupil).

• Reflexes: all reflexes still present. The palpebral, oral, and laryngeal reflexes are beginning to disappear.

• Muscle tone: still evident. A painful stimulus may produce limb movement as well as an increase in heart rate and respiratory rate.

In the dog, yawning may be evident, and even though tracheal intubation will cause reflex coughing and chewing attempts, it is often possible to intubate the dog in plane 1. The cat, however, has greater jaw muscle tone. Thus attempts to intubate at this point can evoke a spastic closure of the mouth and/or serious laryngeal spasm if the vocal cords are touched (see Chapter 5).

Stage III, plane 2 (surgical anesthesia). Characteristics of this stage are:

- Respiration: irregular rate and pattern. Decrease in tidal volume. Respirations may increase during surgical manipulations such as ovary ligation during a routine spay operation. This response is not to be confused with a lightening of anesthesia.
- Circulation: mild decrease in heart rate and blood pressure. Relatively strong pulse (under halothane alone, surgical stimulation may cause a noticeable increase in heart rate, respiration rate, and blood pressure due to the drug's relatively weak analgesic property). Traction applied to abdominal organs during surgery may cause a reflex slowing of heart rate due to stimulation of the vagus nerve, especially if atropine was not administered.
- Eyeball: slight medial rotation, nictitating membrane still prolapsed, nystagmus ceases (with methoxyflurane anesthesia eyeball is centrally fixed)
- Pupil: constricted or moderately dilated; response to light present but diminished in degree; speed of constriction relative to the awake response
- Palpebral reflex: absent
- Corneal reflex: absent or diminished
- Oral reflex: absent in dog, still present in some cats
- Laryngeal reflex: absent in *dog* unless endotracheal tube is placed too deeply

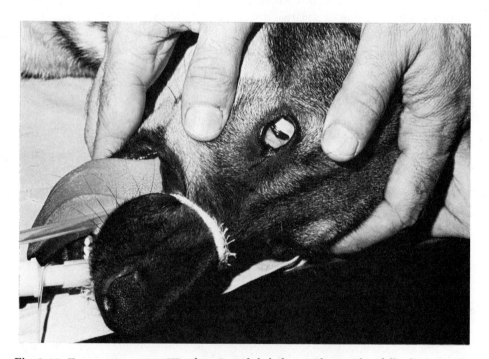

Fig. 2-11. Eye position: stage III, plane I, with halothane. The pupil is difficult to visualize because of prolapse of the nictitans and medial rotation of the eye.

into trachea (intubation of the trachea is easily performed in dogs). Laryngeal spasm may still occur in *cats*. A local analgesic applied to the vocal cords may facilitate intubation in cats. However, if care is taken not to touch the vocal cords, intubation can be performed without the use of a local analgesic spray (refer to Chapter 5).

- Pinna reflex: absent in dogs, still present in many cats
- Pedal reflex: absent
- Patellar reflex: present but diminished in intensity
- Muscle tone: relaxed, permitting abdominal incision in all but massively muscled dogs (methoxyflurane provides a greater degree of muscle relaxation than halothane or enflurane at this plane)

Salivation is still possible in plane 2. This could be a problem as the animal is unable to close its larynx under anesthesia and may aspirate saliva into the trachea. If the animal is positioned with the head higher than the hind end, saliva can course its way down the trachea and into the lungs. If the animal is unable to cough up the saliva, aspiration pneumonitis as well as impaired ventilation could result. Inflation of the endotracheal tube cuff and positioning the head so it is at or below the level of the heart will lessen the chance of aspiration during anesthesia.

Stage III, plane 3. Characteristics of this stage are:

- Respiration: variable pattern, shallow and unequal expansion of the thorax. Tidal volume further decreased. Progressive paralysis of the intercostal muscles causes a "rocking boat" type of breathing due to a greater effort on the part of the diaphragm and abdominal muscles to sustain ventilation.
- Circulation: a slight increase in heart rate at first, then begins to decrease; a weakening of *pulse* as cardiac output drops significantly; a decrease in *blood pressure; neurogenic shock* may occur; *capillary refill* time lengthens beyond $1^1/_2$ to 2 seconds.
- Eyeball: centrally fixed. Nictitating membrane not as prolapsed as in plane 1 or plane 2. Cornea becomes dry (it is advisable to instill a bland ophthalmic ointment in the eyes of all animals as soon after the induction of general anesthesia as possible)
- Pupil: moderately dilated; diminished or absent response to light
- Palpebral reflex: absent
- Corneal reflex: absent
- Oral reflex: absent
- Tracheal reflex: absent or markedly reduced
- Pinna reflex: absent
- Pedal reflex: absent
- Patellar reflex: diminished. May be absent under methoxyflurane due to its greater muscle relaxing property. Loss of the patellar reflex under halothane is a sign of overdosage.
- Muscle tone: greatly reduced, even in large dogs

In the dog and cat under halothane anesthesia, most surgical operations can be performed with the eyeball rotated medially so that about half of the iris and pupil are visible behind the prolapsed nictitating membrane (see Fig. 2-10). Rotation of the eyeball to a centrally fixed position with moderately dilated pupils is a sign of impending halothane overdosage. It should be remembered, however, that methoxyflurane will cause the eyeball to fix centrally at a slightly lighter plane than halothane. With methoxyflurane, the pupil is not as dilated as it is when halothane fixes the eyeball centrally. Most surgical procedures under methoxyflurane are done with the eyeball centrally fixed.

Stage III, plane 4 (overdosage). Characteristics of this stage are:
- Respiration: irregular and very shallow. Nearly complete paralysis of intercostal and abdominal muscles of respiration. Diaphragmatic efforts cause jerky motions of the abdomen. This, coupled with a noticeable movement of the lower jaw, may be falsely interpreted as a lightening of anesthesia. Anesthesia must *not* be increased without checking other vital signs and reflexes since it would lead to an even greater overdosage.
- Circulation: heart rate decreases; pulse decreases; blood pressure decreases, prolonging capillary refill time; skin feels cool; neurogenic shock further decreases blood pressure and cardiac output. Visceral traction may still evoke a reflex slowing of heart rate that would result in a further depression of cardiac function.
- Eyeball: centrally fixed
- Pupil: widely dilated; unresponsive to light
- Reflexes: absent or greatly obtunded
- Muscle tone: practically flaccid. Visceral traction reflex is absent. The cornea is dry and appears dull because of lack of tear production.

This is an extremely dangerous plane of anesthesia. Stage III, plane 4, ends with apnea due to paralysis of all respiratory muscles.

Stage IV (terminal stage)

This is a variable stage in that it represents the time interval between respiratory arrest in stage III, plane 4, and cardiac arrest in stage IV. It is, in actuality, the period of time between respiratory failure due to anesthetic overdosage and death due to cardiac failure from hypoxia. Cardiac muscle and brain tissue are highly dependent on adequate oxygenation of arterial blood. Respiratory and cardiovascular failure causes a rapid decline in arterial oxygen concentration, resulting in brain cell death and myocardial failure (cardiac dysrhythmias or arrest). Once the heart stops, the brain suffers immediate anoxia. If circulation and oxygenation are not restored within a very short period of time, permanent brain damage and/or death results. Stage IV requires immediate resuscitative measures to support respiratory and cardiovascular functions.

MONITORING THE ANESTHETIZED PATIENT

It is important to adopt good habits when first learning how to monitor the anesthetized animal's vital signs and depth of general anesthesia. Vital signs should be evaluated at least every minute during the induction stage. Vital signs and reflexes should be evaluated as often as possible during the maintenance and recovery stages but not less frequently than once every 5 minutes. Respiratory arrest that goes unnoticed for longer than 3 to 5 minutes could result in an unnecessary loss of life or permanent brain damage. Cardiac arrest may occur if respirations cease for longer than 60 seconds. Since cardiac arrest is the ultimate emergency situation, any precautionary measures designed to avoid it will enhance both peace of mind and reputation. Cardiac arrest can occur with little or no warning. The sooner it is recognized and resuscitative measures begun, the greater the chance of saving the animal.

Anesthesia forms

The use of an anesthesia form will help organize the information important for accurate patient monitoring, especially in procedures lasting longer than 30 minutes. Anesthesia forms are also useful in determining the cause of death from anesthesia. In addition, they provide a means for reviewing the total number of anesthetic procedures in a practice, improving anesthetic approaches and eliminating potential hazards.

In a practice where animal owners are given itemized bills, including separate charges for anesthesia, it is advisable to maintain these records for all animals as part of their permanent record. In a multiveterinarian practice, it is essential to have a record of previously used anesthetic drugs and methods as part of an animal's medical and surgical history. Older animals or animals in high risk categories are of particular concern. Records of previous successful anesthetic episodes are of immense value to the veterinarian who may be administering anesthesia to such an animal for the first time.

Two examples of anesthesia forms are presented here. Fig. 2-12 is an example of an extensive form used in most veterinary schools and larger practices. The short form (Fig. 2-13) can be used on an everyday basis in a smaller-volume practice. The anesthesia form should include the following information:
1. Client name or identification number
   - Species of animal
   - Sex of animal
   - Age and name of animal
2. Date
3. Procedure
4. Vital signs
5. Blood chemistry and complete blood count (CBC) values

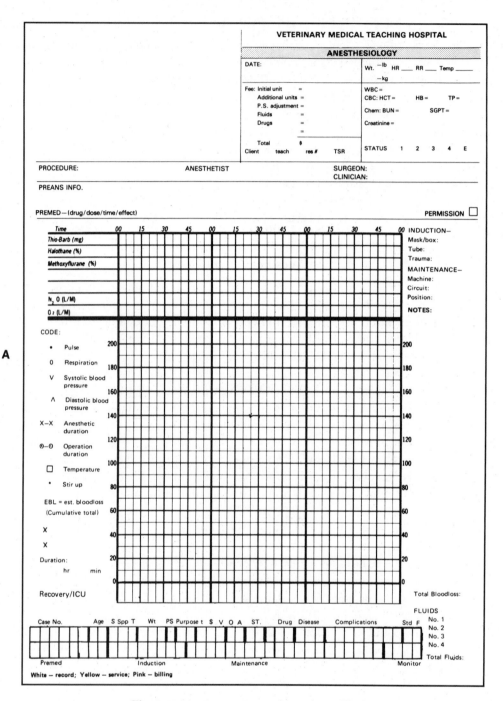

Fig. 2-12. A, Extensive anesthesia form, blank.

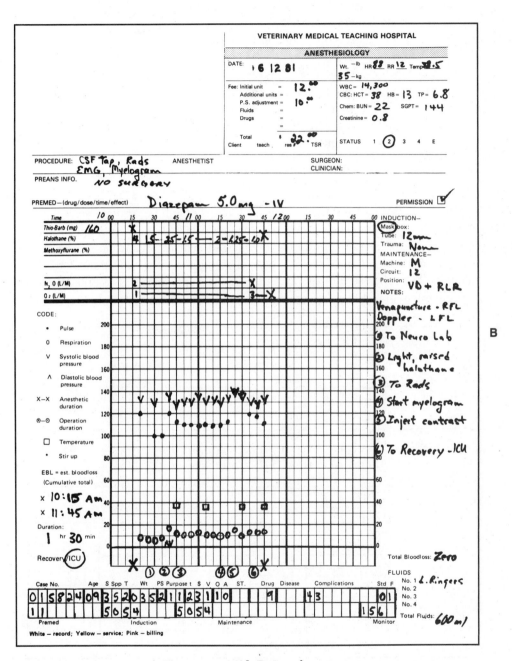

Fig. 2-12, cont'd. B, Sample case.

6. Fluids administered during the procedure
7. Estimated blood loss
8. Method of anesthetic induction and maintenance
9. Venipuncture site(s)
10. Relative concentrations of inhalation anesthetic drug used
11. Drugs administered (including dosages)
12. Additional comments

The vital signs to be recorded should include:

1. Heart rate and/or pulse rate
2. Respiration rate
3. Body temperature
4. Blood pressure (optional)

The vital signs and anesthetic concentrations should be recorded chronologically on a graph to show their progression through the induction, maintenance, and recovery phases of general anesthesia. Preanesthetic drugs should be recorded on a separate space along with their dosage and route of administration. Vital signs should be taken before the administration of any depressant medication, providing a baseline for comparison during general anesthesia. The larger and more detailed

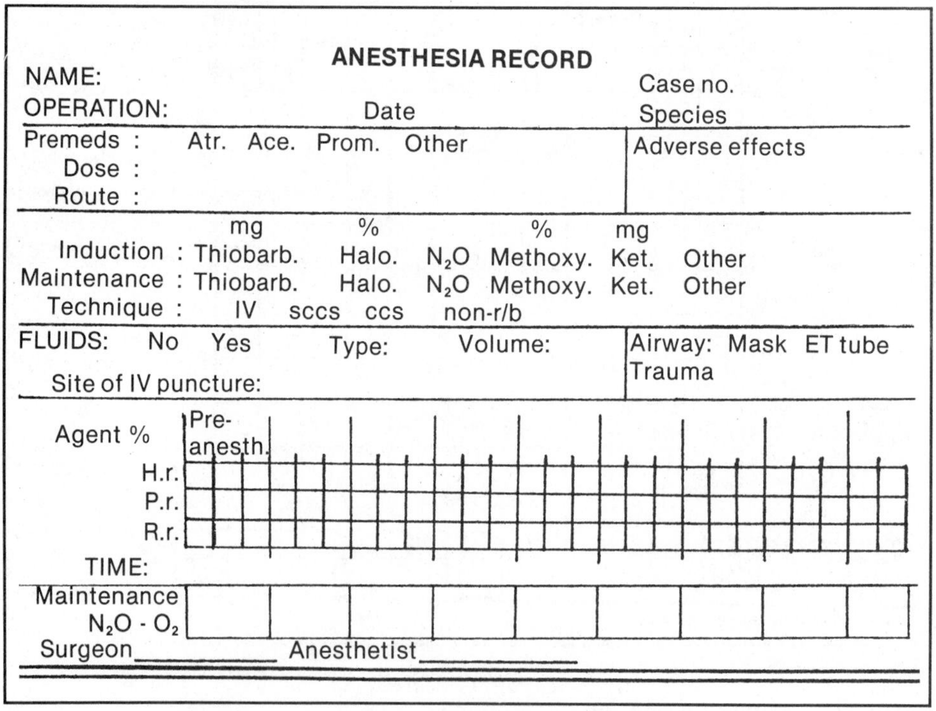

ANESTHESIA RECORD

NAME: Case no.
OPERATION: Date Species

Premeds : Atr. Ace. Prom. Other Adverse effects
   Dose :
   Route :

              mg   %   %   mg
Induction : Thiobarb. Halo. N$_2$O Methoxy. Ket. Other
Maintenance : Thiobarb. Halo. N$_2$O Methoxy. Ket. Other
Technique : IV sccs ccs non-r/b

FLUIDS: No Yes Type: Volume: Airway: Mask ET tube
   Site of IV puncture: Trauma

Agent % Pre-anesth.
   H.r.
   P.r.
   R.r.
TIME:

Maintenance
N$_2$O - O$_2$
Surgeon_____ Anesthetist_____

Fig. 2-13. Short form anesthesia record.

anesthesia forms used by human and veterinary anesthesiologists contain an extensive amount of information in coded form (see Fig. 2-12, A). The purpose of these detailed forms is to store and retrieve as much anesthetic case information as possible. Universal code symbols record such events as the start of anesthesia; the start of surgery; the patient's pulse, respiration, and blood pressure; the end of surgery; and the end of anesthetic administration. All of these events are recorded on a graph-like grid and plotted against time. The use of such a form requires trained staff to maintain the records and transfer the information from the anesthesia form into a data retrieval system. A small, private practice may have no need for such a system and would be better off using a simplified and shorter form.

Keeping anesthesia records focuses attention on the patient's vital signs and helps prevent unnecessary anesthetic overdosage. Since the induction phase of general anesthesia is usually the *most dangerous* period for the patient—the time when respiratory or cardiac arrest is more likely to occur—vital signs and reflexes must be continuously observed in order not to overlook signs of impending danger. There is often little time, especially during this phase, to record such details as vital signs every 1 to 2 minutes. Therefore this information usually is not documented until 5 or 10 minutes into surgical anesthesia when the animal has reached a more stabilized plane. Of course, if a patient begins to demonstrate obvious signs of distress or anesthetic overdosage at any time, immediate action must be taken to remedy the situation. Pertinent notations about a critical situation can be made later.

Patient monitoring

Patients under general anesthesia can be monitored manually and/or mechanically. Manual monitoring, although subject to human error, has the advantage over mechanical devices in that humans demonstrate more flexibility, experience, and knowledge of species' variability. In addition, people do not require electric power to operate and function normally. Electric and mechanical monitoring devices are beneficial in that they enable the monitoring of a greater number of vital signs, constantly checking the anesthetized patient. The major problems are that they require special training to operate and interpret and, because of delicate instrumentation, are subject to malfunction or breakage. Attention to proper manual methods of patient monitoring will prove adequate for all but the most critical patients.

Manual methods of patient monitoring

Manual monitoring requires the following *equipment:*
- Rectal thermometer. Direct reading preferred (esophageal temperatures are more accurate than rectal temperatures)
- Pocket penlight for testing pupil response and observing mucous membrane color

- Percussion hammer for testing patellar reflex (although the handle of a 7 inch bandage scissors will suffice)
- Stethoscope. Esophageal stethoscope preferred but a regular stethoscope should be available at all times (see Fig. 2-14)

An esophageal stethoscope enables evaluation of heart and lung sounds without interfering with surgical drapes to auscultate the chest area. Once the animal is anesthetized, the ballooned end of the esophageal probe is passed a predetermined distance into the esophagus and stopped at the level of the heart (see Fig. 2-15). A small amount of water or lubricating jelly can be placed on the esophageal probe to facilitate its passage into the esophagus. It is easier to pass the stethoscope *after* intubating the trachea. The opening into the esophagus is dorsal and to the left of the opening into the trachea. If an endotracheal tube is already in place, the eso-phageal stethoscope enters the esophagus with relative ease.

Vital signs routinely monitored are:

- Heart rate and rhythm
- Respiratory rate, depth, and rhythm
- Arterial pulse
- Body temperature

- Mucous membrane color
- Capillary refill time
- Pupil size and response to light
- Muscle tone

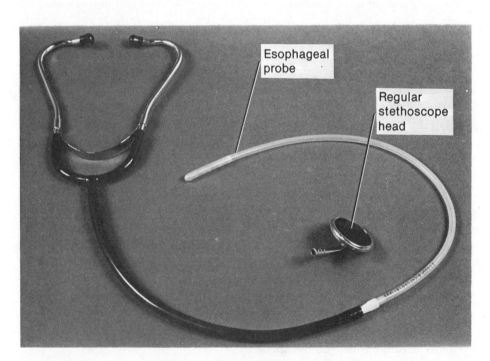

Fig. 2-14. Esophageal stethoscope.

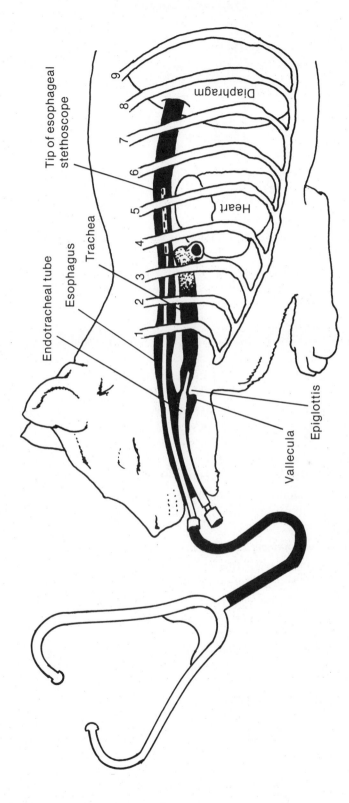

Fig. 2-15. Position of esophageal stethoscope in cat.

Reflexes routinely monitored are:
• Palpebral
• Corneal
• Oral (jaw tension)
• Pupil
• Pinna
• Pedal
• Patellar

Mechanical methods of patient monitoring

Electrocardiogram (ECG). An ECG (see Fig. 2-16) measures electric activity of the heart muscle and provides a visual means for evaluating conduction of impulses through the atria and ventricles. It also measures heart rate and rhythm and allows visualization of cardiac dysrhythmias. The readings may be displayed on an oscilloscope screen or permanently recorded on special ECG paper or both. An ECG provides valuable information during cardiac emergencies to determine asystole from ventricular fibrillation.

Electroencephalogram (EEG). An EEG, which measures electric activity of the brain, is not routinely used in veterinary practice.

Audible esophageal stethoscope. This stethoscope is battery operated and provides audible heart rate and lung sounds (see Fig. 2-17).

Arterial blood pressure cuff. The use of a blood pressure cuff is limited in veterinary patients because of the extreme variability in limb anatomy. However, the use of indirect blood pressure measuring devices continues to show promise (see Fig. 2-18). Arterial blood pressure can be measured from an arterial catheter and displayed on an oscilloscope or recorded on paper. In addition, special recorders are available that can simultaneously display and record many different channels of information. However, these recorders are expensive and used mostly in research laboratories.

Arterial blood gas analyzer. Such a machine can analyze blood taken directly from a peripheral artery (usually the femoral artery) and determine in minutes pH, oxygen tension (PaO_2), and carbon dioxide tension ($PaCO_2$). Monitoring arterial pH, P_aO_2, and P_aCO_2 aid tremendously in assuring proper oxygenation, ventilation, and pH balance during long-term anesthetic procedures or in anesthetizing high risk patients. However, blood gas analyzers are expensive and require skilled maintenance. (See Table 6-1 for normal and anesthetized canine blood gas values.)

Packed cell volume (PCV)* measurement. Sampling venous (or arterial) blood for PCV, using microhematocrit tubes and a centrifuge, gives relative values for the patient's state of hydration, circulating red blood cell volume, and hemoglobin con-

---

*See Tables A-1 and A-2 in Appendix A for normal canine and feline clinical chemistry and CBC values.

Assessing the depth of general anesthesia

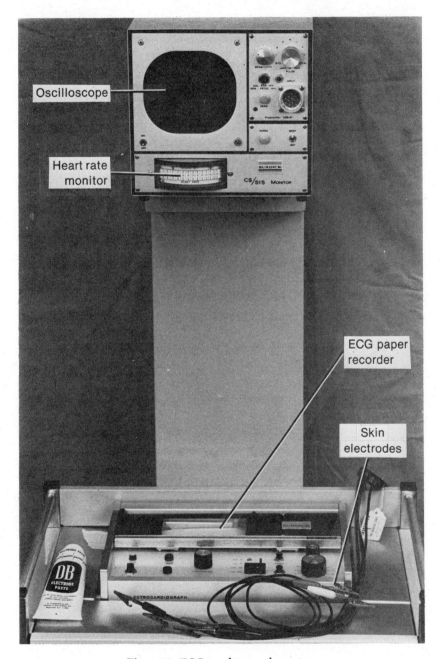

Fig. 2-16. ECG machine and monitor.

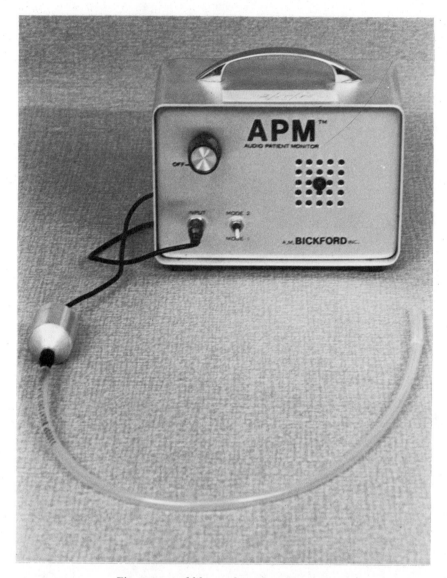

Fig. 2-17. Audible esophageal stethoscope.

centration (dividing the PCV by 3 gives an approximation of hemoglobin concentration). This procedure is valuable when an animal is experiencing major blood loss and/or when large volumes of intravenous fluids are being administered. For example, a PCV of 20% or less is a possible indication for transfusing the patient with whole blood, a normal PCV value in dogs and cats being 35% to 55%. This measurement could also indicate overhydration of the patient with intravenous fluids, resulting in a dilution of PCV and/or plasma protein values.

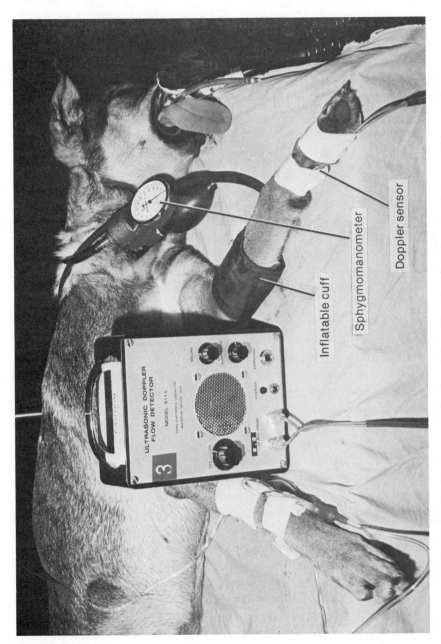

Fig. 2-18. Doppler setup on foreleg of dog. The Doppler also provides an audible monitor of pulse rate and rhythm.

Total plasma protein concentration measurement. Sampling venous or arterial blood for the total plasma protein concentration is another means of evaluating the patient's hydration and nutritional status. A refractometer determines total protein by measuring serum or plasma levels. A normal value for dogs or cats is 5.5 to 7.5 gm/100 ml.

Central venous pressure (CVP) monitor. This device measures the ability of the heart to receive fluids. Although it is not routinely used, it is valuable when the patient is in shock and/or must receive large volumes of fluid intravenously. It is also useful in monitoring cardiac patients for signs of right-sided heart failure. In both dogs and cats, a normal CVP value is under 8 cm H_2O pressure, with a pressure over 12 to 15 cm H_2O considered elevated.

RECOVERY FROM GENERAL ANESTHESIA

Recovery from a state of general anesthesia involves elimination of the anesthetic drug(s) from both the blood and the body tissues. The recovery period is generally defined as the period between discontinuation of anesthetic administration and the animal's regaining of all of its protective reflexes, including its ability to stand and support weight. With *intravenous* anesthetic drugs the length of this period will depend primarily on the amount of time it takes the animal to metabolize and eliminate the active portion of the anesthetic drug. Drug metabolism depends on such factors as liver enzyme activity, body temperature, and kidney function. If body temperature drops below 35° C, enzyme activity throughout the body decreases significantly. It is essential, therefore, to maintain body temperature above 35° to 36° C to avoid a prolonged and exaggerated recovery period. However, a prolonged recovery period from anesthetic drugs can be expected in thin or emaciated animals or animals with liver and/or kidney disease.

The recovery period in the case of *inhalation* anesthetic drugs is generally shorter than for the intravenous drugs. The major portion of an inhalation anesthetic drug is eliminated from the bloodstream by normal ventilation. Some of the inhalation anesthetic drug is also metabolized by liver enzymes and excreted through the kidneys. Generally, the longer the period of anesthetic administration, the greater the amount of body saturation, and the longer the recovery period—no matter what anesthetic drug is used.

In most cases, an animal is said to be recovered from anesthesia when it is able to sit up on its sternum without falling to one side. This is referred to as reaching sternal recumbency. Although there is usually no need for constant monitoring after this point, certain precautions should be taken. For instance, brachycephalic breeds, because of their short muzzles and overly long soft palate, may experience respiratory distress following extubation of the trachea. Such animals must be watched closely until they are fully conscious and able to stand.

As an animal recovers from general anesthesia, it will show characteristic signs of awakening as it emerges from a deeper plane to a ligher plane of unconsciousness. This is sometimes referred to as lightening of anesthesia. Reflexes lost during the induction phase return almost in reverse order of their disappearance—that is, as an animal continues to recover from the anesthetic state, the vital signs observed during the induction phase will undergo a reverse progression before stabilizing at their preanesthetic values. However, during the recovery phase, passage from a deep plane of anesthesia to a lighter plane often occurs more rapidly, and changes in vital signs and reflexes may be more subtle than during the induction phase.

General anesthetics, such as ether and pentobarbital, that cause an exaggerated excitatory stage (stage II) on induction will often produce a similar excitement as the animal passes back through stage II during recovery. The terms used to describe an exaggerated stage II on emergence from general anesthesia are "stormy recovery" or "recovery hysteria." Anesthetics requiring many hours for removal from the bloodstream tend to produce stormier recoveries than those agents that are removed more rapidly. Recovery hysteria may be marked by delirium, hyperventilation, howling, head thrashing, or paddling movements of the limbs. The animal, in a state of semiconsciousness, may seriously injure itself. Disruption of the surgical repair may also occur during a thrashing episode or spastic attempts of the animal to right itself. Padding the recovery cage will help prevent self-induced injury.

The recovery stage is a dangerous period. Constant attention must be paid to the animal to avoid injury, aspiration of fluid, or airway obstruction from the soft palate. If the endotracheal tube is not removed at the proper time or the animal is not closely observed, it may bite through the tube and aspirate the distal portion into the trachea. Often, it is best to sit with the animal if it is delirious and gently stroke its head and neck while talking quietly in a reassuring manner. There is *no substitute* for good TLC (tender loving care) during the recovery period. It is wise to have a quiet recovery area since loud or sharp noises can evoke or enhance delirium and hallucinations. Further, recovering animals must never be left with open cage doors or placed in a cage with food or water.

Recovery signs

General signs of awakening to be observed as an animal progresses from a deeper plane to a lighter plane of general anesthesia are:

1. Increase in respiratory rate and tidal volume
   - Deeper and more rapid breaths
2. Medial rotation of eyeball
   - As anesthesia lightens, the eyeball rotates from its centrally fixed position medially and then back to central again before the animal recovers its swallowing or tracheal reflexes.
3. Return of protective reflexes
4. Shivering

- All anesthetics lower body temperature. As the animal awakens, it may shiver to produce heat from muscle activity. Although this is normal, the muscle activity consumes considerable amounts of oxygen. Thus oxygen should be administered to patients at risk during the recovery period.

5. Spastic movements of the tongue
   - Noticeable especially if the animal has an endotracheal tube in place. As reflexes return, the animal will chew on the tube and attempt to swallow.

6. Attempt to stand
   - Front leg coordination generally returns before the rear limbs are able to support weight. If the animal attempts to stand too soon, it may collapse on its rear legs. The animal will usually settle for sternal recumbency at this stage (see Fig. 2-19). Full recovery from anesthetic drugs does not occur until the animal can stand and walk normally.

During the recovery period it is important that attention be given to the following:

1. Preventing heat loss
   - A circulating warm water heating pad at a temperature between 37° to 38° C should be placed between the animal and the bottom of the cage. Newspapers, towels, or an insulated blanket beneath the animal may be substituted. Plastic bottles containing warm water can also be placed next to the animal for added warmth. The animal should not be overheated. Great care must be taken not to burn the animal's skin if an electric heating pad is used, and an electric heating blanket should be set at the lowest temperature (rapid heating of a hypothermic patient may result in shock and/or third degree burns).
   - The animal should not be placed on a metal surface, which tends to remove body heat and lower the animal's body temperature even further.
   - Heavy blankets should not be laid over the animal's chest or abdomen as this could seriously impair ventilation.

2. Checking vital signs
   - Vital signs should be evaluated at least every 3 to 5 minutes.
   - Close attention should be paid to brachycephalic breeds, animals that are weak or have lost considerable amounts of blood, sick or aged animals, animals with respiratory or cardiovascular disease, and overweight or excessively lean animals, for example, sighthounds.

3. Rotating the animal from side to side once every 10 to 15 minutes unless contraindicated
   - Hypostatic pulmonary congestion of the lower portion of the lung field can develop if the animal lies on one side for longer than 30 to 45 minutes. Blood and fluid tend to gravitate, impairing ventilation and circulation (this may predispose the animal to a postanesthetic pneumonia or pulmonary congestion).

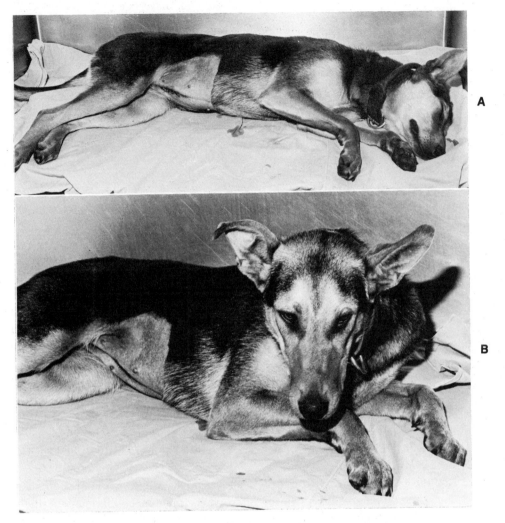

Fig. 2-19. Dog, **A**, in unconscious state and **B**, in sternal recumbency.

Young healthy animals will not necessarily die from neglect if the above precautions are not taken during the recovery period. However, the older or debilitated animal is less able to compensate for such problems as heat loss and respiratory embarrassment. Neglecting these animals during the recovery period could easily lead to an unnecessary death from anesthesia.

Anesthetic deaths due to metabolic acidosis, hypoxia, hypothermia, or respiratory distress can occur even after an animal has reached sternal recumbency. An animal is never totally out of danger until 36 to 48 hours have elapsed and all traces of anesthetic drugs are out of the system. Even then the possibility exists for post-anesthetic complications or death. Examples include the tracheal mucosa necrosis that can occur 3 to 5 days after anesthesia as a result of overinflation of the cuff on the endotracheal tube, inhalation pneumonia secondary to an animal aspirating vomitus or irrigating solution, severely bruised sclera 2 days after an animal thrashed its head into the cage door during a stormy recovery period, and third degree burns that develop 2 to 3 days after the use of an electric heating pad directly on an animal's skin during surgery or recovery (even though an insulated blanket or newspapers would have sufficed). There are numerous examples of post-anesthetic complications—all of which point out the fact that the veterinarian and AHT can never feel completely relaxed and immune from unusual circumstance. Remaining alert to such dangers and monitoring the animal carefully minimizes the incidence of serious complications and make those that do occur more manageable.

ANESTHETIC EMERGENCIES

In spite of all the monitoring devices and precautions used to guard an anesthetized animal's life, anesthetic emergencies will still occur. Medicine is not an exact science. Life and the study of a life science such as medicine must deal with the unexpected. Fortunately, when careful attention is paid to detail, the incidence of "unexpected" anesthetic emergencies is low, and many emergencies can be avoided altogether. Emergencies can occur at any time—from the moment a preanesthetic sedative is administered all the way into the postrecovery period. Certain periods, such as induction and recovery, are considered more dangerous because of the greater number of potentially serious emergencies that can occur, yet there is no period in anesthesia that is completely free from possible complication. It is unwise to assume that anesthetic emergencies occur only in the critically ill or high risk patient.

Routine procedures carried out on healthy animals are not without their share of "unexpected" emergencies. All too often when an animal suffers an anesthetic death the postmortem examination reveals no significant lesions. In many cases the anesthetic death could have been avoided, but occasionally an animal under anesthesia may die with little or no warning, the exact cause of death remaining a mystery. When an animal is under the effects of any anesthetic drug for any reason, its life is at risk. Training for and being prepared for possible emergencies is, in itself, one means of prevention. Should an anesthetic emergency develop, its successful management requires a calm and systematic approach on the part of the technician as well as the veterinarian.

It is not the intent of this chapter to discuss the etiology, treatment, and prevention of each emergency condition. Some are discussed in other chapters while some require supplementary reading. Overdosage from barbiturate anesthetics, for instance, is discussed in Chapter 3, while overdosage due to inhalation anesthetics is discussed in Chapter 5. Shock and cardiac arrest are discussed in Chapter 5 of *Small Animal Surgical Nursing*.[1]

Anesthetic emergencies most likely to occur in a busy surgical and diagnostic small animal hospital are:

1. Respiratory system emergencies
   - Apnea (respiratory arrest)
   - Irregular or diaphragmatic breathing
   - Aspiration of food or fluid
   - Paralysis of respiratory muscles
   - Obstruction to patient's airway or breathing circuit
   - Laryngeal and/or bronchial spasm
   - Ventilation-to-perfusion abnormalities
   - Pneumothorax following open-chest surgery
   - Postanesthetic hypoventilation and/or atelectasis
2. Cardiovascular system
   - Neurogenic shock due to anesthetic overdose
   - Hypovolemic shock due to surgical hemorrhage
   - Cardiac dysrhythmias
   - Cardiac arrest
3. Air embolism
4. Severe hypothermia
5. Anesthetic overdose
6. Vomiting and regurgitation
7. Malignant hyperthermia

Anesthetic overdose

Characteristic signs of anesthetic overdosage due to barbiturate and inhalation anesthetic drugs do not apply to overdosages with dissociative anesthetics. It is important that the technician monitoring the anesthetized animal never make a diagnosis of anesthetic overdose without consulting the veterinarian. It is far better to be overly attentive to any changes in the animal's vital signs and call for help than it is to ignore a warning sign until a real emergency has developed. Anesthetic overdosage must never be diagnosed from a single vital sign or reflex. The total condition of the animal must be considered and many signs evaluated quickly before making a final judgment as to a particular course of action. For example, one should not assume the administration of an overdose of halothane just because the animal has no patellar reflex when, in fact, a muscle-paralyzing drug was previously dispensed, which paralyzed the skeletal muscles of the legs. Reducing the concentration of halothane in this case would render the animal sensitive to pain yet unable to respond.

Another example of the need for constant attention to details is a case where a cat begins to demonstrate signs of awakening from halothane anesthesia 10 minutes after it was induced with an ultrashort-acting barbiturate, intubated, and placed on the inhalation anesthesia machine. Increasing the concentration of halothane and ventilating the cat to deepen anesthesia may do little good without first checking to see if the endotracheal tube was accidentally placed in the esophagus—a common error when intubating cats. Ventilating the esophagus will not induce anesthesia, yet it will cause gastric distention that could lead to other complications, such as abdominal pain, decreased venous return to the heart, vomiting, or pressure on the diaphragm—all of which can lead to more serious complications.

General signs of anesthetic overdose

1. The respiratory system
   - Decreased rate of ventilation (<8 breaths/minute)
   - Decreased tidal volume: lack of chest expansion; air expelled with little or no force; rapid yet shallow respiration
   - Diaphragmatic breathing resulting in a "rocking boat" type of respiratory pattern
   - Apnea that may be intermittent or constant
   - Cyanotic mucous membranes due to insufficient oxygenation of pulmonary blood
2. The circulatory system
   - Decreased heart rate (<70 to 80 beats/minute), decreased pulse rate, and irregular heart rhythm
   - Decreased pulse pressure; pulse becoming erratic or weak and possibly impalpable in lingual or femoral arteries, indicating hypotension
   - Prolonged capillary refill time due to decreasing blood perfusion
   - Pale mucous membranes due to shock superimposed on respiratory depression
   - Irregular or absent (QRS) complexes on ECG, premature ventricular contractions (PVCs), or other conduction disturbances indicative of impending cardiovascular collapse
3. Body temperature
   - Hypothermia causing body temperature to drop below 35° C, increasing the possibility of anesthetic overdosage
   - Mouth, skin, and ears cold to the touch
4. Pupil response to light
   - Decreased (responds slowly or not at all)
   - Widely dilating pupils
5. Reflexes
   - All reflexes greatly diminished or totally absent (loss of the patellar reflex possibly indicating serious anesthetic overdose)

Failure to recognize and respond to these signs can rapidly evolve into a critical anesthetic emergency as the patient becomes increasingly acidotic and hypoxic. Death resulting from anesthetic overdosage with barbiturate or inhalation anesthetic drugs can be an insidious process unmarked by such obvious external signs as muscle tremors or seizures. General anesthetic drugs progressively depress the CNS leading, eventually, to severe hypoxemia, hypotension, and death due to respiratory arrest (apnea) and/or cardiac arrest.

Aspiration emergencies

When an animal is being induced with a general anesthetic drug, the vomiting center of the brain apparently becomes more sensitive to stimulation. Hence the presence of food, water, or air in the stomach will distend the fibers of the stomach wall and may initiate a vomiting reflex. This hyperexcitability of the vomiting center corresponds roughly with stage II of general anesthesia. Vomiting, as opposed to regurgitation, involves an active contraction of the stomach to discharge its contents. Regurgitation is the passive discharge of stomach contents through the esophagus and into the pharynx. It occurs with less force than vomiting and can be as much of a complication as active vomiting. Although vomiting is most likely to occur during induction of general anesthesia, it can also occur during recovery from anesthesia. Some anesthetic drugs, such as diethyl ether, tend to stimulate vomiting more than other anesthetics. Regurgitation is more likely to occur once anesthesia has been induced since it is caused by a relaxation of the cardiac sphincter muscle between the esophagus and stomach. Relaxation of this sphincter allows stomach contents or secretions to course their way up the esophagus, especially when the animal is positioned in dorsal recumbency with the head lower than the stomach. Regurgitation under anesthesia can occur in spite of adequate preanesthetic fasting. Often the only sign of regurgitation maybe a small amount of fluid draining from the animal's mouth or nostrils. Regurgitation may occur under anesthesia whenever external pressure is applied to the stomach—for example, when abdominal packs are used for positioning or the surgeon inadvertently leans on the animal's stomach—or in cases of traction or manipulation of the stomach during abdominal surgery.

Obstruction of the animal's airway can also cause regurgitation as a result of the increased abdominal pressure that accompanies the obstructive breathing pattern under anesthesia. Both vomiting and regurgitation are considered anesthetic emergencies, as either one can lead to serious postanesthetic complications or death. Vomiting can cause aspiration of stomach contents into the trachea, bronchi, or lungs. If a large volume of fluid or food were to lodge in the trachea, asphyxiation could lead to a rapid death unless the obstruction were relieved immediately. Aspiration of either partially digested food into the lungs or of acidic gastric secretions into the trachea or lungs can result in a condition referred to as *aspiration pneu-*

monitis. When sufficient liquid material having a pH of 2.5 or less enters an animal's respiratory tract, it rapidly spreads through the lungs and results in aspiration pneumonitis.

The word pneumonitis connotes an acute inflammation of lung tissue. Aspiration pneumonitis is characterized by three cardinal signs: cyanosis, tachycardia, and tachypnea (excessively rapid breathing).

These signs of aspiration pneumonitis may not develop for several hours after the fluid or semidigested food material was inhaled. Other clinical signs include wheezing, harsh inspiratory and expiratory noise, fever, and pulmonary edema. When the material is first aspirated, hypotension and bronchospasm usually occur immediately. Whenever aspiration of stomach secretions or vomitus is suspected, radiographs should be taken as soon as possible to visualize any pulmonary changes. Subsequent daily chest radiographs should be taken to follow the progress of the pneumonitis.

Prevention of aspiration pneumonitis

Even when an animal has been denied food and water for an appropriate time before induction, reactions such as lethargy, fear, pain, or excitement may delay the passage of food from the stomach and upper small intestine. Gastric torsion, pregnancy, or abdominal masses can also delay gastric emptying. When an animal is in shock or traumatized and must undergo emergency surgery, it is best to assume that the stomach still contains food or water. Whenever an animal is suspected of having a full or partially full stomach, anesthesia should be induced rapidly and the trachea intubated immediately with a cuffed endotracheal tube. Suction should be readily available. The animal should be positioned on the operating table so it may be tilted head down in the event vomiting or regurgitation should occur. In that case the mouth, pharynx, and endotracheal tube require immediate suctioning until they are free from vomitus. Should aspiration occur, the bronchi and trachea may require suctioning by direct bronchoscopy. In addition, 100% oxygen should be delivered to prevent cyanosis. (These precautions are also necessary whenever large amounts of blood are present in the oral or nasal passageways.)

The anesthetist should be prepared for potential aspiration problems when anesthetizing animals that may have a full stomach or are undergoing oral, nasal, or dental surgery. A suction apparatus with sterile catheter is a requirement as is tracheal intubation to be used with a properly functioning endotracheal tube cuff and 100% oxygen.

Treatment for aspiration pneumonitis

Unfortunately, once fluid or vomitus has been aspirated into the lungs it spreads so rapidly that attempts to remove it or wash it out are usually of little avail. Aspiration pneumonitis will almost always develop if the pH of the inhaled material is less than 2.5 and the volume exceeds 0.5 ml/kg. The treatment is basically supportative and may involve:

- Oxygen therapy delivered through a nasal catheter or oxygen cage
- Broad-spectrum antibiotics
- Corticosteroids to reduce the severe inflammation in the lungs
- Bronchodilating drugs to reduce brochospasm and allow the animal to cough up material that could not be suctioned
- Respiratory therapy using positive end expiratory pressure (PEEP)

In severe cases, when the animal is unable to be oxygenated via the nasal passage due to soft palate or laryngeal swelling, the animal may require a *tracheostomy* in order to maintain adequate ventilation and oxygenation. Surgically opening the trachea requires an aseptic approach and insertion of a special tracheostomy tube. The technician should be familiar with the care and management of these tubes to prevent them from:

- Becoming obstructed with blood or secretions
- Becoming contaminated with materials such as bacteria, hair and feces
- Being dislodged either by the animal or during normal handling procedures

(For a discussion of emergency tracheostomy, refer to Chapter 5 of *Small Animal Surgical Nursing.*[1])

Airway obstruction

There are a number of possible causes for respiratory failure in animals. Anything that can interfere with the animal's normal ability to breathe (ventilate) and exchange oxygen and carbon dioxide from lung alveoli to pulmonary blood can lead to respiratory failure. The most common cause for respiratory failure in small animal patients is inadequate ventilation, which can be attributed to anything that interferes with the passage of air (or gas) into and out of the lungs. Obstruction of the air passageways is but one of many possible causes for inadequate ventilation. For example, an animal's ability to expand its chest wall and draw gas into the lungs is commonly impaired by such factors as (1) preanesthetic sedatives, barbiturates, or inhalation anesthetic drugs, (2) obesity, (3) excessively heavy draping material during surgery or use of sandbags for positioning, (4) inadvertent leaning on the chest wall during surgery, (5) excessively tight chest bandaging, (6) heavy-handed restraint, (7) use of muscle-paralyzing drugs, and (8) improper positive pressure ventilation due to manual or mechanical artificial ventilation.

Failure to adequately ventilate the lungs results in lowered oxygen tension in the blood (hypoxemia) and elevated carbon dioxide tension (hypercapnia). Ventilation failure leads to respiratory failure, which in turn can lead to respiratory arrest (apnea). In the anesthetized animal, respiratory apnea quickly leads to cardiac arrest and profound hypoxia. Anesthetic drugs by themselves depress ventilation. Thus it is imperative that any situation that impairs ventilation or results in respiratory arrest under general anesthesia be considered an immediate emergency. The essential goals of any respiratory emergency are:

- To establish an open airway to the lungs *immediately*
- To ensure an adequate oxygen supply to the lungs
- To ensure adequate carbon dioxide removal from the lungs
- To support ventilation with positive pressure breathing (that is, artificial ventilation) through the use of an Ambu bag (see Fig. 2-20)

The upper airway of the respiratory tract consists of all air passageways from the nostrils to the bronchioles: external nares, nasal passages, mouth, pharynx, oropharynx, larynx, trachea and bronchi. If any one or more of these air passageways becomes partially or totally obstructed, inadequate ventilation results. The severity of ventilation failure depends on whether the obstruction is *partial* or *total* and the location of the obstruction. If, for instance, a cat has both nostrils totally obstructed with mucus and purulent debris, the degree of ventilatory failure is not as severe as if the cat were to experience an irreversible laryngospasm during tracheal intubation. Totally occluded nostrils would still allow the cat to breathe through its mouth. Severe laryngospasm, however, would be an acute and total obstruction to ventilation requiring immediate action in order to prevent cardiac arrest.

Signs

Clinical signs of impaired ventilation in the anesthetized animal are usually not as obvious as in the awake animal. *Partial obstructions* to the oral cavity, pharynx, nostrils, or larynx dictate a rapid induction of general anesthesia and placement of an endotracheal tube. Once the animal is intubated, ventilation is improved, since air bypasses the obstruction via the endotracheal tube. The danger comes during recovery when the endotracheal tube must be removed from a semiconscious animal. The original cause of the obstruction can lead to serious ventilation problems during the recovery period. Brachycephalic breeds of dog or cat are especially prone to obstructions of the soft palate or external nares after extubation of the endotracheal tube. Partial obstructions to breathing may go unnoticed during general anesthesia, especially when the animal's trachea is intubated. Clinical signs of a partially obstructed airway, although less obvious than signs for complete airway obstruction, can be equally life threatening. An animal weakened by a circulatory or respiratory disease, if its airway is partially obstructed, can progress into a severe state of hypoxemia and hypercapnia, especially if allowed to breath room air instead of 100% oxygen. The effort a weakened animal must expend to work at ventilating its lungs can quickly lead to exhaustion even under anesthesia. In the awake animal *partial* airway obstruction is characterized by noisy breathing such as snorting, snoring, and/or open-mouth breathing. If the partial obstruction is deeper in the larynx or trachea, signs would increase in severity to include:

- Labored breathing (dyspnea)
- Increased rate and effort of breathing

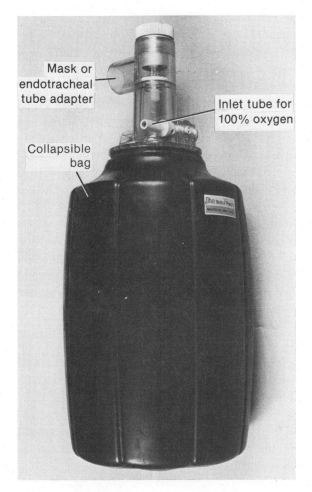

Fig. 2-20. Ambu resuscitation bag.

- Decreased tidal volume
- Coughing to expel any foreign material causing the obstruction
- Increased use of diaphragmatic muscle for breathing, resulting in abdominal breathing

Cyanosis is sometimes a sign of airway obstruction but should not be used as a determining factor for action. Cyanosis can be misleading in that its presence (or absence) is not always a true sign of hypoxemia. In addition, the mucous membranes of the mouth may appear cyanotic if the animal is hypothermic even though the animal is not hypoxemic but merely cold.

In the anesthetized animal the above responses to partial airway obstruction may be hard to observe since deep anesthesia diminishes the body's ability to respond to inadequate ventilation. Often the only clue to airway obstruction is stertorous breathing and a noticeable resistance to positive pressure ventilation. The obstruction, whatever its cause, also interferes with uptake and elimination of the inhalation anesthetic drug. Airway obstruction must be considered in cases of unusually prolonged anesthetic induction or recovery or when an animal demonstrates signs of awakening during the maintenance period of inhalation anesthesia. *Total* airway obstruction is marked by excessive breathing efforts and choking noises in addition to those signs already listed. Exhaustion from the increased effort of breathing can quickly lead to apnea if the cause for the obstruction is not corrected immediately.

The most accurate means for determining the adequacy of ventilation in the awake or anesthetized patient is to measure the arterial concentrations of oxygen, carbon dioxide, and pH. Unfortunately, most private practitioners do not routinely perform blood gas analysis, and it is rarely available for acute emergency situations. Determination of ventilation failure must therefore rely on a careful clinical assessment of the patient.

Causes

Partial or complete upper airway obstruction can result from a variety of causes, natural or mechanical. Most of those naturally occurring causes of airway obstruction under anesthesia may be circumvented by intubation of the trachea.

Natural causes
- Accumulation of secretions, vomitus, or blood in the mouth, pharynx, or trachea as well as the potential danger of aspiration of an extracted tooth or water into the trachea during dental procedures
- Soft tissue obstruction of the glottis due to relaxation of an overly large soft palate or tongue under general anesthesia (a major problem in brachycephalic breeds)
- Space-occupying tumors of the mouth, pharynx, nasal sinus, or trachea (large tumors in the neck or esophagus may partially compress and/or deviate the trachea as well)
- Collapsing trachea syndrome (usually seen in toy breeds and brachycephalic dogs)
- Inflamed tonsils or everted lateral laryngeal ventricles causing obstruction of the glottis
- Laryngospasm (seen predominantly in cats)

In addition, airway obstructions or impaired ventilation may result from mechanical errors during anesthesia.

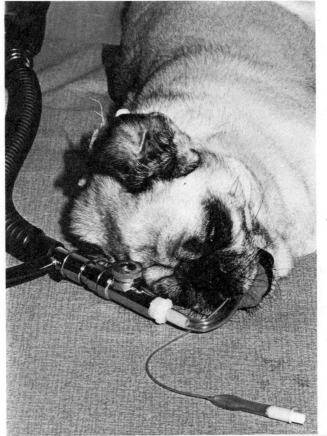

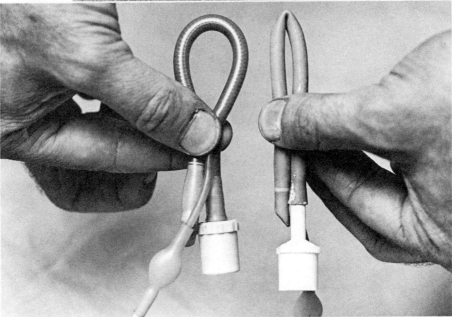

Fig. 2-21. A, Kinked endotracheal tube in dog, and **B,** kinked vs. coiled ET tube. Tube on left contains an inner coil.

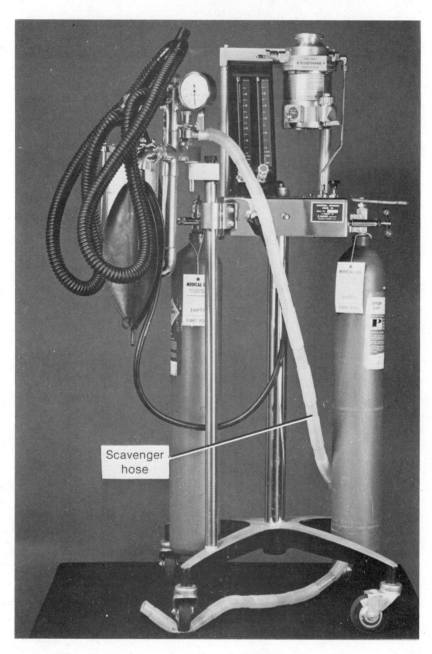

Fig. 2-22. Occlusion of scavenger hose by anesthesia machine.

Mechanical causes

Endotracheal tube. The endotracheal tube itself is a major cause for airway obstruction and must be monitored for signs of kinking (see Fig. 2-21); occlusion from secretions, blood or vomitus; overinflation of the cuff; or using cuff of too small a diameter (see Chapter 5).

Anesthesia machine. Some potential causes of impaired ventilation when an anesthesia machine is used to deliver oxygen to the anesthetized animal are:

- Dislodgment of the endotracheal tube by the weight of the breathing tubes
- Occluded or constricted breathing tubes
- Sticky inhalation or exhalation valves
- Overinflated breathing bag due to a closed "pop-off" valve or occlusion of the exhalation valve on a nonrebreathing bag
- Insufficient fresh gas flow causing collapse of the breathing bag
- Accidental disconnection of the fresh gas inlet tube
- Significant leaks in the patient breathing circle
- Insufficient supply of compressed oxygen
- Excessive vacuum applied to scavenger system, causing collapse of patient breathing bag or occlusion of the scavenger hose (see Fig. 2-22)
- Incorrect assembly of anesthetic breathing circuit

Improper positioning. Any positioning of the animal for surgery or diagnostic procedures should be done in as near a normal position as possible. Excessive head or neck flexion can lead to tracheal obstruction. Positions that compress the chest or diaphragm can impair the ability of the animal to expand its thorax, thereby decreasing ventilation. Tilting of female dogs and cats during routine spay operations is discouraged for this reason.

Occlusive drapes. When an animal is not connected to an anesthesia machine, cloth or other heavy, nonporous surgical draping material must not occlude the endotracheal tube, nostrils, or mouth of the anesthetized animal. The presence of draping material over these parts causes the animal additional effort to ventilate its lungs. Further, exhaled carbon dioxide may accumulate beneath the draping material where it could be rebreathed. Airway obstructions must be treated by immediate support of ventilation and elimination of the causative factor.

REFERENCE

1. Tracy, D.L., editor: Small animal surgical nursing. In Warren, R.G., series editor: Mosby's fundamentals of animal health technology, St. Louis, 1983, The C.V. Mosby Co.

3

Injectable anesthetic drugs

PERFORMANCE OBJECTIVES

After completion of this chapter, the student will:

- Differentiate, using examples, the classification of barbiturate anesthetic drugs according to their duration of action

- List and discuss the respiratory and cardiovascular effects associated with a barbiturate overdosage

- Discuss the etiology, treatment, and prevention of a barbiturate skin slough

- List the disadvantages of pentobarbital associated with its sole use as a routine general anesthetic drug

- Describe the term "given to effect" as it concerns the administration of a barbiturate drug for the purpose of producing a surgical plane of anesthesia

- Describe the basic differences in the general anesthetic state produced by conventional anesthetic drugs and that produced by cataleptoid anesthetic drugs

- Discuss the classification and usage of steroid anesthetic drugs in small animal patients

- List and describe the methods for administering local analgesic drugs to small animal patients

BARBITURATES
Classification

Barbiturate drugs are routinely classified according to the speed of onset and duration of their action (see Table 3-1). Those barbiturate drugs used for producing general anesthesia in animals are either *short-acting* or *ultrashort-acting*. Barbiturates classified as *long* or *intermediate* in action are not used for general anesthesia. Instead, they are used as sedatives, hypnotics, or anticonvulsants and are usually administered by the oral or intramuscular route.

All barbiturate drugs have similar chemical structures related to the barbituric acid molecule. The barbiturates employed for general anesthesia are also classified as *oxybarbiturates* or *thiobarbiturates*, according to the presence of either an oxygen or a sulfur atom on the barbituric acid molecule (see Fig. 3-1). All thiobarbiturates are ultrashort in action; however, not all ultrashort-acting barbiturates are thiobarbiturates. Methohexital, for instance, is an oxybarbiturate that is classified as an ultrashort-acting barbiturate. Long- and intermediate-acting barbiturates are also oxybarbiturates. Barbiturate drugs act by depressing the central nervous system (CNS) and are considered relatively weak analgesics.

General use of barbiturate drugs

Barbiturate drugs have three general *therapeutic* uses in dogs and cats:
1. *General anesthesia*. Barbiturates are used more for anesthesia than any other single purpose (exclusive of their use for euthanasia purposes).
2. *Anticonvulsant therapy*. Intermediate- and short-acting barbiturates are sometimes used to suppress seizures caused by conditions such as poisoning, hypocalcemia, and epilepsy. Phenobarbital is the classic drug in this category.
3. *Sedation*. Before the introduction of tranquilizer drugs in the early 1950s, barbiturates were used extensively for their sedative, hypnotic, and sleep-inducing actions. Drugs such as phenobarbital, barbital, secobarbital, and hexobarbital are still used in humans for their sedative effects and are usually administered by the oral route.

All barbiturate drugs, especially the intermediate- and short-acting ones, are capable of producing physical and psychologic dependence. As a result of their addictive quality, they come under the restrictions of the Controlled Substance Act. The majority of barbiturate drugs belong to Schedule II and therefore require federal licensing, purchase forms, strict record keeping, and storage in a special Class II safe. Ultrashort-acting barbiturate anesthetics are presently classified as Schedule III controlled substances, which allows for a lesser degree of control and record keeping because of their decreased potential for abuse. The AHT should become familiar with the laws and restrictions pertaining to these and other commonly used Schedule II drugs (see Chapter 1).

TABLE 3-1

Classification of barbiturates by name, structure, duration of action, and excretion route

Generic name	Trade name	R_1	R_2	R_3	X	Duration of action	Organ of excretion and/or metabolism*
Phenobarbital	Luminal Phenobarbitone	Ethyl	Phenyl	H	Oxygen	Long	I
Barbital	Veronal Barbitone	Ethyl	Ethyl	H	Oxygen	Long	I
Amobarbital	Amytal	Ethyl	Isoamyl	H	Oxygen	Intermediate	III
†Pentobarbital	Nembutal	Ethyl	1-Methyl-butyl	H	Oxygen‡	Short	III
Secobarbital	Seconal	Allyl	1-Methyl-butyl	H	Oxygen	Short	III
†Methohexital	Brevane	Allyl	1-Methyl-2-pentynyl	CH₃	Oxygen	Ultrashort	IV
†Thiopental	Pentothal	Ethyl	1-Methyl-butyl	H	Sulfur‡	Ultrashort	IV
†Thiamylal	Surital	Allyl	1-Methyl-butyl	H	Sulfur	Ultrashort	IV

Modified in part from Goodman, L.S., and Gilman A., editors: The pharmacological basis of therapeutics, ed. 5, New York, 1975, Macmillan Publishing Co., Inc., Table 9-1; and Lumb W.V. and Jones E.W.: Veterinary anesthesia, Philadelphia, 1973, Lea & Febiger, Table 12-7.

*I: Excreted mainly by kidneys, II: Metabolized in the liver and excreted by kidneys, III: Metabolized in the liver, IV: Absorbed by fat, metabolized in the liver, and excreted by kidneys.

† Drugs most often employed in veterinary anesthesia.

‡ NOTE: These two drugs differ only with respect to the inclusion of an oxygen or a sulfur atom in the "X" position of the general structure of barbiturates.

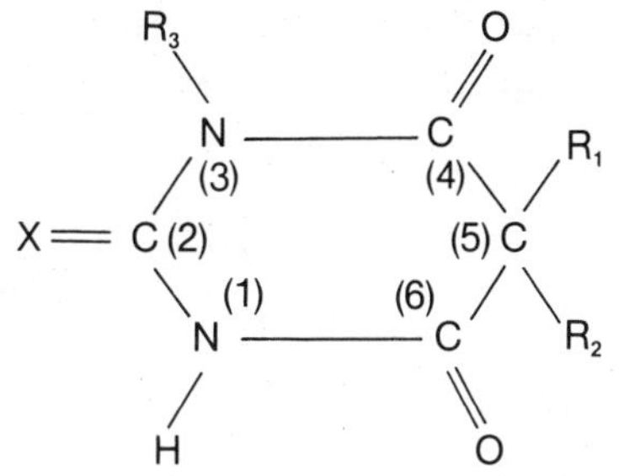

Fig. 3-1. General chemical structure of barbiturates. The "X" position contains an oxygen or a sulfur group.

General mode of action for barbiturate anesthetics

All barbiturate drugs used for anesthetic purposes have a depressant effect on the respiratory and cardiovascular systems. They progressively depress the CNS according to the sequence presented in Chapter 2. The ultrashort-acting thiobarbiturates owe their relatively rapid action and short duration of action to increased lipid solubility and rapid redistribution from the brain to muscle and fat tissue. Short-acting barbiturates, of which pentobarbital is the primary example, owe their relatively slow onset and longer duration of action to a decreased solubility in fat and therefore to a slower redistribution away from brain tissue. Barbiturate anesthetics, in general, gain entrance into the patient's bloodstream by direct intravenous injection. The concentration needed for depression of the CNS to the point of Stage III anesthesia is calculated and administered as a single intravenous injection. Once the desired plane of anesthesia is achieved, it is maintained with additional injections of the barbiturate as needed. Barbiturates, like most injectable anesthetic drugs, cannot be eliminated from the body until the drug has been metabolized by the liver and excreted through the kidneys—a relatively slow process.

Dynamics of barbiturate anesthesia

Once a barbiturate anesthetic is injected into the bloodstream, it is immediately distributed throughout the body. The drug then penetrates cell walls of various organs and will, if the animal is pregnant, also cross the placenta into the fetus. General anesthesia depends on the degree to which the barbiturate permeates the brain cells and depresses CNS activity. The speed of anesthetic induction, its depth and maintenance, and the length of time it takes to recover from the barbiturate drug are related to the following factors:

1. pH of the blood and tissue
2. Plasma protein binding
3. Relative dose and route of administration
4. Solubility in fat
5. Redistribution into nonnervous tissues
6. Rate of liver detoxification and renal excretion

It is important to understand these six interrelated factors since, after a barbiturate is injected into the animal, there is no way to retrieve the drug. Overdosage with barbiturate anesthetics is a major cause of anesthetic deaths in small animals. The AHT should never administer any anesthetic drug without prior knowledge of its pharmacologic actions and general precautions concerning the drug. These essential six factors mentioned will be discussed as each relates to the uptake, distribution, and elimination of barbiturate anesthetics in the animal's body.

pH of blood and body tissues

Blood and tissue fluid in the body of most warm-blooded animals is slightly alkaline (pH of 7.34 to 7.43). The term "pH" is a numerical expression of the relative acidity or alkalinity of a fluid. A pH of 7.0 is considered neutral. When an animals' blood has a pH of less than 7.34 (for example, 7.13), it is referred to as *acidosis*. If the blood has a higher than normal pH (for example, 7.52), it is termed *alkalosis*. Most metabolic diseases cause the blood pH to drop and lead to a *metabolic acidosis*. Any respiratory disease that interferes with removal of CO_2 from the lungs leads to a buildup of CO_2 in the blood that combines with water to form carbonic acid:

$$\underset{\text{Carbon dioxide}}{CO_2} + \underset{\text{Water}}{H_2O} \rightleftharpoons \underset{\text{Carbonic acid}}{H_2CO_3 \text{ (weak acid)}} \rightleftharpoons \underset{\substack{\text{Hydrogen} \\ \text{ion}}}{H^+} + \underset{\substack{\text{Bicarbonate} \\ \text{ion}}}{HCO_3^-}$$

Therefore respiratory diseases often lead to a *respiratory acidosis* due to an accumulation of hydrogen ions. Hyperventilation results in a *respiratory alkalosis* due to excessive removal of CO_2 from the lungs, thereby lowering its concentration in blood and, as a consequence, lowering the relative concentration of hydrogen ions.

All barbiturates used for intravenous anesthesia are manufactured as sodium salts to facilitate their going into solution. Sodium bicarbonate is also added to the thiobarbiturates to keep them in strongly alkaline solution (pH 9.5 to 10.5)—hence the source of irritation and skin sloughing if it is accidentally injected outside the vein (see pp. 129-130). Once a thiobarbiturate enters the bloodstream, it equilibrates into two forms—the unionized form (salt or acid) and ionized form:

$$\underset{\text{Na} - \text{B}}{\text{Unionized salt}} \rightleftharpoons \underset{\text{B}^- + \text{H}^+}{\text{Ionized form}} \rightleftharpoons \underset{\text{H} - \text{B}}{\text{Unionized acid}}$$

The pH at which equal amounts of a drug exist in the ionized and unionized form is taken as the "dissociation constant" (pKa) for that particular drug (see Table 3-2). In order for a barbiturate to cross the lipid cell membrane, it must be in the unionized form (B-Na), be it a brain cell, a muscle cell, or a fat cell.

Dosages used for general anesthesia assume the pH of the patient's blood to be within normal range. However, when actually administering anesthetics on a daily basis to a variety of animal species, both sick and healthy, one cannot make such an assumption. Changes in the pH of blood can lead to significant alterations in the

TABLE 3-2

Physical properties of three barbiturate anesthetics

	Thiopental	Pentobarbital	Methohexital
Dissociation constant (pKa)*	7.6	8.1	7.9
Percent of molecule in the nonionized (diffusible) form at physiologic pH = 7.4*	61%	83%	76%
Percent of molecule bound to plasma protein at pH = 7.4*	75%	40%	75%
Effective brain/blood partition coefficient (that is, lipid solubility)*	2.0	0.042	Low
pH of prepared solution	2.5% = 10.5-11	6.0% = 10-10.5	5.0%-10-11
Onset of action†	20-30 seconds	30-60 seconds	10-30 seconds
Duration of action following single dose†	10-20 minutes	1-2 hours	5-10 minutes

*Information from Eger, E.I., II: Anesthetic uptake and action, Baltimore, 1981, The Williams & Wilkins Co. p. 88.
†From data compiled by Dornette, W.H.L., and published by Ohio Medical Products, with additions from Lumb, W.V., and Jones, E.W.: Veterinary anesthesia, Philadelphia, 1973, Lea & Febiger.

depth of barbiturate anesthesia. Any condition that results in a respiratory or metabolic acidosis will shift the equilibrium to the left and increase the unionized form of the drug in the bloodstream. This would allow for more of the drug to penetrate into cells of the CNS and lead to a deepening of anesthesia. All barbiturates cause a degree of respiratory depression that leads to an increase in the level of CO_2 in the blood (hypercapnia). Hypercapnia then causes the pH to decrease and results in a respiratory acidosis, usually within about 5 to 30 minutes, depending on the degree of respiratory depression. It should now be evident why barbiturate anesthesia can be so dangerous. It perpetuates a degree of respiratory acidosis that tends to increase the unionized form of barbiturate, thereby increasing the depth of anesthesia with time and with repeated injections of the drug. The rate and depth of anesthetic depression will be considerably greater in sick, debilitated, or dehydrated animals that are already acidotic—unless the dose administered is reduced by 50% to 90%. On the other hand, if the blood is alkalotic—as may occur with hyperventilation (natural or artificial) or administration of sodium bicarbonate—the depth of barbiturate anesthesia may lighten. Alkalosis causes the equilibrium to shift toward the right and cause a relative decrease in the amount of unionized barbiturate available for cell penetration. Animals that receive barbiturate anesthesia in a state of alkalosis will require a longer induction period and a relatively larger dose of the drug than the normal healthy animal.

Plasma protein binding

Proteins dissolved within blood plasma form a chemical bond with the barbiturate molecule. The major portion of the binding is to the plasma protein albumin. At normal pH not all the barbiturate molecules in the blood are bound to proteins. However, those that are bound can no longer cross cell membranes, which means the drug is essentially "tied up" and unable to act on the CNS. The bond between plasma albumin and the barbiturate molecule is reversible according to the pH of blood. Maximum binding of barbiturate to albumin occurs when the pH is between 7.5 and 8.1. When the blood becomes acidotic (<7.3), less barbiturate is bound to protein, thereby allowing for more of the barbiturate to be free and become unionized in the blood. Since it is the unionized and unbound form of the drug that is capable of crossing cell membranes, a decreasing blood pH will lead to an increase in the depth of barbiturate anesthesia because of the release of additional barbiturate molecules from plasma protein (hence more will be available to depress the CNS). In addition, certain drugs such as aspirin and phenylbutazone can displace the barbiturate from its plasma protein binding site.

Thiobarbiturates, such as thiamylal and thiopental, are more soluble in fat and lipid then are oxybarbiturates. The fat soluble barbiturates are more highly bound to plasma proteins at a given pH. Therefore, if an animal becomes acidotic during thiobarbiturate anesthesia, there will be a relatively greater amount of the drug released from protein and available to further depress the CNS as compared with pentobarbital anesthesia. It should be remembered that, in routine dosages given for barbiturate anesthesia, it is assumed that the animal is healthy, is not acidotic, and has a normal amount of protein in its plasma.

Caution must be exercised and the dosage reduced in animals that are acidotic and/or have a greater or lesser than normal level of albumin present in the blood. An approximation of the animal's protein level can be determined from the total amount of proteins present in a sample of serum or plasma. A small amount of serum or plasma can be used to make the total protein determination if a refractometer is available. The plasma remaining in the microhematocrit tube may be used for total protein determination once packed cell volume (PCV) has been recorded. A total protein of less than 5 gm/100 ml would indicate *hypoproteinemia*, and barbiturates as the sole anesthetic should either be eliminated or the dosage considerably reduced. Induction of anesthesia with an inhalation anesthetic would decrease the chance for anesthetic overdosage in animals that are hypoproteinemic.

Relative dose and route of administration

The initial speed of anesthetic induction and degree of CNS depression are related to the dose of barbiturate injected, the route by which it is administered, and the speed with which it is injected. Since it is difficult to compute all the factors affecting barbiturate anesthesia, the dose and method of administration are the only factors over which the anesthetist has any degree of control. If the dose administered is too great for the particular animal, the effect will be noticed in the form of an overdosage or prolonged recovery time. A common error when first learning how to administer barbiturate anesthesia occurs during the initial induction period, even when a correct dosage has been calculated. If the animal jumps or struggles during the initial intravenous injection of the barbiturate, the needle may dislodge from the vein while the injection continues. A small volume of barbiturate may be accidentally injected subcutaneously around the vein causing a swelling to appear in the area of the injection. If the amount of barbiturate given intravenously prior to the dislodging of the needle was insufficient to cause unconsciousness, the animal may show exaggerated stage II excitement. In order to overcome this, there is usually a hurried attempt to complete the induction by injecting additional barbiturate into another vein, forgetting about the drug that was accidentally given subcutaneously. Unfortunately, this subcutaneous volume will be absorbed slowly into the bloodstream over a period of 10 to 20 minutes, in which case an overdosage may follow due to the additional barbiturate absorption. Diluting the subcutaneous barbiturate to prevent a skin slough will do nothing to prevent its eventual absorption into the blood. For this reason an intravenous catheter should be placed into the vein (*intravenous* being the preferred route of administration for barbiturate anesthetics) *before* administering the barbiturate solution.

The barbiturate dosage is generally given "to effect," meaning that only about one-third to one-half of the total calculated dosage for anesthesia is administered relatively rapidly in order to get the animal through stage II rapidly and with minimal excitement. After waiting sufficient time for the drug to act on the CNS and checking the animal's vital signs and reflexes, additional amounts of the barbiturate are given in small doses "to effect" until a surgical plane of anesthesia has been obtained. The period of time over which this injection should take place is longer (5 minutes) for the short-acting barbiturates than it is for ultrashort-acting barbiturates (1 to 2 minutes). In order to maintain the surgical plane of anesthesia small doses of the barbiturate are given "to effect" at intervals as needed, remembering that once injected, the drug will continue to accumulate in the blood and body tissues until it is metabolized by the liver.

An overdosage can occur if the calculated dosage of barbiturate is administered too rapidly via the intravenous route. If the entire dosage is not given "to effect," a large bolus of barbiturate can directly depress both the heart and CNS, resulting in serious cardiovascular and respiratory collapse. If too small a dose of barbiturate is injected or the initial injection is made too slowly, the animal may experience unnecessary excitement. Additional barbiturate over and above the calculated dosage will then be needed to overcome stage II excitement and produce the desired plane of anesthesia. However, this can lead to an overdosage and will increase the length of time it takes the animal to recover from the barbiturate.

The amount of barbiturate required to produce a surgical plane of anesthesia in an animal is affected by many factors including the breed, age, weight, nutritional status, relative obesity, physical status, and anxiety level of the animal. Administration of preanesthetic sedatives will also reduce the amount of anesthetic drug required.

The dosages presented here for barbiturate anesthetics should be considered only guidelines for use with dogs and cats. Care and caution must be a routine matter when administering any depressant drug, especially when the drug is administered via the intravenous route. The lower end of the dosage range is recommended when performing a slow anesthetic induction. The upper end of the dosage range is used when attempting a rapid ("crash") induction in order to insert the endotracheal tube as rapidly as possible. These recommended dosages for barbiturate anesthetics must be reduced accordingly when preanesthetic sedatives are used and when the animal is ill or considered an anesthetic risk. Generally, the dosage should be reduced by one-third to one-half when using preanesthetic sedatives and one-half to three-quarters when administered to seriously ill or at risk animals.

Solubility of barbiturate in fat tissue

The ultrashort-acting thiobarbiturates are extremely soluble in fat as compared to the oxybarbiturates. The brain is composed of large amounts of lipid, which is similar to fat. Due to their high solubility in fat, thiobarbiturates are able to penetrate brain tissue and produce CNS depression rapidly—that is, in 20 to 30 seconds. Oxybarbiturates are less soluble in fat and require a longer period of time to pass across the blood-to-brain lipid barrier and produce CNS depression (2 to 5 minutes). Thiobarbiturates, because of their high fat solubility, are considered more potent than the oxybarbiturates. Apnea due to respiratory depression is more likely to occur during induction with a thiobarbiturate, especially if the drug is administered rapidly. The apnea that results is usually of short duration (1 to 3 minutes) and is managed by artificially ventilating the animal until spontaneous respirations return. Apnea due to a short-acting barbiturate is usually of longer duration and may require artificial ventilation throughout the anesthetic period (1 to 2 hours).

The short duration of surgical anesthesia (10 to 30 minutes) and the rapid recovery period (1 to 2 hours) associated with thiobarbiturates are also related to their high solubility in muscle and fat tissue. The dosage recommended for thiobarbiturate anesthesia assumes that the animal has a normal proportion of lean body tissue to fat body tissue. *Caution* must be exercised when administering thiobarbiturates to dogs or cats that are extremely thin or emaciated or that have a disproportionately large amount of lean muscle tissue. The racing greyhound and other thin breeds of dog (for example, the Afghan, saluki, whippet, and borzoi) require much less thiobarbiturate due to their lack of body fat. Since little of the thiobarbiturate is able to leave the blood for fat, the level within the blood remains high in thin

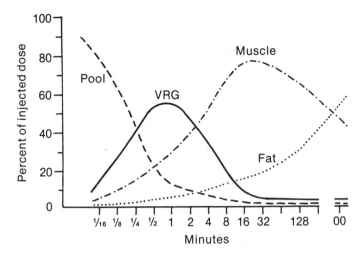

Fig. 3-2. Redistribution curve for thiopental in different tissues at various times following intravenous injection. Notice that lean tissue (muscle group) contains about 80% of the injected dose after 20 minutes, while fat tissue does not begin to play a role until after almost 2 hours. Redrawn with permission from Price, H.L., et al.: The uptake of thiopental by body tissues and its relation to the duration of narcosis, Clin. Pharmacol. and Ther. 1(1):16, 1960.

animals and results in a sustained level of CNS depression. In such animals thiobarbiturates should be eliminated or used in greatly reduced dosages for anesthetic induction and intubation only. Inhalation anesthesia should be used for maintenance in order to prevent a prolonged recovery from the thiobarbiturate.

Redistribution into nonnervous tissue

Induction of anesthesia with barbiturate drugs depends primarily on the dosage and speed of administration, the blood supply to the brain, and the solubility of the barbiturate in fat. So long as the initial level of the barbiturate in plasma is sufficiently high, anesthesia will be induced. The duration of anesthesia and the time required for an animal to regain all of its protective reflexes are dependent on the length of time it takes for the plasma concentration of anesthetic drug to drop below its respective CNS depressant level. As the plasma concentration begins to fall, so too will the concentration within the brain, since anesthetic molecules tend to diffuse from an area of higher concentration into an area of lesser concentration. The longer duration of anesthesia and recovery seen with short-acting barbiturates is caused by the failure of plasma level to drop significantly until a major portion of the drug has been metabolized by the liver. The relatively short duration of anesthesia and recovery periods seen with the ultrashort-acting barbiturates results from a rapid decline in their plasma level due to redistribution from the blood and brain into nonnervous tissues, initially muscle and then fat (see Fig. 3-2).

Redistribution of the barbiturate is dependent on its solubility in muscle or fat and the relative blood supply to tissues other than the brain. Oxybarbiturates are not redistributed to the extent that are thiobarbiturates because of their low solubility in fat (see Table 3-2).

The tissues of the body can be divided into four general groups according to their relative blood supply (see Table 3-3):

1. The vessel-rich group (VRG): brain, heart, kidneys, and liver
2. The muscle group (MG): skin and muscle
3. The fat group (FG): all fatty tissue
4. The vessel-poor group (VPG): bone, cartilage, tendons, and ligaments

The vessel-poor group has little effect on the induction, maintenance, or recovery phases of barbiturate anesthesia since its blood supply is minimal and does not tend to concentrate the drug.

During the first 5 to 10 minutes after a barbiturate is injected into the general circulation, most of the drug is distributed to the vessel-rich group. These tissues normally receive about 70% of the cardiac output. In the first 2 to 5 minutes there is a rapid uptake of barbiturate by those organs receiving the greatest portion of the cardiac output. The brain alone receives about 10% to 15% of the cardiac output, yet it is only about 1% to 2% of the animal's total body weight (see Table 3-3). At the same time that the VRG organs are taking the anesthetic out of the blood, the lean body tissues are also absorbing anesthetic molecules—only at a slower rate due to their lesser blood supply. Combined skin and muscle account for about 25% of the cardiac output. The degree to which the muscle and skin remove anesthetic from the blood depends on the anesthetic's solubility in these tissues (the thiobarbiturates are more soluble in lean tissue than are the oxybarbiturates). The lean body tissues reach their maximum saturation with barbiturate about 15 to 30 minutes after injection (see Fig. 3-2). In the case of thiobarbiturates this coincides with the initial recovery after a single surgical intravenous dose because of a decline in the plasma concentration of the thiobarbiturate. The lean tissues of the body tend to contain the anesthetic for the next 1 to 2 hours. During the induction of anesthesia with any barbiturate, it is important to realize the effect of cardiac output* and blood volume on anesthetic induction and recovery.

When an animal is in shock, a greater percentage of the cardiac output is diverted to the brain (and heart) even though the total cardiac output decreases. The circulation of blood to nonvital tissues is dramatically reduced in shock, which means that less of the anesthetic is redistributed to nonnervous tissue. The brain can receive an unusually large portion of the injected dose of barbiturate in shocky

---

*Cardiac output (CO) is the volume of blood pumped from the left ventricle in 1 minute. Normal values vary according to the weight and surface area of the body. An approximate value can be obtained by multiplying the weight of the animal (in kg) by 100 ml. For instance, a 12 kg dog would have a CO of about 1200 ml per minute.

TABLE 3-3

Tissue group characteristics for humans

	Vessel-rich group (VRG)	Muscle group (MG)	Fat group (FG)	Vessel-poor group (VPG)
Body mass (%)	9	50	19	22
Volume (L) in a 70 kg human	6	33	14.5	12.5
Perfusion—taken as % of cardiac output	75	18.1	5.4	1.5

NOTE: Although the data is for humans, some extrapolation can be made for animals—particularly that the VRG composes only 9.0% of the total body mass, yet it receives 75% of the cardiac output. In shock, this may rise to even more than 75% as cerebral and cardiac perfusion are maintained at the expense of the other three tissue groups.

From Eger, EI., II: Anesthetic uptake and action, Baltimore, 1974, The Williams & Wilkins Co., Table 4-3, p. 88.

animals and, as a consequence, induction is extremely rapid while recovery is markedly delayed. General anesthetic drugs alone can decrease cardiac output by as much as 40% to 50%. In shocklike states barbiturates must be administered with extreme caution and at a greatly reduced dosage.

When an animal is excited, fearful, or unusually active, blood flow to the muscles is increased, thereby decreasing the portion of the cardiac output that would normally go to the brain. Its effect is to delay the speed of induction. Animals that are excited or anxious during anesthetic induction require more anesthetic to reach stage III, which creates a situation conducive to an anesthetic overdosage. Preanesthetic sedation decreases the likelihood of this occurring by calming the animal and reducing the amount of anesthetic required to reach a suitable plane of surgical anesthesia.

Even though thiobarbiturates are highly soluble in fat, they do not begin to concentrate in fat until about 1 to 2 hours after the initial injection. The reason for the delay in uptake by fatty tissue as compared to lean body tissue is a result of the relatively poor blood supply to adipose tissue (5% to 6% of cardiac output). Fat does not play a significant role in reducing the level of thiobarbiturates in plasma until after the second hour of anesthesia. An animal with excess fat will probably not be affected by anesthetic induction or recovery when a single injection of barbiturate is administered. If, however, thiobarbiturates are repeatedly injected to maintain the anesthetic state beyond 30 to 60 minutes, the amount of fatty tissue present can have a considerable influence on the length of time it takes the animal to recover all its protective reflexes. Because thiobarbiturates tend to concentrate heavily in fat tissue, the plasma level will tend to drop faster in a fat animal than in a lean animal once the thiobarbiturate has been discontinued. When multiple doses of thiobarbiturates are used for anesthesia, a fat animal will usually recover reflexes sooner than will a thin animal. Or, to put it another way, a thin animal will experience a longer recovery period than a fat animal when multiple doses of thiobarbiturate are used to maintain anesthesia beyond 30 to 60 minutes. In effect, the muscle and fat act to extract the thiobarbiturate from the blood and hence the brain—allowing for a more rapid return of reflexes. It is theoretically possible to give a large enough dose of thiobarbiturate over a long enough period that all body tissues, including blood and fat, become saturated. In such a case the animal would not begin to show signs of recovery until the greater portion of thiobarbiturate underwent metabolism and excretion—a period of time usually in excess of 4 to 6 hours.

Rate of liver metabolism and renal excretion

Recovery from short-acting oxybarbiturates depends almost entirely on the length of time required for the body to break down the active barbiturate molecule and remove it from the bloodstream. The process of metabolism (biotransformation) takes place primarily in the liver and is the result of enzyme activity on the barbiturate molecule. The breakdown products from the liver are released into the circulation and subsequently removed by the kidneys and excreted from the body via the urine. In young healthy dogs and cats with properly functioning liver and kidneys, this process (totally removing the active form of the barbiturate drug from the plasma) takes about 6 to 8 hours.

Recovery from a single intravenous dose of an ultrashort-acting barbiturate in most dogs and cats begins within 20 to 30 minutes. Complete return of all reflexes and ability to stand and walk usually takes 1 to 2 hours. However, the drug itself has only been redistributed out of the bloodstream. It still must undergo metabolism by the liver and elimination through the kidneys—a process requiring the same amount of time as for a short-acting barbiturate. Animals with impaired liver or renal function will require a considerably longer period of time to recover all reflexes following administration of either a short-acting or an ultrashort-acting barbiturate drug.

When an animal's body temperature drops below 34° to 35°C, the activity of liver enzymes is markedly reduced. Hypothermia therefore tends to prolong anesthetic recovery, especially with barbiturate anesthesia. General anesthetic drugs normally cause a drop of 1° to 2°C in body temperature. When a surgical procedure involves excision of a body cavity, such as the abdomen or thorax, additional body heat is lost into the room air. The longer an animal is under general anesthesia, the greater will be the degree of hypothermia. Body temperatures of 31° to 32°C are possible during long surgical procedures. It is important that an animal's body temperature be maintained between 36° to 38°C while under general anesthesia in order to prevent an excessively long recovery period and/or serious depression of cardiopulmonary functions.

Signs of barbiturate overdosage

All barbiturate drugs depress respiration and directly depress the myocardium. Certain barbiturates depress one more than the other. Overdosage with any barbiturate will lead to signs of both respiratory and cardiovascular failure.

Respiratory effects

Ventilation is impaired by the depressant action of barbiturates on the respiratory center within the CNS. Both tidal volume and rate of breathing are reduced, thereby decreasing the animal's respiratory minute volume. The depression on ventilation increases as anesthetic depth increases. With an overdosage respiratory arrest (apnea) may occur (barbiturate apnea is usually a response to an overly large or rapid intravenous injection of the drug). Thiobarbiturates will depress ventilation during induction more than oxybarbiturates. When apnea occurs on induction, further injection of the barbiturate should be halted until spontaneous respirations return and artificial ventilation given until the animal resumes a normal respiratory rate and depth. The most common cause of death in animals anesthetized for long periods with short-acting barbiturates, namely pentobarbital, is progressive respiratory depression in the absence of ventilatory support.

The ability of the respiratory center to respond to rising levels of arterial carbon dioxide is depressed by barbiturate drugs. Normally the respiratory center will initiate a breath when the carbon dioxide level in the blood supplying the brain rises above 40 to 45 mm Hg (see Chapter 5). Under barbiturate anesthesia the respiratory center does not respond until the carbon dioxide tension becomes much higher, that is, 60 to 70 mm Hg. This respiratory depression is dose related. With moderate to deep levels of anesthesia, a respiratory acidosis occurs. As respiration becomes progressively more depressed, hypoxia develops in addition to the hypercapnia until eventually the heart and brain are impaired. When the animal is under a deep plane of barbiturate anesthesia, it is best to artificially ventilate it in order to adequately control oxygenation and CO_2 removal. Pure oxygen administered to an animal spontaneously breathing room air under barbiturate anesthesia can, on some occasions, cause apnea by eliminating the respiratory center's ability to sustain ventilation in response to lowered arterial oxygen levels. If 100% oxygen is administered during barbiturate anesthesia and the animal becomes apneic, ventilation should be controlled by the anesthetist.

Summary of overdosage signs associated with ventilation
- Decreased rate of breathing
- Decreased tidal volume
- Hypercapnia*
- Respiratory acidosis*
- Hypoxia*

*A blood gas analyzer is required in order to determine the precise degree of hypercapnia, hypoxia, and respiratory acidosis.

Cardiovascular effects

Barbiturate anesthetic drugs, like inhalation anesthetic drugs, cause a direct depression of the myocardium. The degree of myocardial depression is greatest during the induction stage of anesthesia and for 5 to 10 minutes following intravenous injection. Signs of myocardial depression may be seen in the form of:

- Decreased cardiac output
- Decreased blood pressure
- Tachycardia
- Ventricular dysrhythmias (most often premature ventricular contractions [PVCs] with bigeminal rhythm)

One of the most common causes of anesthetic death during the induction phase of barbiturate anesthesia is circulatory collapse, most often resulting from too rapid an injection of a thiobarbiturate. A relatively large and rapid intravenous injection allows a bolus of the barbiturate to reach the myocardium where it can result in severe depression and cardiac arrest within seconds to minutes. The dose of thiobarbiturate required to cause cardiac arrest in a healthy animal is usually greater than the dose that will arrest respiration. The potential for severe circulatory depression during induction with thiobarbiturates can be decreased if the drug is administered slowly and to effect—in dilute concentrations of 2.0% to 2.5%.

When a barbiturate anesthetic is injected slowly by the intravenous route, the decrease in cardiac output and blood pressure is relatively mild and of short duration. Within a few minutes after injection the cardiac output, blood pressure, and heart rate return to near normal values. In many animals the heart rate and blood pressure may increase slightly once the major portion of the injected barbiturate has been distributed to the muscle and various body organs.

When barbiturate anesthetics are used in animals with cardiovascular disease, the precautions to be taken are basically the same as with any other general anesthetic. A diseased or stressed myocardium is extremely sensitive to the depressant effects of anesthetic drugs. The diseased heart that may be functioning maximally to maintain life is less able to compensate for changes in blood pressure, cardiac output, and heart rate. A dosage of barbiturate that can be tolerated by a normal healthy animal may cause severe cardiovascular depression in a weakened or diseased heart. Barbiturates create a secondary insult to the heart as a result of their effects on respiration. The respiratory acidosis, hypercapnia, and hypoxemia associated with barbiturate anesthesia can further depress the cardiovascular system unless the animal's ventilation is controlled or assisted throughout the anesthetic period.

General precautions and/or complications

In general, the use of barbiturates for anesthesia involves the same precautions as would accompany the use of any general anesthetic. Careful observation of vital signs, reflexes, and overall effects of the barbiturate must accompany the usual amount of caution when animals undergo anesthesia for one or more of the following conditions:

- Cardiovascular disease
- Shock
- Hemorrhage
- Dehydration
- Pulmonary disease
- Impaired ventilation caused by such conditions as diaphragmatic hernia, pneumothorax, collapsing trachea, and fractured rib
- Thoracic or abdominal trauma
- CNS depression due to organic disease, trauma to the head, or over-sedation from other sedative drugs
- Very old or very young animals
- Extremely thin or lean animals
- Hypothermia
- Hyperthermia
- Metabolic or respiratory acidosis
- Hypoproteinemia
- Anemia
- Impaired liver function
- Impaired kidney function
- Obstruction to urine outflow
- Fearful, excited, or nervous animals

Obviously, precaution and careful observation of the patient should be practiced with all patients, including the normal healthy animal. Administration of anesthesia must never become so routine that, should a complication arise, one loses a sense of precaution at the expense of the patient. Barbiturates should never be used when equipment for artificial ventilation and resuscitation is unavailable.

Skin slough

An additional complication that may accompany the use of barbiturate drugs for anesthesia is that of tissue irritation following a perivascular injection. When some or all of a barbiturate injection is accidentally deposited outside the vein, the solution (because of its alkaline pH) can cause a severe inflammation of the surrounding skin. The irritation may not appear until 1 to 2 days after the injection. When an alkaline barbiturate solution is deposited subcutaneously, the resulting skin irritation may be so severe that the skin cells are killed, resulting in necrosis and a sloughing of the affected skin 2 to 4 days later. If the barbiturate solution is highly concentrated (greater than 4.0% to 5.0%, a skin slough may occur with a relatively small volume). The irritation that follows a perivascular injection of barbiturate solutions may also cause the animal to lick, chew, or even mutilate the affected limb. Skin sloughs are unsightly, irritating to the animal, and extremely upsetting to the owners—especially if they are the first to notice the problem. Once a skin slough has occured it is impossible to reverse the effect. The raw skin must be treated as a severe abrasion with antiseptic soaks, systemic antibiotics, and bandages until it has healed. Most sloughs require 2 to 4 weeks to heal. The hair rarely returns and the animal may be left with a scar for life. Often the animal must be tranquilized or an Elizabethan collar placed around its head to discourage licking and chewing while the wound heals.

Accidental perivascular injections can usually be prevented by placing an indwelling catheter in the vein before administering the barbiturate. The additional small cost of the catheter is well worth the aggravation that can be prevented should an upset owner seek retribution for a permanently scarred pet or show animal. Skin sloughs are less likely to occur if the barbiturate injection is made up as a dilute solution (2.5% or less).

If a barbiturate is accidentally injected perivascularly, a slough may be avoided if the area is immediately infiltrated with 3 to 5 ml of saline containing 1 to 2 ml of 2.0% procaine (the procaine must not contain epinephrine). The subcutaneous tissue surrounding the barbiturate site is injected with the saline-procaine mixture and massaged to ensure dilution of the barbiturate. Despite this precaution the owner should be alerted to the possibility of a skin irritation developing 1 to 2 days later.

Examples of commonly used barbiturates

Following is a brief discussion of four barbiturate drugs commonly used for general anesthesia in dogs and cats:

- Pentobarbital
- Thiamylal
- Thiopental
- Methohexital

Each barbiturate will be discussed as to its (1) general classification, (2) usage in dogs and cats, (3) concentration and intravenous dosage, (4) method for administration, (5) speed and duration of action, (6) advantages and disadvantages, and (7) precautions and/or complications.

Pentobarbital sodium

Classification. Pentobarbital is a short-acting oxybarbiturate.

Usage in dogs and cats. As a rule pentobarbital is no longer routinely used as the sole anesthetic for surgery in a small animal hospital due to its prolonged recovery period and tendency to cause excitement during the induction and recovery period. Because of its unfavorable attributes it is rarely used in cats. Inhalation

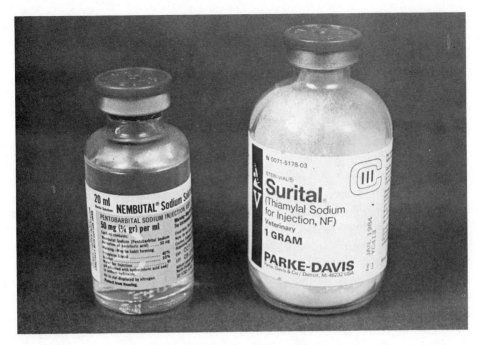

Fig. 3-3. Pentobarbital and thiamylal containers.

anesthetics and thiobarbiturates have largely replaced pentobarbital as the sole anesthetic for short-term as well as long-term procedures in dogs and cats. On occasion pentobarbital may be used as the sleep-producing part of a balanced anesthesia for certain types of cardiac surgery, such as repair of a patent ductus arteriosus (PDA) or a long-term cardiac catheterization study. When used as part of a balanced anesthesia, pentobarbital is diluted to make a 1.0% to 2.0% solution and administered in low doses along with a neuroleptanalgesic, nitrous oxide, and oxygen.

Concentration and intravenous dosage. Supplied as a clear 6.0% or 6.5% solution in a multidose vial (see Fig. 3-3), pentobarbital is soluble and relatively stable in water at room temperature. A 6% solution contains 60 mg/ml of pentobarbital, and a 6.5% solution contains 65 mg/ml of pentobarbital. For both dogs and cats the intravenous dosage is computed on the basis of weight: 25 to 30 mg/kg if pentobarbital is used as the sole anesthetic, 5 to 10 mg/kg with balanced anesthesia.

Pentobarbital is always given to effect. The dosage must be reduced by 30% to 50% whenever preanesthetic sedatives are used.

Method for administering pentobarbital intravenously. When administering pentobarbital for surgical anesthesia in healthy dogs or cats, the anesthetist should:

- Aseptically withdraw the calculated dosage (25 to 30 mg/kg) of pentobarbital from the vial into an appropriate size syringe. An additional 50% of the dosage can be added to the syringe to accommodate procedures lasting more than 60 minutes. When preanesthetic sedatives are used, the calculated dosage should be reduced by 30% to 50% or more.

- Perform aseptic venipuncture of a cephalic or lateral saphenous vein using a 20 or 22 gauge needle (see Fig. 3-7)
- Inject one-third to one-half of the calculated dosage intravenously over a period of 3 to 5 seconds. Allow 1 to 2 minutes to elapse before giving additional increments of pentobarbital
  - Check animal's vital signs and reflexes (if the animal shows signs of stage II excitement, give an additional small volume to get the animal through the excitatory phase).

When signs of stage III become evident, smaller dosages are given to effect until the desired level of surgical anesthesia is obtained, allowing 1 to 2 minutes between incremental doses at this point to assess the drug's effect on vital signs and reflexes. The time from initial injection to surgical anesthesia is usually 5 to 10 minutes. The trachea should be intubated at this point and the tube secured to prevent dislodgement during surgical preparation and positioning. Additional increments are given on the average of every 30 to 60 minutes to maintain a surgical level of anesthesia; however, this will vary among individual animals. Additional dosage should be avoided until the animal exhibits clinical signs of awakening from the pentobarbital.

When used with cats or small dogs, the stock solution of pentobarbital should be diluted with an equal volume of sterile water or saline to provide a 3.0% solution of pentobarbital. In sick or debilitated animals an even weaker solution should be used to lessen the chance of overdosing the animal. Whenever possible a sterile indwelling catheter should be placed in the vein to administer the barbiturate (see Fig. 3-4).

Speed and duration of action
- Induction time: 5 minutes
- Duration of surgical anesthesia: 30 minutes to 2 hours
- Recovery time: 6 to 24 hours

Advantages
- Inexpensive
- Can be used in a variety of different species
- Does not require specialized equipment
- Provides a long anesthetic period
- Useful as part of a balanced anesthesia technique

Disadvantages
- Tends to exaggerate excitement during induction and recovery periods
- Analgesic properties poor to fair; often necessitates having to deepen anesthesia in order to maintain a motionless patient
- Difficult to control depth of anesthesia

- Relatively long induction period (5 to 10 minutes)
- Clinical recovery period 6 to 24 hours or longer
- Must be used with caution in animals with conditions such as head injuries, head or neck surgery, or orthopedic surgery, where a stormy recovery could result in additional trauma to the head and/or surgical site
- Necessity to control or assist ventilation if hypercapnia and hypoxia are to be avoided
- Classified as a Schedule II controlled substance

Precautions and/or complications The precautions and complications that accompany the use of pentobarbital sodium for general anesthesia are essentially the same as those listed for all barbiturate anesthetic drugs (see pp. 128-130).

Thiamylal sodium

Classification. Thiamylal is an ultrashort-acting thiobarbiturate.

Usage in dogs and cats

- As the sole anesthetic for surgical or dental procedures lasting 10 to 30 minutes. Additional incremental doses may be given for up to 60 minutes of surgical anesthesia.
- As an induction agent to facilitate tracheal intubation. When used for a slow induction or a rapid ("crash") induction, it is usually followed by maintenance with an inhalation anesthetic drug administered via the endotracheal tube.
- As the sole anesthetic for relief of pain and/or immobilization during short-term diagnostic procedures such as radiology and biopsy

Concentration and intravenous dosage. Thiamylal is supplied as a sterile crystalline powder in sealed multi-dose vials containing 1, 5, or 10 gm of the drug (see Fig. 3-5). Thiamylal powder is soluble in water but is relatively unstable once it is mixed with water or saline, especially when exposed to atmospheric air. In order to stabilize thiamylal, a buffer, sodium carbonate, is added that results in a strong alkaline solution. When the powder is diluted to prepare a working solution, sterile saline or sterile water is added to the multidose vial to make a 2% or 2.5% solution. A 2% solution contains 20 mg/ml of thiamylal, and a 2.5% solution contains 25 mg/ml of thiamylal.

Since thiamylal is more potent than thiopental but less potent than methohexital sodium, dosages for thiamylal will be slightly lower than for thiopental. For both dogs and cats the intravenous thiamylal dosage is computed on the basis of weight:

- For surgical anesthesia of short duration: 10 to 25 mg/kg
- For rapid induction to allow tracheal intubation: 6 to 10 mg/kg
- For a slow induction to allow inhalation anesthesia by face mask: 4 to 8 mg/kg

In all of these cases thiamylal is administered to effect, taking into account all those variables that exist to alter the effect of the drug in different animals under different situations. Dosages should be reduced by 30% to 80% for preanesthetic sedation and/or debilitated animals.

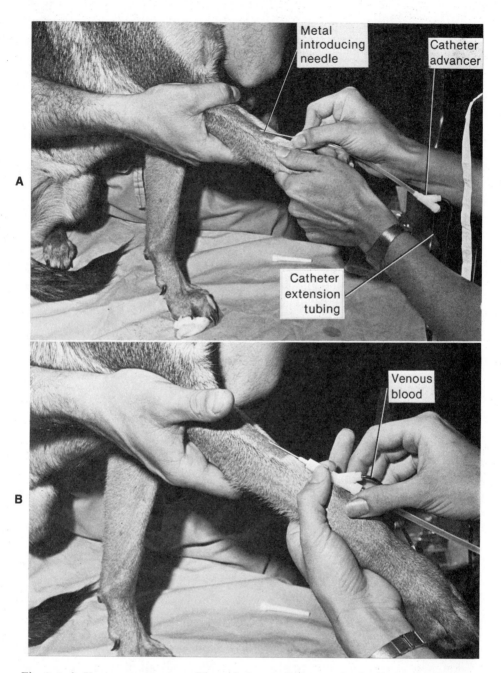

Fig. 3-4. A, Venipuncture using a "through-the-needle" type of indwelling catheter. **B,** Advancement of catheter into the cephalic vein. Note that the dark-colored venous blood present in the catheter extension tubing serves as a verification of proper placement. The person restraining the animal must remember to release pressure over the vein before advancing the catheter.

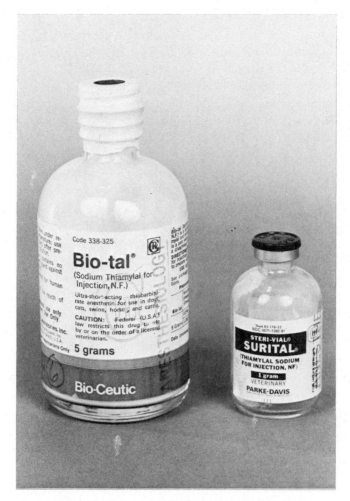

Fig. 3-5. Thiamylal multidose vials in two sizes.

To retard aging and prevent deterioration, thiamylal solutions should be stored away from light and refrigerated at about 5°C. When allowed to stand at room temperature, the solution may age more rapidly and become cloudy or form crystals, which indicates that the solution has lost its potency and a fresh bottle should be prepared. Any unusable barbiturate solution should be immediately discarded by flushing it down a sink. Unattended barbiturate invites theft and/or accidental use. Room air should not be injected into the thiamylal solution as it adds carbon dioxide to the solution, decreasing its pH, which causes thiamylal to precipitate out of solution (precipitated barbiturate solutions should never be injected intravenously).

Preparing the thiobarbiturate solution

Since preservatives are not included in the dry crystals of thiamylal, thiopental, or methohexital, aseptic technique must be used to prevent contamination of the multidose vial during reconstitution. The volume of sterile saline or sterile distilled water used as a diluent for the powdered barbiturate depends on the working concentration desired and the amount of dry powdered barbiturate contained within the vial. The 5.0 and 10.0 gm bottles are more economical in practices with a large anesthetic caseload—that is, 10 to 20 cases per day. The 1.0 gm bottles, although more expensive on a unit volume basis, may be more economical for small volume practices with an anesthetic caseload of less than five cases per day. Once the powdered barbiturate is made into solution, it should be discarded after 2 to 3 days as anesthetic potency begins to decline with aging of the solution.

Following are the procedures for preparing a 2.5% working solution of thiamylal (see Fig. 3-6). The procedure assumes use of a 5.0 gm multidose bottle and applies to all powdered barbiturates:

1. Remove the protective cap from stoppered end of vial. Be careful not to remove the entire rubber cap. Swab rubber injection cap with alcohol. Set multidose vial upright on table surface.
2. Aseptically remove a little less than 200 ml of sterile saline, and inject it into the 5.0 gm bottle of powder so that the final solution contains 5.0 gm of thiamylal in a *total* volume of 200 ml. (A 2.5% solution of thiamylal is defined as 2.5 gm of thiamylal in every 100 ml of solution—hence 5 gm/200 ml = 2.5 gm/100 ml.)
3. While injecting the sterile saline into the thiamylal vial, allow the pressure created to escape so the rubber cap is not exploded off the vial. Inserting a 22 gauge needle through the cap (while injecting the saline through a 19 or 20 guage needle) will allow the pressure to equalize with room air. The 22 gauge needle should be removed as soon as the correct volume of diluent has been added to avoid spilling or contaminating the solution.
4. Gently rotate the vial to hasten the dissolving of thiamylal powder.
5. *Label the vial with the percent solution and date of reconstitution.*
6. Refrigerate the solution when not in use.
7. When aspirating thiamylal solution, do not inject air into the multidose vial for pressure equalization as this may cause the solution to precipitate.

Methods for administration

For surgical anesthesia

1. Make sure that all equipment and supplies are in readiness and the animal has been cleared for premedication and general anesthesia by the attending veterinarian. Allow sufficient time for preanesthetic sedation to take effect.
2. Aseptically remove the calculated dose of thiobarbiturate from the multidose vial into a syringe.

3. Perform venipuncture of the cephalic or lateral saphenous vein with a 20 to 22 gauge needle, or introduce an indwelling catheter (see Fig. 3-7).

4. Administer one-third of the calculated dose over 10 to 15 seconds. Allow 15 to 30 seconds before giving any additional thiamylal. Secure needle and syringe (or catheter) to limb (see Fig. 3-8).

5. Monitor vital signs and reflexes before giving additional increments. Administer the remaining thiamylal to effect until the desired level of surgical anesthesia is obtained. Monitor respiration, pulse rate, and heart rate very closely at this stage, and be prepared to ventilate the animal if apnea occurs.

6. Intubate the trachea and secure the endotracheal tube in place to prevent dislodgement during surgical preparation and positioning (see Chapter 5).

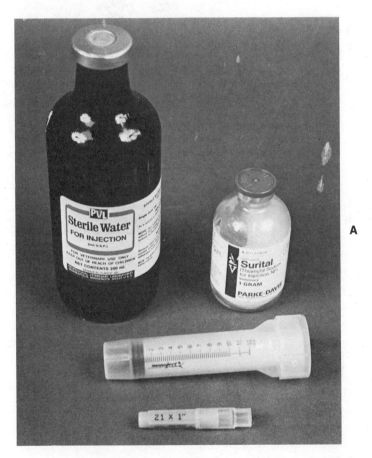

A

Fig. 3-6. Preparation of thiobarbiturate solution. **A,** Supplies needed.

Continued.

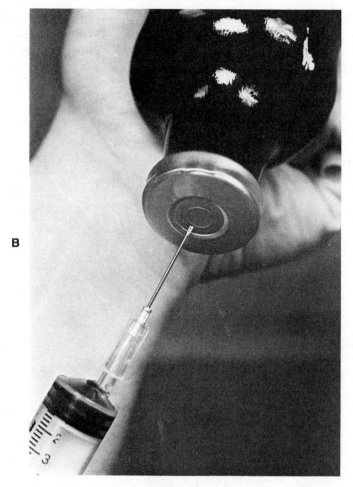

Fig. 3-6, cont'd. B, Close-up of correct needle entry into multidose vial.

Additional doses of thiamylal may be administered to effect, as needed, to prolong the anesthetic period. It is not advisable to prolong the anesthetic period beyond 45 to 60 minutes as this greatly increases the chances for overdosage and prolongs anesthetic recovery.

For rapid ("crash") induction sequence with thiamylal

1-3. Same except for calculated dosage (6 to 10 mg/kg)

4. Administer the calculated dose as a single injection over a period of 10 to 15 seconds. Allow 30 to 45 seconds to monitor vital signs and critical reflexes while the thiamylal is acting on the CNS.

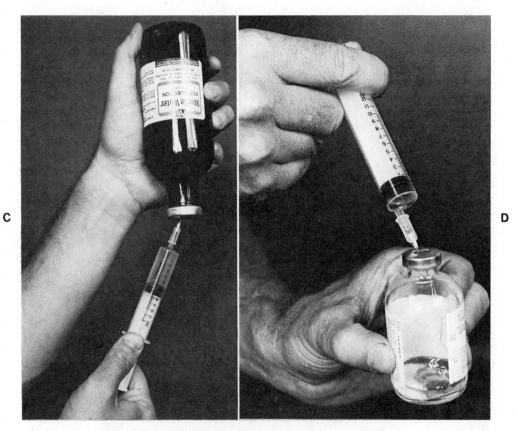

Fig. 3-6, cont'd. C, Aspirating sterile diluent. **D,** Injecting diluent to prepare a 4% solution.
Continued.

5. Intubate the trachea promptly and secure the tube in place. Connect the tube to the inhalation anesthesia machine. *Watch animal carefully for signs of apnea and/or cardiovascular instability.*

The dose of thiamylal in this case will generally fall short of producing a surgical level of anesthesia. Surgical anesthesia is provided by the inhalation anesthetic drug and maintained throughout the remainder of the procedure. It is important to be aware that transitory apnea can occur from the barbiturate injection, and the animal should be ventilated. Apnea prevents the uptake of oxygen as well as inhalation anesthetic gases and leads to hypercapnia. Rapid injection of a barbiturate drug is not advised in sick or debilitated animals.

A rapid induction sequence is desirable when anesthetizing brachycephalic animals or animals with any form of ventilation difficulty such as a swollen tongue, fractured jaw, head injury, or collapsing trachea. Rapid induction is also advisable with an animal that has recently eaten. The intent of a "crash" induction is to allow

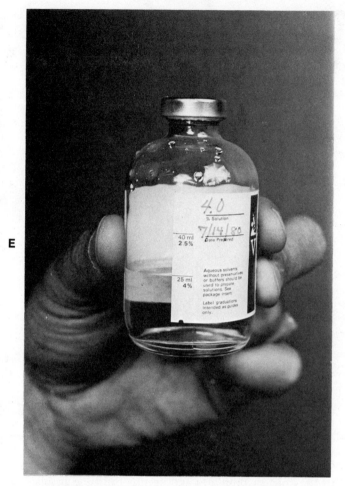

E

Fig. 3-6, cont'd. E, Completed and labeled solution of thiamylal.

rapid control of the animal's airway through tracheal intubation. Rapid barbiturate induction must never be performed until all equipment and supplies are ready. Since difficulty with intubation may be experienced, the use of a laryngoscope is recommended. If the animal is suspected of having a full stomach, the trachea should be intubated as rapidly as possible after the initial barbiturate injection. The endotracheal tube used should have a functional cuff for inflation to assist in artificial ventilation and prevent aspiration of saliva or stomach contents into the lungs. *Always check the inflatable cuff to assure it is operable before starting the induction sequence.*

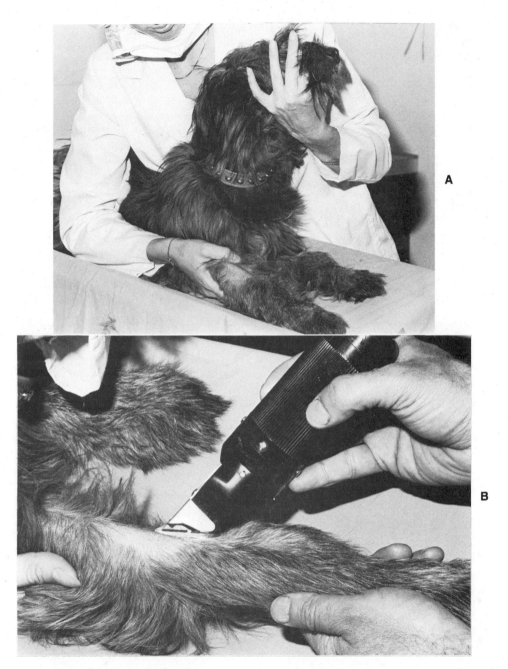

Fig. 3-7. Cephalic venipuncture and intravenous injection sequence in dog. **A,** Leg and head restraint. **B,** Clipping foreleg.   *Continued.*

C

D

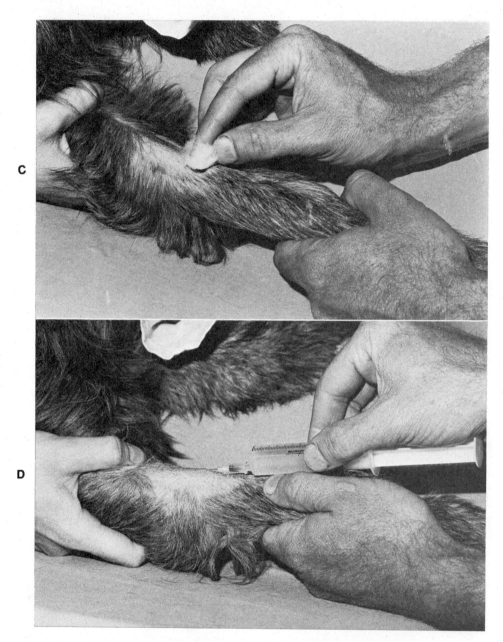

Fig. 3-7, cont'd. C, Applying alcohol to site. **D,** Entering vein.

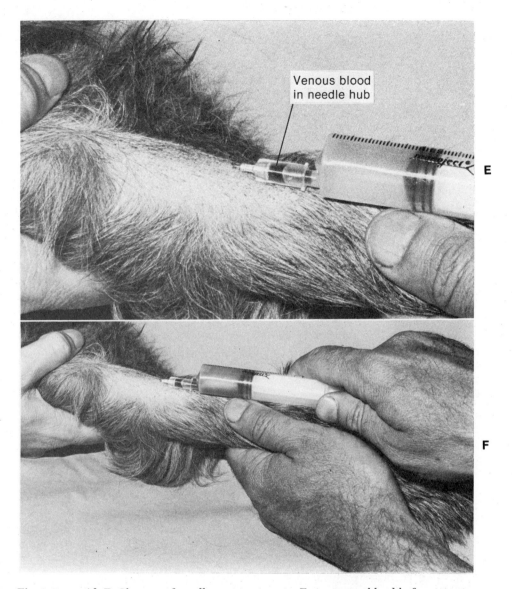

Venous blood
in needle hub

E

F

Fig. 3-7, cont'd. E, Close-up of needle position in vein. **F,** Aspirating blood before injection.

Continued.

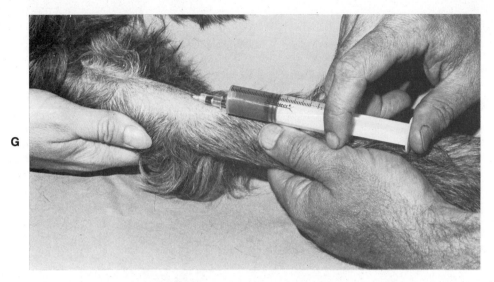

Fig. 3-7, cont'd. G, Injection.

For slow induction sequence

Ultrashort-acting barbiturates, unlike pentobarbital, can be administered slowly to effect. After adequate preanesthetic sedation, stage II excitement and apnea are usually minimal. This induction process employs the use of inhalation anesthesia by face mask to complete the transition from sleep into a surgical level of anesthesia. Slow inductions are risky in animals with impaired ventilation as the process requires several minutes during which the animal could vomit or have its airway obstructed due to relaxation of an overly large soft palate or tongue.

Following is the sequence recommended for a slow induction in most dogs and cats:

1.-3. Same except that calculated dose is reduced by 4 to 8 mg/kg, assuming that the animal has received preanesthetic sedation

4. Administer the calculated dose slowly to effect over a period of 30 to 60 seconds. When the animal shows signs of borderline unconsciousness, yet is not totally anesthetized, discontinue the barbiturate injection and introduce the face mask gradually until accepted by the animal (see Fig. 3-9). Since the animal is still semiconscious, the face mask must not be pushed quickly over the muzzle. Allow the animal to begin breathing nitrous oxide (except where contraindicated) and oxygen (see Chapter 4).

5. Once the animal has accepted the face mask, begin adding halothane to the nitrous oxide–oxygen mixture. Monitor vital signs and reflexes to determine the proper depth of anesthesia necessary to perform tracheal intubation (the animal may be intubated once a surgical plane of anesthesia has been obtained).

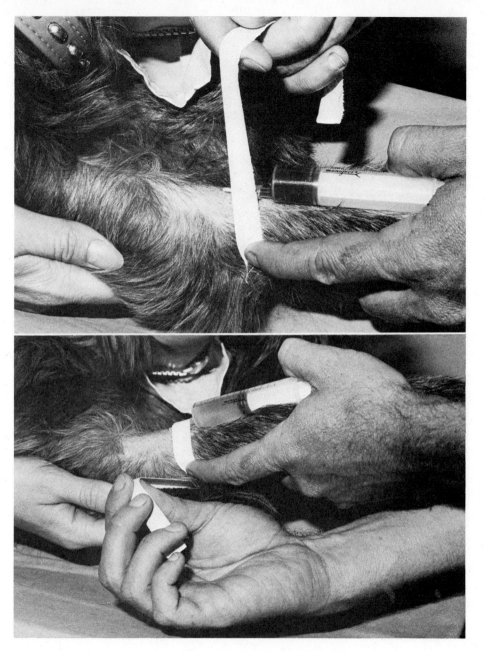

Fig. 3-8. Procedure for taping syringe to leg. *Continued.*

6. Intubate the trachea and secure the endotracheal tube. Inflate endotracheal tube cuff if necessary to prevent gas leakage around the outside of the tube. Connect tube to anesthesia machine.

7. Maintain the desired level of anesthesia with the inhalation anesthetic machine.

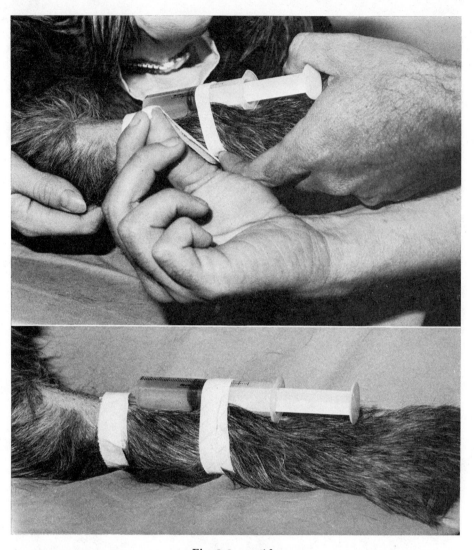

Fig. 3-8, cont'd.

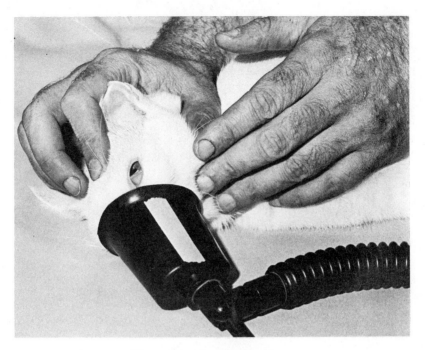

Fig. 3-9. Mask induction of cat.

Speed and duration of action
- Induction time: 1 to $1\frac{1}{2}$ minutes
- Duration of surgical anesthesia: 10 to 20 minutes
- Recovery time: 1 to 2 hours

Recovery time will be prolonged with multiple doses. If thiamylal is used for longer than 60 minutes, recovery will depend on liver detoxification (as with pentobarbital) and can be for as long as 6 to 24 hours.

Advantages
- Inexpensive
- Does not require specialized equipment
- Can be used with a variety of different species
- Rapid induction with minimal excitement
- Relatively short recovery period with minimal delirium
- Good for short procedures
- Good for induction and tracheal intubation prior to inhalation anesthesia
- Not a Schedule II drug. Ultrashort-acting barbiturate anesthetics are classified as either Schedule III or IV controlled substances, which means they are not subject to the strict federal regulations of purchase, use, and storage as are Schedule II substances.

Disadvantages
- Poor analgesic properties
- Difficulty in controlling anesthetic depth
- Respiratory depression greatest when injected rapidly (apnea common on induction)
- Cardiovascular depression when injected rapidly as a large bolus
- Possibility of cardiac dysrhythmias, especially during induction
- Must be used cautiously in extremely thin cats or dogs
- Need for assisting or controlling ventilation when used as a general anesthetic for procedures exceeding 20 to 30 minutes
- Requires reconstitution before use
- Once reconstituted, effective shelf life only 2 to 3 days (requires refrigeration)
- Prolonged recovery with repeated doses
- Requires special DEA order forms and records relative to Schedule III or IV substances

Precautions and/or complications. The precautions and complications that accompany the use of thiamylal are essentially the same as those listed for all barbiturate anesthetic drugs (see previous discussion).

Thiopental sodium
Classification. Thiopental is an ultrashort-acting thiobarbiturate.

Usage in dogs and cats. Identical to thiamylal.

Concentration and intravenous dosage. Thiopental has actions similar to thiamylal. It is supplied as a dry powder, must be reconstituted with sterile saline or water, and requires refrigeration once made into a solution. Like thiamylal it will deteriorate after 2 to 4 days and must be discarded when the solution becomes cloudy or forms a precipitate. The concentrations used for anesthesia or induction are the same as for thiamylal. The pH of a 2.5% solution of thiopental, like thiamylal, is between 9.5 and 11.0.

The intravenous thiopental dosage for dogs and cats is computed on the basis of weight:
- For surgical anesthesia: 20 to 30 mg/kg
- For tracheal intubation: 8 to 10 mg/kg

The dosage for thiopental is slightly higher than thiamylal since thiamylal is approximately $1^{1}/_{2}$ times as potent as thiopental. It is rare for a small animal hospital to stock both thiamylal and thiopental in that their actions are practically the same. Most of the small and large animal veterinary practitioners in the United States use thiamylal primarily because it was first marketed for veterinary use while thiopental is marketed for human use. For practical purposes, thiopental is used at about the same dosage as thiamylal.

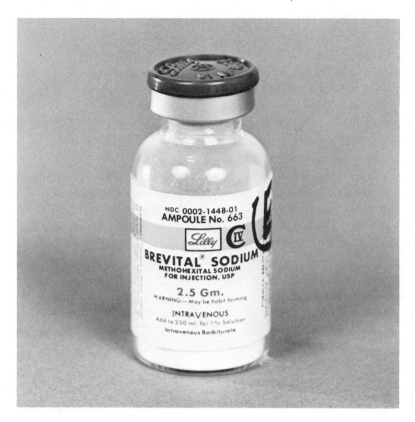

Fig. 3-10. Methohexital vial.

Method of administration. Like thiamylal, thiopental can be administered rapidly or slowly to effect for short-term general anesthesia or induction and intubation prior to inhalation anesthesia.

Speed and duration of action. Similar to thiamylal.

Advantages and disadvantages. Similar to thiamylal.

Precautions and/or complications. Similar to thiamylal.

Methohexital sodium

Classification. Methohexital is an ultrashort-acting oxybarbiturate (see Fig. 3-10).

Usage in dogs and cats. Methohexital is more potent than either thiamylal or thiopental. Its speed of induction is somewhat faster than thiamylal and thiopental. The duration of action and recovery period are also shorter due, in part, to a more rapid rate of liver metabolism.

Methohexital is used primarily as a rapid induction agent in dogs and cats to facilitate tracheal intubation prior to inhalation anesthesia. It is especially useful in extremely thin and/or muscular dogs (such as greyhounds, Afghans, and whippets) for induction and intubation of the trachea. One injection is usually sufficient to render the animal unconscious and allow for tracheal intubation. It is not recommended as the sole drug for surgical anesthesia as the recovery period is often characterized by excitement, struggling, and muscle tremors. When inhalation anesthetics are used to maintain anesthesia after methohexital induction, these recovery signs are usually not observed.

Concentration and intravenous dosage. Methohexital is supplied as a sterile dry powder in multidose vials containing 2.5 gm of the drug. It is generally made up as a 1% or 2% solution for use in dogs and cats. Unlike thiamylal and thiopental, solutions of methohexital are quite stable even at room temperature with a shelf life of about 6 weeks. The pH of a 2.5% solution is about 10 to 10.5.

The recommended intravenous dosage for rapid induction in dogs and cats is 4 to 8 mg/kg.

Method of administration
1-3. Same as for other thiobarbiturates (see previous discussion)
4. Approximately 50% to 75% of the calculated dosage is administered intravenously (as a rapid bolus) over 5 to 15 seconds.
5. Vital signs and reflexes are evaluated. If, after waiting 30 seconds, additional drug is needed, it is given to effect. Continue evaluation of vital signs and reflexes. Be prepared for apnea and/or muscle tremors during induction.
6. Intubate the trachea and secure the endotracheal tube in place. Inflate the endotracheal tube cuff if necessary and attach the endotracheal tube to the inhalation anesthesia machine. *Watch animal closely for signs of apnea and/ or cardiovascular instability.*
7. Maintain the desired level of anesthesia using the inhalation anesthesia machine.

Speed and duration of action
• Induction time: 15 to 60 seconds
• Duration of surgical anesthesia: 5 to 10 minutes
• Recovery time: 25 to 30 minutes

Advantages
• Long shelf life; refrigeration not essential
• Does not require specialized equipment
• Rapid induction
• Extremely short recovery period (30 minutes)
• Classified as Schedule IV controlled substance

Disadvantages

In addition to those already listed for thiamylal and thiopental, methohexital is:

- Extremely potent. Since the lethal dosage is only 2 to 3 times the anesthetic dosage, a 1% solution is recommended. Lethal dose results in respiratory and/or cardiac arrest.
- Inappropriate for use as the sole anesthetic drug
- Marked by muscular tremors and/or stormy recovery period. Not recommended for short procedures where recovery excitement could result in trauma to the animal or the surgical site. Unsuitable for use in animals with a seizure history

Precautions and/or complications. The precautions and complications that accompany the use of methohexital sodium are essentially the same as those listed for all barbiturate anesthetic drugs (see previous discussion).

CATALEPTOID ANESTHETIC DRUGS (dissociative anesthesia)
Classification

The *cyclohexamines* are a grouping of closely related drugs that have recently been introduced into human and veterinary anesthesia. There are three drugs presently of anesthetic interest: phencyclidine, ketamine, and tiletamine. Of these, phencyclidine is the original parent compound from which the other two are derived. Phencyclidine received a brief period of clinical use in humans in the mid 1950s; however, it was soon discontinued because of its excessive stimulation of excitatory and hallucinatory episodes. Ketamine is presently the most widely used cyclohexamine derivative in clinical human and veterinary anesthesia. When clinical trials of ketamine's anesthetic, analgesic, and immobilizing properties began in 1965, the term "dissociative anesthesia" was coined as a means for distinguishing its signs of anesthesia from the more conventional anesthetic drugs. The term implies an electroencephalographic dissociation of CNS activity whereby the patient is no longer responsive to normal physical stimuli such as pain, pressure, and heat.

The cyclohexamine anesthetic drugs, in general, produce an atypical anesthetic state characterized by:

1. Profound analgesia
2. Cataleptic immobility of the limbs
3. Loss of responsiveness to external physical stimuli
4. Amnesia

General use of cataleptoid anesthetic drugs in cats

Presently, ketamine hydrochloride is the only cyclohexamine approved for clinical use in veterinary or human patients. Within the small animal veterinary field, ketamine is approved by the Food and Drug Administration (FDA) only for use in cats and nonhuman primates. It is *not* approved for clinical use in dogs since ketamine commonly produces seizures in that species during recovery.

Ketamine has the following uses with cats:

- To provide short-term anesthesia for minor surgical or diagnostic procedures (20 to 30 minutes)
- To provide immobilization and restraint for purposes of examination and/or treatment of intractable cats. Because it can be administered intramuscularly, it can facilitate venipuncture in cats that are difficult to handle.
- To provide preanesthetic sedation and chemical restraint prior to induction of surgical anesthesia with another anesthetic drug. Ketamine is compatible with most other anesthetic drugs and has a wide margin of safety. However, the dosage of other general anesthetic drugs should be reduced by 50% to 75%.
- To facilitate ophthalmic examination of the retina (ketamine produces a centrally fixed eye with dilated pupil)

General mode of action

Clinical signs of anesthesia with ketamine are completely different from those for inhalation agents. General anesthesia produced by the conventional anesthetic drugs (the barbiturates and inhalation anesthetic drugs) results from a progressive depression of the CNS, as represented by Stage III of Guedel's four classic stages. Anesthesia produced by ketamine results instead from a *stimulation* of the CNS as represented by Guedel's Stage II. Cataleptoid anesthetic drugs never produce Stage III CNS depression. Rather they progressively excite the CNS until they finally produce overdosage signs in the form of spastic limb movements or tonic-clonic convulsions. These drugs produce a form of general anesthesia through excitation of the CNS rather than depression. As is the case with other general anesthetic drugs, the exact mechanism of cyclohexamine's action on the CNS is unknown.

A typical sign of anesthesia from cyclohexamine-type drugs is catalepsy, noted especially in the front limbs (see Fig. 3-11). The rigid posture that is produced causes an inability to locomote and loss of the righting reflex as well as of jaw muscle action, abnormal postures, and occasional random movements of the head or limbs. The random movement of limbs during anesthesia with ketamine can occur even without surgical stimulation. It is important not to confuse these movements with a "lightening" of the anesthetic state. To the contrary, they may indicate a relative overdosage. Under conventional anesthesia with a drug such as halothane, patient movement is usually considered a sign that anesthesia is becoming light. With cataleptoid anesthesia random movements of the animal should not be interpreted as a sign that more of the drug is needed. Additional doses are ineffective in eliminating these movements and only add to the length of recovery and/or possibility for producing serious convulsions.

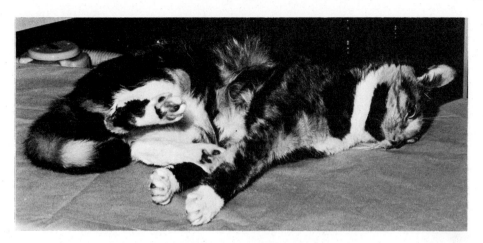

Fig. 3-11. Ketamine-induced catalepsy in cat.

It is difficult to totally eliminate the muscle rigidity that accompanies the use of the cyclohexamines. Premedication or admixture of the cataleptoid drug with a tranquilizer (acepromazine or diazepam) will lessen the degree of rigidity but will not eliminate it altogether. For this reason ketamine is not a good anesthetic to use in cats for orthopedic surgery where large muscle masses must be traversed to expose the surgical site. Catalepsy is indicative of a suitable level for minor surgery. Deep-seated pain, however, associated with surgical procedures involving the bones, abdominal organs, or thorax may not be obliterated by ketamine or related drugs. To some degree the animal is unable to respond to pain due to its immobile state. Therefore these drugs are, at present, not recommended as the sole anesthetic drug for surgical procedures in these areas. When a cat is beginning to lighten from cataleptoid anesthesia and experiences a painful stimulus, it often growls even though it may still be cataleptic and unable to move from the stimulus.

Much of the research into the exact location and mechanism of action for cataleptoid anesthesia involves the use of an electroencephalograph machine (EEG) to study the effect of the drug on electric activity within the brain and cranial spinal cord regions. Investigations of this nature have shown evidence that the cyclohexamines act on the CNS by exciting the region of the brain known as the hippocampus.[1] Originally it was thought that these drugs acted primarily on lower regions of the brain and spinal cord in the area of the limbic system. In order to more accurately categorize cataleptic anesthesia, stage II has been further divided into three phases: A, B, and C[1]:

Stage II

Phase A. Characterized clinically by salivation, mydriasis, hyperactivity, and hallucinations

Phase B. Continued pupillary dilation, decreased responsiveness to physical stimuli, centrally fixed eyes, increased muscle rigidity, incoordination, and loss of aggressive behavior

Phase C (cataleptic state). Analgesia, amnesia, loss of responsiveness, dilated pupils, centrally fixed eyes that remain open, fixed stare, extensor rigidity of skeletal muscles with occasional random muscle jerks. This is the stage under which minor surgical procedures can be performed.

Testing the traditional reflexes to monitor animals under cataleptoid anesthesia is an inappropriate method for assessing anesthetic depth. Instead vital signs should be used routinely to determine the animal's state of health and approximate depth of stage II anesthesia.

Phase C of stage II is different from conventional general anesthesia in that:
• The eyes remain open.
• Pharyngeal and laryngeal reflexes are *not* completely abolished.
• Muscles are rigid rather than relaxed.
• There is minimal respiratory depression.
• There is stimulation rather than depression of the cardiovascular system as evidenced by (1) increased heart rate, (2) increased blood pressure, and (3) increased cardiac output.

As a result of the eyes remaining open during anesthesia, the cornea can become excessively dry, leading to corneal irritation or postoperative ulceration. Therefore a blank ophthalmic ointment of mineral oil should be placed in both eyes as soon as the cat becomes immobilized (see Fig. 3-12).

Cyclohexamine drugs usually cause considerable salivation, which can interfere with the animal's capacity to maintain a clear airway in spite of its ability to swallow. Aspiration pneumonitis is still a possibility during anesthesia with these drugs, especially if the trachea is not intubated. Unfortunately, tracheal intubation is difficult following intramuscular ketamine injection, and laryngospasm may result. Ketamine and related drugs do not seem to stimulate or predispose the animal to vomit, even with a full stomach. For this reason they are particularly useful in cats suspected of having food or water in the stomach.

Means for elimination of cyclohexamine drugs

Cyclohexamine drugs are eliminated from the body in two ways: through liver metabolism and through elimination of the unmetabolized drug along with its active and inactive metabolites by the kidneys. Consequently, these drugs should be avoided in animals with liver or kidney disease. The length of time required for *complete* recovery from intramuscular ketamine anesthesia in cats is variable but averages about 4 to 6 hours in normal healthy adults. Immature cats may recover more rapidly while older cats or cats with impaired liver and/or kidney function may require 24 hours or longer. Recovery time following an intravenous dose of ketamine is considerably less.

Recovery period

Hallucinations, spastic incoordination, and hyperexcitability are relatively common side effects during the recovery period with cyclohexamine drugs. After this form of anesthesia, animals should be placed in a quiet and darkened area since noise and bright light tend to exaggerate the hallucinations attributable to these drugs. Animals must still be observed closely during their recovery from cataleptic drugs for signs of hyperexcitability, convulsions, or contorted body positions that may compromise respiration or cause trauma to the surgical site. The usual precaution of withdrawing food and water from an animal until it has *fully* recovered from anesthesia must also be observed.

Signs of overdosage

Signs of overdosage from cyclohexamine drugs are related primarily to overstimulation of the CNS and include (1) tonic-clonic convulsions, (2) hyperexcitable action, and (3) hypothermia. Overdosage is more likely to occur when large doses are administered to overly aggressive cats by rapid intramuscular injection, especially if the injection is accidentally given into a vein. Convulsions due to ketamine can be treated with intravenous diazepam.

When ketamine or related drugs are administered, it is important to forewarn the owner that the cat may possibly require overnight hospitalization until it has

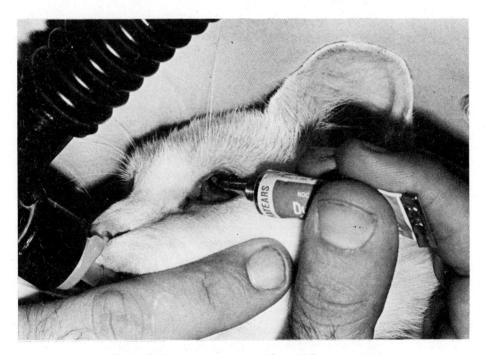

Fig. 3-12. Protecting cornea with eye lubricant in cat.

fully recovered from the anesthesia. Injury could result if the cat leaves the hospital in a disoriented state since most owners are unaware of the dangers associated with tending to an animal that is not in full control of its reflexes. Discharging an animal that is not fully recovered from *any* anesthetic drug could be grounds for a legal suit, should the animal injure itself as a direct result of its disoriented state.

Precautions and/or complications

The cyclohexamine anesthetic drugs, namely ketamine, are considered to have a wide margin of safety within the species for which their usage is cleared by the FDA. However, *caution* must be observed and dosages either reduced or eliminated with:

- Animals with kidney or liver impairment, especially when the serum glutamic-pyruvic transaminase (SGPT), blood urea nitrogen (BUN), or creatinine values are markedly elevated
- Older animals
- Debilitated or dehydrated animals
- Animals suffering injuries to the head, face, or spinal column
- Animals with known or suspected seizure disorders
- Animals undergoing surgical or diagnostic procedures involving the head or spinal cord where postoperative seizures may result
- Extremely aggressive or excitable animals
- Animals with clinical signs or medical histories indicating possible intoxication from insecticide preparations or ingestion of poisonous substances that act on the CNS, including such compounds as strychnine, organophosphates, amphetamine, mescaline, marijuana, alcohol, and aspirin
- Animals with cardiac disease involving a reduced cardiac reserve or irregularities in cardiac conduction and rhythm

Complications associated with the administration of phencyclidine anesthetic drugs occur primarily in the form of:

- Excessive stimulation of the CNS that produces excitement, agitation, muscle tremors, jerking movements, or tonic-clonic convulsions. Excessive CNS stimulation is seen more with intravenous administration and/or large intramuscular dosages of these drugs.
- Irregular breathing pattern with breath holding. This is often observed when administering inhalation anesthesia by face mask following a preanesthetic dose of ketamine. Breath holding on the part of the cat delays the uptake of oxygen and anesthetic gases from the lungs, thereby prolonging the induction of surgical anesthesia. Respiratory acidosis and hypoxemia may also follow this irregular respiratory pattern referred to as *apneustic* breathing.
- Excessive salivation, which may predispose the animal to aspiration pneumonitis or partial airway obstruction due to accumulation of secretions in the

posterior pharynx and trachea. Accumulation of secretions may necessitate the use of suction to remove the offending fluid and relieve any respiratory embarrassment. Premedication with atropine (or glycopyrrolate) lessens the severity of drug-induced salivation.

- Predisposition to corneal damage due to drying or spillage or irritating solutions, since eyelids do not close. Use of a bland ophthalmic ointment or mineral oil in the eyes is recommended whenever these drugs are used.

- Exaggerated muscle tumors, ataxia, agitation, and intermittent tonic-clonic muscle spasms may occur during recovery. These signs are thought to be the result of ketamine's hallucinogenic effect on the CNS. The incidence of such undesirable side effects are fewer with ketamine than phencyclidine. External stimuli from noise and bright light tend to precipitate these hallucinogenic side effects, which are difficult to reverse. Placing the animal in a dark and quiet recovery cage is one good means for reducing the incidence of hallucinations. The animal must not be neglected, however, just because it is in a dark room. Observation on a periodic basis for several hours is necessary to check vital signs and surgical sites. Occasionally, an animal may develop serious convulsions or extreme excitement following the use of a cyclohexamine drug, which cannot be controlled by altering the environment.

- Prolonged recovery period, especially in older animals or animals with renal or hepatic impairment. Additional doses of the drug to maintain anesthesia will lengthen the recovery period and tend to enhance the hallucinogenic side effects.

Examples of cyclohexamine drugs for anesthesia

Ketamine hydrochloride

Since ketamine is presently the most widely used cyclohexamine drug, it will be discussed in greater detail than phencyclidine or tiletamine. Ketamine is one of the most popular anesthetic drugs presently being used in feline practice. In combination with a tranquilizer such as acepromazine, ketamine is often employed for minor surgical procedures, restraint, and diagnostic procedures. The tranquilizer helps to lessen muscle rigidity and allows for a reduction in the dosage of the ketamine. Most of ketamine's popularity has been achieved during the 1970s. Recently, xylazine has been used in combination with ketamine for surgical procedures in cats.

Derivation. Phencyclidine.

Availability. Ketamine is commercially supplied as a clear solution in multidose vials containing 10, 50, or 100 mg/ml. The concentration most often used for cats is the 100 mg/ml solution. Ketamine is relatively stable at room temperature but may deteriorate if exposed to excessive light or heat.

Route of administration. Ketamine is most often administered to cats by intramuscular injection (see Fig. 3-13), which affects their coordination and righting reflexes. Within 5 minutes they are unable to move, scratch, or bite and they lie still with open eyes and mildly dilated pupils. The palpebral, corneal, laryngeal, and swallowing reflexes remain. The skeletal muscles become rigid and extensor tone is exaggerated, especially in the muscles of the forelimbs. Salivation occurs in most cats and may warrant the use of atropine in low dosages to prevent excessive salivation.

Ketamine may be administered by the intravenous route in lowered dosages; however, this may lead to an increased potential for adverse effects on blood pres-

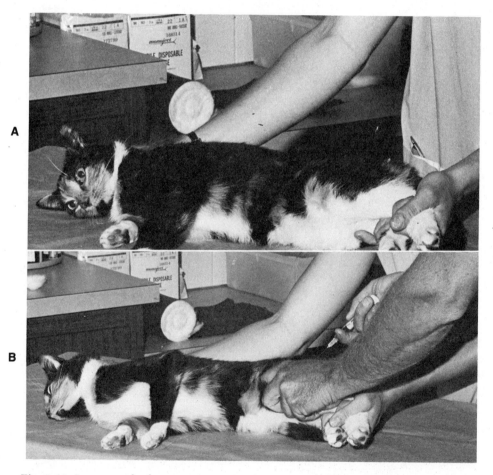

Fig. 3-13. Intramuscular ketamine injection. **A,** Assistant holds cat by the skin of the neck and both rear legs. **B,** Injection is made into the muscle of the left hind leg while assistant stretches the cat slightly in order to gain control of the head and all four legs.

sure and cardiac rhythm. Accidental injection of an intramuscular dosage into a vein is one cause of ketamine-related death. Ketamine has a poor effect when given subcutaneously. After intramuscular injection of ketamine it is advisable to return the cat to its cage or place it on the floor and observe it closely during the induction phase. If the cat is left unattended during the first few minutes of induction, signs of overdosage may go unnoticed. Further, since cats lose their righting reflexes within minutes after an intramuscular injection, they must never be left unattended since serious injury could result if the cat were to fall from a table or counter top.

Dosages for cats
Intramuscular
- Preanesthetic sedation and/or chemical restraint: 5 to 10 mg/kg
- Minor surgical procedures: 10 to 30 mg/kg

Intravenous
- Preanesthetic sedation and/or chemical restraint: 1 to 2 mg/kg
- Minor surgical procedures: 2 to 4 mg/kg

Speed and duration of action
Intramuscular
- Induction time: 3 to 5 minutes
- Duration of surgical anesthesia: 20 to 30 minutes
- Recovery time: 4 to 6 hours

Intravenous
- Induction time: 30 to 60 seconds
- Duration of surgical anesthesia: 5 to 15 minutes
- Recovery time: 1 to 3 hours

Advantages
- Inexpensive compared to inhalation anesthesia
- Does not require specialized equipment
- Provides good analgesia, restraint, and effective light surgical anesthesia by intramuscular injection (in cats)
- Rapid induction following intramuscular injection
- Wide margin of safety in cats when given intramuscularly
- Can be combined with other anesthetic drugs and allows for a reduced dosage of the general anesthetic drug
- Particularly suited for ophthalmic examinations of the retina due to its mydriatic action on the pupils
- Minimal respiratory depression
- Stimulatory effect on heart rate, blood pressure, and cardiac output
- Can be used in cats with full stomachs since it does not stimulate vomiting
- Swallowing and laryngeal reflexes are maintained, thereby lessening the chance for aspiration of secretions under anesthesia.

At the present time, ketamine is under no special federal control. However, this situation is expected to change in the near future because the hallucinogenic nature of ketamine-like drugs makes them potentially addictive and subject to abuse.

Disadvantages

- Undesirable hallucinogenic and excitatory effect on the CNS
- Not suitable for use in dogs due to a high incidence of convulsions during the recovery period
- Does not provide muscle relaxation
- Can stimulate tonic-clonic convulsions during the recovery period, especially when stimulated by noise or bright lighting
- Does not lend itself to long-term anesthesia cases since additional doses tend toward convulsive activity
- Inappropriate for surgical procedures involving abdominal or thoracic organs of orthopedic repair
- Variability of complete recovery after an intramuscular dose (can extend up to 24 hours or longer)
- Difficult to control or assess the depth of anesthesia
- Vulnerability of eyes (that remain open) to corneal damage due to drying or possibility of spillage of such preparations as iodine, alcohol, and soap into the eyes
- Increased potential for overdosage and/or prolonged recovery in cats with renal or hepatic impairment

The potential for illegal use invites theft. Ketamine and related drugs should be locked up, along with Schedule II drugs, as a safeguard against their abuse.

Precautions and/or complications. Those associated with ketamine are the same as with all cyclohexamine drugs.

Phencyclidine hydrochloride

The two other cataleptoid anesthetics, phencyclidine and tiletamine, are rarely, if ever, used in cats or dogs. Phencyclidine was abandoned for use in humans shortly after it was introduced, due to its strong hallucinogenic and agitative effects. Until 1978 phencyclidine was marketed for use only in nonhuman primates although it was also being used as an immobilizing drug for a variety of wildlife species. The drug was taken off the market altogether in 1978 because of its relatively low sales potential and hallucinogenic properties. Before that time the illegal use of phencyclidine, in the form of "PCP" or "angel dust," was responsible for numerous drug overdosages and drug-related deaths, especially in those people unfamiliar with its hazardous CNS-stimulating effects. Intramuscular dosage of phencyclidine for nonhuman primates was 0.5 to 2 mg/kg.

Tiletamine hydrochloride

Tiletamine is the most recently introduced cyclohexamine anesthetic drug. It is still undergoing clinical investigation as an anesthetic and preanesthetic drug for domestic cats and nonhuman primates. In cats the duration of anesthesia from a single intramuscular injection is 1 to 2 hours, as compared to 30 minutes for ketamine. There is marked variation in response to tiletamine's anesthetic potential and a recommended dosage is still under investigation. The apneustic breathing pattern and hyperrigidity of skeletal muscles common to tiletamine and other cyclohexamines can be decreased by combining it with a low dose of tranquilizer—for example, 0.1 mg of acepromazine or 0.5 mg of promazine. Intravenous diazepam (0.5 mg) may also be administered before the tiletamine to reduce muscle rigidity; however cats may still exhibit breath holding during inspiration.

Intramuscular dosage

For cats

• Immobilization or preanesthetic sedation: 1.0 to 5.0 mg/kg
• For minor surgical anesthesia: 10 to 40 mg/kg

For nonhuman primates

• Immobilization and restraint: 1 to 4 mg/kg

STEROID ANESTHESIA FOR USE IN CATS

Steroid anesthetic drugs have been used for clinical anesthesia in countries other than the United States since the early 1970s. Their approval for use with cats in the United States is expected shortly. The steroid product most often used for feline anesthesia in Great Britain is Saffan.* Most of the information regarding steroid anesthesia relates to clinical investigations with this drug. Although the steroid anesthetic drug that is eventually released on the American market will be similar to Saffan, it may carry a different trade name.

Classification. The steroid anesthetic drug is composed of two derivatives of the steroid pregnanedione: alphaxalone (the primary active ingredient) and alphadolone acetate. The preparation is clear and somewhat viscous due to the presence of castor oil and saline to dissolve the steroid. The drug combination provides good muscle relaxation and has a wide margin of safety.

Usage. Steroid anesthetics are presently cleared for use only in cats. Their use in dogs is not recommended due to an apparent histamine release attributable to the solubilizing agent (castor oil). The duration of anesthesia in cats is directly related to the dose administered. Steroid anesthesia can be used alone for sedation or for general anesthesia lasting 10 to 20 minutes. When administered intravenously, supplemental doses can be given during the procedure to maintain the

*Glaxo Laboratories Ltd., Greenford, Middlesex, England.

desired level and duration of anesthesia. Steroid anesthesia may also be used for tracheal intubation in conjunction with inhalation anesthesia. Alphaxalone is compatible with other preanesthetic and anesthetic drugs commonly administered to cats.

Concentration and route of administration. Saffan is presently marketed in 5 and 10 ml ampules containing 12 mg/ml of total steroid, which consists of 9 mg/ml alphaxalone and 3 mg/ml alphadolone acetate.

Steroid anesthetics can be administered to cats by intravenous or intramuscular injection:

- Intramuscular: recommended for sedation or light anesthesia to facilitate handling and certain diagnostic or therapeutic procedures such as radiography, teeth cleaning, and superficial wound or abscess repair. Can be used for preanesthetic sedation at low dosage
- Intravenous: suitable for short procedures that are not associated with a high degree of pain—for example, castration or dental extraction—or as an induction agent for use with another general anesthetic drug. For procedures lasting more than 5 to 10 minutes the steroid anesthetic can be given in small incremental doses to maintain the anesthetic state. Use of an indwelling intravenous catheter is recommended when administration of the steroid drug by repeated injection is anticipated.

Steroid anesthetics are ineffective when administered by subcutaneous injection. Perivascular injection of the steroid preparation is *not* associated with irritation or necrosis.

Dosage

Intramuscular

- Preanesthetic sedation: 4 mg/kg
- Mild sedation: 9 mg/kg
- Deep sedation: 12 mg/kg
- Light anesthesia: 18 mg/kg

Intravenous supplementation of the steroid may be given to induce and/or maintain anesthesia following an intramuscular dose. Incremental doses do not significantly lengthen recovery time.

Intravenous. A single dose (9 mg/kg) is given rapidly as a bolus injection. In aged or debilitated cats, 50% of the dosage should be given rapidly while the remaining portion is given to effect by slow injection. Supplemental doses of 3 mg/kg can be administered to maintain anesthesia beyond 5 to 10 minutes.

Speed of onset and duration of action

Intramuscular

- Maximum effect after injection: 7 to 12 minutes
- Duration of action: 5 to 20 minutes
- Recovery of reflexes: variable, depending on dosage (3 to 6 hours)

These times are more variable when the steroid drug is administered by the intramuscular route, depending on the muscle used for injection. The drug should be given by deep intramuscular injection into a muscle that is relatively thick and free from fascia. The belly of the quadriceps femoris muscle (located anterior to the femur) is a preferred site of injection.

Intravenous

- Onset of action (induction): 10 seconds
- Maximum effect: 30 seconds
- Duration of action (following a single 9 mg/kg dose): 10 minutes
- Recovery of righting reflex: $1\frac{1}{2}$ to 2 hours

Duration of action and the time to full recovery are directly related to the intravenous dosage administered. In general, normal behavior can be expected within 3 to 4 hours following the first (or final) intravenous injection.

Advantages. Although steroid anesthetic drugs have not yet received clinical sanction in the United States the following lists are based on the use of Saffan in Great Britain:

- Large safety margin allows for variable dosage under different clinical situations.
- It provides good sedation with muscle relaxation when administered by intramuscular or intravenous injection.
- It causes negligible tissue irritation when given intramuscularly or inadvertently injected perivascularly. Due to its poor absorption from subcutaneous tissue, any perivascular injection of the drug can be disregarded concerning its cumulative effect on the CNS.
- It requires no expensive equipment, although the drug itself is relatively expensive at the present time.
- It is especially suited for short-term procedures or sedation when a rapid full recovery is desired.
- Supplemental doses can be used to maintain anesthesia without prolonging recovery and with little chance for producing toxicity.
- Rapid clearance from plasma allows for rapid recovery and metabolism of the active drug, thereby lessening the likelihood of overdosage due to cumulative effects.
- Respiration is well maintained and cardiovascular stability is minimal at dosages of 9 mg/kg or less.
- It can be used to induce general anesthesia and allows for endotracheal intubation.
- It is compatible with other general anesthetic drugs and most preanesthetic sedatives (potent phenothiazine tranquilizers such as acetylpromazine may act to prolong anesthetic duration and recovery).
- It is useful in cats when peripheral veins are too small or difficult to locate

since deep sedation or light anesthesia is obtained from a single intramuscular injection.

• It does not induce vomiting.

• It does not have a high potential for abuse and therefore is unlikely to require the regulations and restrictions of a Schedule II controlled substance.

Disadvantages

• It is unsuitable for use in dogs.

• It is a relatively expensive drug compared to ketamine or thiamylal.

• Its solubilizing agent tends to cause histamine release, which can result in a transient swelling of the cats' paws and/or ears.

• It is associated with a significant decrease in mean aortic blood pressure and mild tachycardia, especially after intravenous injection and even at dosages as low as 1.2 mg/kg. These cardiovascular effects occur within 1 minute of injection and usually return to normal values within 2 to 5 minutes.

• It may produce twitching, paddling, or muscle tremors during the recovery period. Physical disturbances or rough handling of the cat during the early recovery period can result in exaggerated or violent movements.

• It must be used with caution in cats with a full stomach. An 8 to 12 hour fast is recommended before its use as an anesthetic.

LOCAL ANALGESIA
Classification

Local analgesic drugs act directly on sensory and motor nerves to produce a temporary loss of pain sensation and muscle relaxation. The term "local analgesia" will be used throughout this text instead of "local anesthesia," primarily as a means for differentiating these drugs from those anesthetic drugs that have their primary site of action in the brain.

Local analgesic drugs act directly on peripheral and spinal nerves to block transmission of nerve impulses along the nerve fiber. The block is reversible with time as the drug is removed from the nerve site by venous circulation and metabolized by enzymes in the blood and liver. Nerves that conduct impulses from a peripheral organ toward the spinal cord are called "afferent" nerves. These nerves are sensory in nature and respond to pressure, heat, touch, and pain. Nerves that conduct impulses away from the spinal cord and toward an organ are called "efferent" nerves. Nerves that conduct impulses to skeletal muscle to produce motion or tone are termed "efferent motor" nerves or simply "motor" nerves.

The CNS consists of the brain, spinal cord, and nerves connecting with the spinal cord that are both efferent and afferent in nature (see Fig. 3-15). The spinal cord also contains sympathetic fibers belonging to the autonomic nervous system. These nerves conduct impulses to the heart and blood vessels to maintain (1) heart rate and smooth muscle tone for blood pressure, (2) smooth muscle contraction of internal organs such as the esophagus, stomach, and digestive tract, and (3) sweat glands of the skin. When a local analgesic drug is injected into or around the spinal cord, impulse conduction in all these nerve fibers will be affected, resulting in a block of sensory, motor, and sympathetic nerve function. Blockage of sympathetic fibers is an undesirable yet unavoidable side effect of epidural and spinal nerve block techniques. A serious complication of sympathetic blockade due to a local analgesic drug takes the form of hypotension and bradycardia.

Local analgesia was first used clinically in the mid 1880s when cocaine became widely used for desensitizing the eye. Within a few years local analgesic drugs were being used in humans for dentistry and local skin blocks. When general anesthetic techniques became more sophisticated in the early 1900s, local analgesia began to decline in popularity, especially in veterinary medicine. Local analgesic techniques are regaining popularity in human anesthesiology but are used infrequently in dogs and cats, primarily because of overdosage problems related to the small size of the patient, the uncooperative nature of animal patients, and a general lack of familiarity with the techniques for administering local analgesic drugs. Since all local analgesic drugs are potentially dangerous when absorbed (or injected) into the bloodstream, they must always be used in the lowest possible concentration and volume. Local analgesic drugs should *never* be injected intravenously by mistake as they can cause convulsions or immediate cardiac arrest. Local analgesics used for epidural injection can cause paralysis of the diaphragm and intercostal muscles if the drug travels too far toward the cranium, resulting in apnea and the need for controlled ventilation.

Drugs routinely employed for local analgesia are classified according to their chemical bond as either an *ester* grouping or an *amide* grouping. Some common examples of local analgesic drugs are:
1. Ester group
   a. Cocaine (no longer available as a local analgesic)
   b. Procaine
   c. Tetracaine
   d. Chlorprocaine
2. Amide group
   a. Lidocaine
   b. Dibucaine
   c. Mepivacaine

Uses of local analgesia in dogs and cats

Local analgesia is generally reserved for use in older animals for minor surgery of the skin or in animals that are at risk with general anesthesia due to uncompensating diseases of the liver, kidney, respiratory, or cardiovascular systems. Local analgesia is sometimes used in conjunction with a light level of general anesthesia to enhance the effects of analgesia and muscle relaxation that would be possible only with deeper planes of the general anesthetic drug. (see "Methods of administration" for more specific mention of the uses of local analgesics in dogs and cats.)

Epinephrine is often added to the local analgesic solution for its vasoconstrictive action on local blood vessels in the area of injection. The reason for incorporating epinephrine is twofold: (1) it enhances the blockade by slowing the rate of absorption of the local analgesic drug into the bloodstream through its constricting action on nearby blood vessels (the net effect is a prolongation of action) and (2) it decreases the chances for rapid absorption of the local analgesic drug into the circulation by slowing the absorption rate into regional blood vessels, which lessens the likelihood of the development of toxic blood levels. When incorporated into a local analgesic injection, epinephrine should be used at a concentration of 1:200,000 (5 μg/ml).*

Any drug clinically employed for local analgesia should exhibit as many of the following characteristics as possible:
- Low toxicity when absorbed into the general circulation
- Action confined to nerve tissue
- Nonirritating to local tissues
- Complete reversibility within a clinically acceptable time period
- Short latency period (the time required from injection to onset of action)— that is, 5 to 10 minutes
- Relatively long duration of analgesia (45 to 90 minutes)
- Compatibility with epinephrine
- Solubility in water or saline
- Stability at room temperature and unaffected by light

When repeated doses of a local analgesic drug are used to sustain a nerve block, a decreased response may occur with time, rendering the block ineffective. The term applied to a decrease in response following consecutive injections of a drug at short intervals is "tachyphylaxis." With local analgesic drugs the cause, it is believed, is a decreased pH within the region of the injection, rendering the drug less effective.

Mechanism of local analgesic action

The exact mechanism by which a local analgesic drug molecule effectively blocks impulse transmission within the neuron is beyond the intent of this text (refer to *Principles of Pharmacology*).[2] The process is complex and incompletely understood even by experts in neurophysiology. The student should realize that the site of action is at the neuron itself and not within the brain. The local analgesic drug must diffuse through several physical barriers before it reaches individual neurons within a peripheral nerve. The larger the nerve, the longer it will take the drug to diffuse

---

*A 1:200,000 concentration would be equivalent to 1 mg of epinephrine diluted into 200 ml of saline.

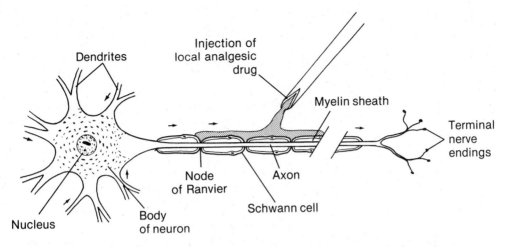

Fig. 3-14. Diagram of a motor neuron (nerve) showing myelinated sheath and nodes of Ranvier. Solid arrows indicate pathway for normal nerve conduction.

into the center of the nerve fiber and complete the blockade. Obstacles, such as fat, fibrous tissue, large blood vessels, scar tissue, edema, or hemorrhage in the area of the injection, tend to impede the diffusion of the local analgesic drug toward and into the nerve.

Local analgesic drugs are never purposely injected directly into a nerve. To do so would elicit considerable pain. Instead, the drug is deposited around the desired nerve or nerves and allowed to diffuse into the nerve bundles of the individual nerve fibers. It is this diffusion process that determines the latency period for onset of action with local analgesic drugs. In most instances when a local analgesic drug is injected, a minimum of 3 to 5 minutes must pass before any analgesic or muscle relaxing effect is obtained.

In addition to these physical barriers of diffusion, there is also a continuous process of analgesic drug removal by absorption into nearby capillaries and lymphatic vessels. Absorption tends to lower the concentration of the analgesic drug within and around the nerve while raising its concentration in circulating blood. Once the local analgesic drug is absorbed from the area around the nerve, its effect on the nerve is also removed and the nerve recovers its function. In the case of myelinated nerves the areas of penetration by the local analgesic drug are between the nodes of Ranvier (see Fig. 3-14), which add a further delay to onset of analgesia.

The toxic effect of a local analgesic drug is related to its concentration in the blood. It is desirable, therefore, to prevent sudden or high blood levels from occurring. This can be achieved by constricting blood vessels within the area of injection and using the lowest possible concentration and volume of drug. Some local analgesic drugs are considered more toxic than others once they are absorbed into the bloodstream. Cocaine, for instance, is rarely used as an injectable local analgesic due to its highly toxic action on the CNS once it is absorbed into the blood-stream.

Methods for administering local analgesic drugs

Local analgesic drugs are administered to dogs or cats by one of four general methods (see Fig. 3-15): topical application, local infiltration, regional injection, and intravenous regional analgesia.

Topical application

Anesthesia of the skin, eye, or mucous membranes can be achieved by applying a local analgesic drug directly onto the area. Very few drugs are able to penetrate the skin and produce a desensitization of the cutaneous nerves. Temporary analgesia of the skin lasting 30 to 60 seconds can be achieved by spraying *ethyl chloride* liquid directly onto a small area of skin. Analgesia is achieved by the rapid evaporation of ethyl chloride, which causes a freezing of the skin and nerves. Since ethyl chloride is extremely volatile and flammable, care must be taken not to use it in the presence of heat, open flames, or sparks. Overzealous use of ethyl chloride to freeze skin could result in permanent damage due to skin necrosis. When the drug is used in humans, the thawing of the skin following its use can be pruritic and painful. Such a sensation in animals could lead to undesirable chewing or licking of the previously anesthetized region. *Butacaine* is a local analgesic drug commonly used in over-the-counter skin lotions for relief of pain and itching caused by such irritations as poison ivy, insect bites, or sunburn.

Local analgesic drugs in the form of sprays, gels, or paste can be used to produce a desensitization of the eye or mucous membranes of the mouth, nasal passages, larynx, external ear canal, or urethra. Duration of action is relatively brief (10 to 30 minutes). Following are some local analgesic drugs commonly used for topical anesthesia of the eye and/or mucous membranes.

Cocaine. Cocaine is used for desensitization of the cornea and conjunctiva. Due to its toxic effects on the CNS and potential for abuse, cocaine is rarely used today (cocaine is classified as a Schedule I controlled substance). It is difficult to prepare a sterile water-soluble solution and its long-term use may damage the cornea.

Tetracaine. A topical anesthetic solution to desensitize the cornea and conjunctiva for ophthamologic procedures, it is also used to desensitize other mucous membranes. A 0.2% to 1% solution is generally employed for topical application.

Lidocaine. Lidocaine is used as a topical anesthetic solution, gel, or cream to desensitize mucous membranes of the nose, mouth, larynx, and urethra. It is often used for cats before tracheal intubation to desensitize the vocal cords and decrease laryngospasm. A concentration range of 2% to 10% is generally used for topical application.

Cetacaine. Cetacaine is used as a topical anesthetic spray to desensitize skin and mucous membranes of the mouth and larynx.

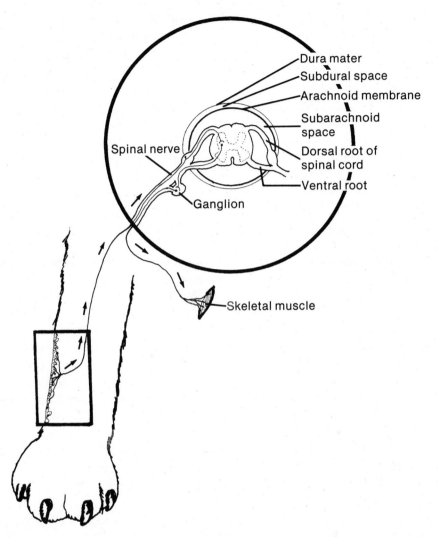

Fig. 3-15. Sites for blocking nerve fiber transmission from spinal cord to carpus. Rectangular area represents site for a local infiltration block.

Localized infiltration

The local analgesic drug is injected around sensory nerve fibers using a hypodermic syringe and small gauge needle (23 or 25 gauge). Infiltration is generally done at the distal end of sensory nerves to produce a very localized area of analgesia without blocking motor nerves to skeletal muscles of the limb. The local analgesic drug can be injected intradermally, subcutaneously, or between muscle layers. The injection is limited to the area of surgery, and care must be taken to prevent accidental injection of the drug into the nerve and/or a local blood vessel.

Infiltration analgesia may be used for minor surgical procedures in dogs and cats, including suturing of skin lacerations, removal of small warts or skin tumors, amputation of puppy tails, and skin biopsies. Combining the sedative effects of a tranquilizer and/or narcotic with local infiltration allows for a greater degree of analgesia and less physical restraint. Animals that are considered too sick or depressed to withstand general anesthesia are candidates for surgery under local infiltration with or without sedation.

Some veterinarians prefer infiltration of the ventral abdomen with a local analgesic drug (combined with neuroleptanalgesia and nitrous oxide–oxygen) for cesarean sections in depressed dogs or cats. This technique avoids the use of general anesthetic drugs, which may depress the newborn. Once the fetuses are removed from the uterus, the remainder of the surgical procedure can be completed with nitrous oxide–oxygen and an inhalation anesthetic drug such as halothane or enflurane.

With infiltration anesthesia a period of 5 to 10 minutes must elapse after injection before the nerves supplying the skin are sufficiently desensitized to allow incision. Epinephrine at a concentration of 1:50,000 or 1:200,000 is added to local analgesic solutions used for infiltration in order to prolong the effect and prevent rapid absorption into the systemic circulation.

Following are some examples of local analgesic drugs commonly used for infiltration anesthesia in dogs and cats.

Procaine. One of the original drugs used for local analgesia in both humans and animals, procaine is used as the standard of reference for all other local analgesic drugs. A concentration range of 0.5% to 2% is generally used for infiltration analgesia.

Lidocaine. Somewhat more potent and toxic than procaine, lidocaine can also be used for topical and regional analgesia. It is one of the most widely used local analgesic drugs in veterinary practice. Lidocaine also possesses significant antiarrhythmic effects on the heart and is often used for controlling ventricular dysrythmias. When lidocaine is used for infiltration analgesia, a concentration of 0.5% to 2% is generally employed.

Chlorprocaine. A combination of an ester and an amide, chlorprocaine is slightly more potent than procaine, yet has a shorter duration of action. Concentrations used for infiltration analgesia range from 0.5% to 3%.

Regional injection

Regional anesthesia is produced when a local analgesic drug is injected either around the spinal cord or within the area of a major nerve plexus. The most commonly employed method in dogs and cats is to inject the local analgesic into the epidural space between the last lumbar vertebrae and the sacrum (see Fig. 3-16). Regional analgesia may be used in any of the following forms:

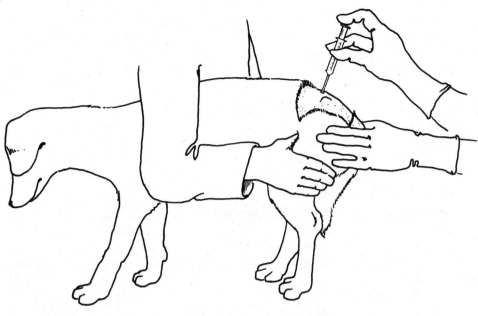

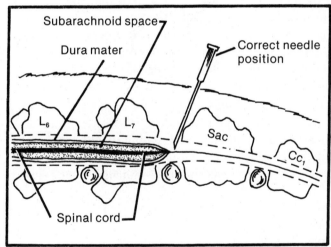

Subarachnoid space

Dura mater

Correct needle position

L_6 L_7 Sac Cc_1

Spinal cord

Fig. 3-16. Epidural injection showing location and position of needle. Insert shows schematic diagram of correct needle placement in epidural space.

- *Epidural blockage* (also called peridural or extradural anesthesia). Provides muscle relaxation
- *Spinal blockade* (also called subarachnoid anesthesia). A form seldom used in dogs and cats
- *Plexus blockade*. Local analgesic is injected into a region such as the brachial plexus, causing desensitization and muscle relaxation of the forelimb distal to the elbow. This form of regional anesthesia is seldom practiced in veterinary anesthesia.

Epidural blockade is a relatively simple technique that may be used when general anesthesia is considered too risky for the animal. It can be employed for most surgical or diagnostic procedures of the posterior abdomen, urethra, rectal area, or rear limbs. Epidural blockade can be used for cesarean section in dogs and/or used in combination with a light level of general anesthesia. Because the local analgesic drug is injected around the spinal cord, smaller volumes are needed than for infiltration analgesia. Epinephrine, without preservatives, can be added to the analgesic drug just before administration. Whenever epidural or spinal blockade is used, it is *extremely important* to position the animal so that gravitation of the drug toward the head is prevented. The animal should be positioned or restrained so that the head end of the body is slightly higher than the spinal cord. If this precaution is not observed, it is possible that the local analgesic drug will drift too far cranially and block the phrenic nerve as it exits the spinal cord around the level of the third to sixth cervical vertebrae. Respiratory depression occurs as the anesthetic drug reaches the mid-thoracic portion of the spinal cord due to blockade of the nerves supplying the intercostal muscles. Total apnea will occur if the phrenic nerve to the diaphragm is blocked. In addition, sympathetic nerves to the heart and blood vessels can be blocked if the local analgesic drug travels as far as the mid-thoracic level of the spinal cord. Sympathetic blockade results in bradycardia, decreased cardiac output, and serious hypotension. Death may result from respiratory and/or cardiovascular depression. When local analgesic drugs are used for epidural blockade, one must be prepared to intubate the trachea and administer artificial ventilation should apnea or hypoventilation occur.

Following are some local analgesic drugs commonly used for epidural, spinal, or plexus blockade. The concentration and volume of each drug will vary according to the level and duration of blockade desired and the size of the animal. With epidural and spinal anesthesia a polyethylene catheter may be inserted for continuous administration of the local analgesic drug as needed. The concentrations for each drug is for epidural anesthesia:

- Lidocaine (Xylocaine): 0.5%-2%
- Chlorprocaine (Nesacaine): 1%-2%
- Bupivacaine (Marcaine): 0.25%-0.75%
- Etidocaine (Duranest): 0.25%-1.5%
- Tetracaine (Pontocaine): 0.1%-0.5%
- Procaine (Novocain): 2%-4%
- Mepivacaine (Carbocaine): 0.5%-1.5%

Intravenous regional analgesia

Intravenous regional analgesia is a relatively recent technique designed for short-term procedures, particularly of the front limbs. It is often used in human anesthesia to anesthetize an extremity for procedures such as laceration repair, surgery of tendons or nerves, and reduction of fractured bones. Onset of analgesia occurs within 5 to 10 minutes after the local analgesic drug is injected into a distal vein. The procedure involves placing a tourniquet on the proximal portion of the limb, exsanguinating the limb distal to the tourniquet, and then injecting the local analgesic drug into a previously placed venous catheter that is also distal to the torniquet. The tourniquet is left in place, and duration of anesthesia time is governed by the length of time the tourniquet is in use (not longer than 90 minutes). To prevent toxic blood levels from occurring, the tourniquet should not be released within 20 to 30 minutes after injecting the local analgesic drug. Anesthesia of the limb disappears within 5 to 10 minutes of releasing the tourniquet pressure. A stepwise releasing process is recommended to prevent toxic reactions due to an excessive amount of local analgesic drug entering the circulation within a short period of time. Lidocaine (0.5%) without epinephrine, at a dosage of 3 mg/kg, is the drug of choice for this technique. Presently this technique is not very popular in veterinary medicine.

Toxicity of local analgesic drugs

Deaths due to injection of local analgesics are rare in animals. Toxic reactions are seen more in very young, small, diseased, or older animals. Toxic reactions to the use of local analgesic drugs are of two categories: *local* and *systemic*.

Local toxicity

Localized damage to a nerve or nerves may result from the accidental injection of the drug directly into a nerve fiber. It may also be caused by localized tissue irritation due to the pH of the drug or carrier substance being injected in combination with the local analgesic. Such local toxicity is rare and usually results in temporary damage to the nerve; however, permanent nerve damage is not impossible. Damaged peripheral nerves result in a loss of sensory or motor function to the affected skin or muscle for a variable length of time (2 days to 2 months), depending on the severity of nerve tissue damage.

Systemic toxicity

Whenever a local analgesic drug is injected, it will eventually be absorbed into the bloodstream. Once absorbed into the systemic circulation, local analgesic drugs affect other body systems. The CNS and cardiovascular system are particularly sensitive to toxic blood levels of a local analgesic. When local analgesics are used correctly, a toxic reaction is rare. Toxic reactions are most often due to a rapid absorption of a relatively large dose of the local analgesic drug. In addition, a delayed rate of drug metabolism (detoxification) can predispose an animal to a toxic reaction.

CNS toxicity. CNS toxicity is seen more often following clinical doses of a local analgesic than is cardiovascular toxicity. As the blood level of the analgesic drug increases, signs of CNS toxicity may be manifested by muscular twitching or sedation. In severe cases convulsions may occur. The seizures are usually self-limiting; however, the animal's respiration can be depressed, leading to hypoxia and hypercapnia. If apnea occurs, respiratory stimulants, such as doxapram, should be avoided as they may aggravate CNS stimulation. Intubation of the trachea should be performed immediately and the animal ventilated with 100% oxygen. Once the toxic blood level of local analgesic is decreased, the seizures will subside anywhere from 5 to 60 minutes. Diazepam is presently the drug of choice for treating CNS excitability due to local analgesic toxicity. However, support of ventilation with 100% oxygen is also essential during a toxic reaction.

Cardiovascular system toxicity. With the exception of an accidental intravenous injection of a local analgesic, cardiovascular toxicity is unlikely to occur. Large amounts of the analgesic drug must be absorbed before cardiovascular effects are seen. Epidural and spinal blocks are more apt to result in cardiovascular instability from the effect of the local analgesic drug on sympathetic nerves leaving the spinal cord. Sympathetic innervation of the heart may be impaired, resulting in bradycardia and hypotension, especially if the drug travels above the mid-thoracic level of the spinal cord. Treatment is designed to restore blood pressure and heart rate with the use of atropine, intravenous fluids, and vasoconstrictive drugs and to correct any positioning errors. Local analgesic drugs also have a direct effect on the heart, depressing impulse conduction and stabilizing electric membranes. In extreme cases this myocardial depression could result in cardiac arrest.

•   •   •

Occasionally an animal may exhibit an allergic reaction to a local analgesic drug, usually procaine or one of the other ester-type local analgesics. Allergy may manifest itself in the form of a skin rash, hives, or, if severe enough, anaphylactic shock. Allergic reactions to lidocaine or other amide-type local analgesic drugs are less common. When an animal demonstrates an allergic reaction following a penicillin injection, it may actually be reacting to the procaine incorporated into the penicillin suspension.* In animals with a history of allergy to procaine penicillin, it is advisable either to inject a small test dose of procaine intradermally before using it for local analgesia or to use an amide analgesic drug in place of the procaine.

*Procaine acts as a salt to delay the absorption of penicillin from muscle tissue, thereby sustaining plasma level.

REFERENCE

1. McCarthy, T.C.: The phencyclidine anesthetics: their effects on central nervous, cardiovascular and respiratory function, Veterinary Anesthesia 3(1):49-56, 1976.
2. Giovanoni, R.: Principles of pharmacology. In Warren, R.G., series editor: Mosby's fundamentals of animal health technology, St. Louis, 1983, The C.V. Mosby Co.

4

Principles of inhalation anesthesia

A.I. WEBB and ROGER G. WARREN

PERFORMANCE OBJECTIVES:

After completion of this chapter, the student will:

- Explain the concept of anesthetic partial pressure and its relationship to solubility and uptake of an inhalation anesthetic drug

- List those physical and physiologic parameters that affect the uptake, distribution, and elimination of inhalation anesthetic drugs

- Describe how alterations in these parameters affect anesthetic induction and recovery

- List the common inhalation anesthetic drugs as well as qualitative descriptions of their solubility, anesthetic strength, and clinical indications

- Describe the advantages and problems relating to the use of the common inhalation anesthetic drugs in dogs and cats

- List four methods by which anesthetic pollution can be controlled in the operating room environment

Chapters 1 through 3 deal with methods of introducing anesthetic drugs into the bloodstream by intravenous, intramuscular, or subcutaneous injection. They also describe the process by which injectable anesthetic or preanesthetic drugs remain in the body until they are metabolized by the liver and/or excreted by the kidneys. Chapters 4 through 6 are concerned with those anesthetic drugs that exist as gases (or vapors) and can be administered to an animal via its lungs—hence the term "inhalation" or "gas" anesthesia. Inhalation anesthetic drugs are eliminated from the body almost entirely by the lungs.

The concentration of an inhalation anesthetic drug in an animal's bloodstream can be changed merely by altering the concentration delivered to the animal for inspiration—thus providing a means for controlling the depth of general anesthesia. Since anesthetic depth is so readily altered, the need for a knowledgeable and well trained anesthetist becomes essential. The duty of careful patient monitoring and control of anesthetic gas mixtures must, of necessity, be the responsibility of someone other than the surgeon.

Safe administration of inhalation anesthesia requires a constant awareness of the moment-by-moment changes that can occur during this period. The speed with which anesthetic depth can be changed is related to both the anesthetic drug itself and the patient's physical and physiologic status. The intent of this chapter is to introduce the student to the fundamental principles of inhalation anesthesia. The first section deals with the general principles of uptake and distribution of inhalation anesthetic drugs and recovery from them. There is then a discussion of individual inhalation anesthetic drugs from a pharmacologic and clinical point of view and the possible pollution problems these drugs present. The commonly used inhalation anesthetic drugs to be discussed in this chapter are:

- Nitrous oxide (N_2O)
- Diethyl ether (ether)
- Halothane
- Methoxyflurane
- Enflurane
- Isoflurane

PRINCIPLES OF INHALATION ANESTHETIC UPTAKE, DISTRIBUTION, AND ELIMINATION

Most theories that attempt to explain how inhalation anesthetic drugs work are based on the premise that the brain is the primary organ involved in producing unconsciousness, CNS depression, and analgesia. The exact mechanism whereby the cells within the gray matter of the brain are "desensitized" by the anesthetic drug is still controversial and subject to a multitude of theories.

Regardless of the hypothesis it appears that a critical number of molecules must reach the sites of anesthetic action in the brain. To do this, the molecules must first be dissolved in the animal's blood so the anesthetic drug molecules can reach the brain. The mechanism for gas dissolving in liquid (and tissues) relies on pressure. Each molecule of a gas or vapor exerts a pressure because of its random movement within a finite volume—in fact, 6×10^{23} gas molecules in a volume of 22.4 L at $0°$ C create a pressure equal to that of the atmosphere (760 mm Hg). If 10% of a mixture of gas molecules were of a particular gas (A), they would contribute 10% of the mixture's total pressure (that is, 76 mm Hg), which is termed the *partial pressure* (P_P) for that gas. If this gas mixture were dissolved in water, the molecules in the water would exert the same pressure as when they were in the gaseous form. Thus gas A would have a pressure of 76 mm Hg, which is the same as the gas mixture. However, the number of molecules with a partial pressure of 76 mm Hg will not be the same for every gas dissolved in water because different gases have differing solubilities in water. Even the same gas has different solubilities for different liquids or tissues. The more soluble a gas is in a particular liquid, the more molecules will be dissolved (that is, molecular density) in that liquid at any specific partial pressure.

Solubility coefficient of a gas or vapor

A gas mixture may consist of only two gases or vapors (for example, A = 10% of the mixture and B = the remaining 90%). If this mixture is left to dissolve in a beaker of water and oil that separate into two layers (see Table 4-1), the partial pressures for vapor A are 76 mm Hg in each of the three layers (that is, gas, water, and oil). The technical term for these layers is *phases*. Similarly, the partial pressures for vapor B in the three phases will all be the same:

$$P_B = 760 \text{ mm Hg} \times 90\% = 684 \text{ mm Hg}$$

However, the number of molecules per volume (molecular concentration or density) is not the same in each phase for either A or B because the two gases have differing solubilities in each of the phases. In the case of gas A, the molecular densities in the gas and water phases differ by a factor of 2 (0.26 vs 0.52). This factor is called the *solubility coefficient* (λ) and is calculated as the ratio of the vapor's concentration in the gas to its concentration in water (hence the value of 2).

$$\lambda = \frac{\text{Concentration in water}}{\text{Concentration in gas}} = \frac{0.52 \times 10^{19}}{0.26 \times 10^{19}} = 2.0$$

On the other hand, the water/gas solubility coefficient for B is 0.5 because of its differing concentrations when it is a gas and when it is dissolved in water. Thus vapor A is more soluble in oil than water, with an oil/gas solubility coefficient of 20:

$$\frac{5.2 \times 10^{19}}{0.26 \times 10^{19}}$$

or, when compared with water, an oil/water solubility coefficient of 10:

$$\lambda = \frac{\text{Concentration in oil}}{\text{Concentration in water}} = \frac{5.2 \times 10^{19}}{0.52 \times 10^{19}} = 10$$

The molecular concentration of vapor B in oil is lower than in gas. Therefore, the oil/gas solubility coefficient is 0.5:

$$\lambda = \frac{\text{Concentration in oil}}{\text{Concentration in gas}} = \frac{1.21 \times 10^{19}}{2.42 \times 10^{19}} = 0.5$$

This relationship among pressure, solubility, and concentration was discovered by William Henry in 1803, whose work is honored with his name. *Henry's* law states that the amount of gas dissolved in a given volume of liquid is directly proportional to the partial pressure of the gas:

$$V = \lambda \times P_P$$
where V = volume of gas dissolved
λ = solubility coefficient
P_P = partial pressure of the gas

TABLE 4-1

Pressures and molecular densities for a gas mixture (10% gas A and 90% gas B) dissolved in a biphasic mixture of oil and water at atmospheric pressure

| | Total pressure = 760 mm Hg Molecular density = 2.68×10^{19} molecules ml^{-1}* | | | | |
| | A (10%) | | B (90%) | | |
Phase	*Partial pressure (mm Hg)*	*Molecular density (molecules ml^{-1})*	*Partial pressure (mm Hg)*	*Molecular density (molecules ml^{-1})*	
Gas	76	0.26×10^{19}	684	2.42×10^{19}	
—Water/gas	$\lambda = 2$		$\lambda = 0.5$		
Water	76	0.52×10^{19}	684	1.21×10^{19}	
—Water/oil	$\lambda = 10$		$\lambda = 1$		
Oil	76	5.2×10^{19}	684	1.21×10^{19}	

*Superscript ml^{-1} means 1/ml or molecules/ml.

Minimum alveolar concentration

Other examples can be substituted for gas A. Table 4-2 shows the concentration of various inhalation anesthetic drugs in blood and brain when they are fully equilibrated with 1% of the drug (1 drug molecule/100 molecules of total gas mixture). Because concentrations of different anesthetic drugs exert the same partial pressures, they do not necessarily produce the same degree of anesthesia. Those that do produce the same degree of CNS depression are shown below. The common reference value is, traditionally, the alveolar concentration at which 50% of subjects respond to pain and 50% do not. This is called the "minimum alveolar concentration" or (MAC).

Minimum alveolar concentrations for common inhalation anesthetic drugs in the dog

Anesthetic	MAC
N$_2$O	188
Ether	3.04
Halothane	0.87
Methoxyflurane	0.23
Enflurane	2.2
Isoflurane	1.5

MAC values for a particular anesthetic drug can be changed by a number of physical and environmental factors. A decrease in MAC means an animal is more sensitive to an anesthetic and will require a lower concentration to produce anesthesia. Factors that can *decrease* the MAC value are:

- Severe hypotension
- Circadian rhythm (at night in diurnal animals)
- Hypothermia
- Aging

Species, sex, duration of anesthesia, or acid-base disorders do not affect MAC.

If the MAC values above and Tables 4-4 are compared, it can be seen that MAC correlates with oil solubility. This is important because anesthetic drugs concentrate in tissues with high lipid or fat content, such as the brain. They will also accumulate in other tissues and organs, depending on their lipid content and vascularity. This incorporation can be explained by considering uptake of inhalation anesthetic drugs as an hydraulic model, such as proposed by Mapleson in 1961.[1] In Fig. 4-1, when water tank A is kept filled to the top, water will flow into tank B through the connecting pipe C. The rate of flow into B is governed by the pressure difference

TABLE 4-2

Partial pressure and concentration of six common inhalation anesthetic drugs when a 1% mixture of each drug equilibrates with human blood and brain tissue

Media	N₂O			Ether			Halothane			Methoxyflurane			Enflurane			Isoflurane		
	P.P.*	λ†	Conc‡	P.P.*	λ†	Conc‡	P.P.*	λ†	Conc‡	P.P.*	λ†	Conc‡	P.P.*	λ†	Conc‡	P.P.*	λ†	Conc‡
Inspired gas	7.6	—	2.0	7.6	—	3.3	7.6	—	8.8	7.6	—	7.4	7.6	—	8.2	7.6	—	8.2
Blood	7.6	0.47	0.9	7.6	12.1	39.9	7.6	2.4	21.2	7.6	13.0	96.2	7.6	1.9	15.6	7.6	1.4	11.5
Brain	7.6	0.50	1.0	7.6	13.0	42.9	7.6	6.7	59.0	7.6	24.2	179.1	7.6	2.9	23.8	7.6	2.6	21.3

*Partial pressure in mm Hg.
†Tissue/gas solubility coefficient.
‡Concentration in mg/dl.

Hydraulic model

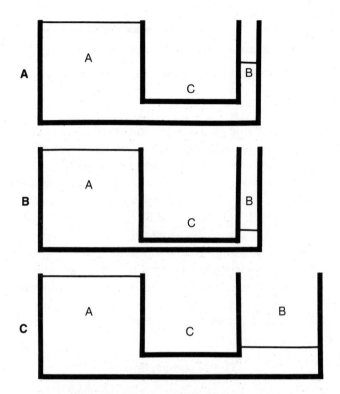

Fig. 4-1. Principles of the hydraulic model.

(pressure gradient) between each end of pipe C (that is, flow ∝ pressure at bottom of A − pressure at bottom of B). This concept can be seen when emptying a bathtub, which empties more rapidly at first because it is full. Its emptying rate slows when the water level falls and the pressure at the drain becomes less. In Fig. 4-1 tank B will fill less rapidly as its water level approaches the level of the full A tank—that is, the pressure difference between the two tanks decreases.

Also affecting the filling rate is the diameter of pipe C and the size of tank B. The French physicist Poiseuille showed that, as the cross section of a pipe doubles, the flow through it increases sixteenfold (flow ∝ diameter^4). The converse is shown in Fig. 4-1, **B,** where the diameter of pipe C decreases. However, if tank B increases in size, it will take longer to fill (that is, doubling of the tank radius quarters its rate of filling). Thus three factors are involved in the filling rate of tank B:

1. Pressure gradient between the two tanks
2. Size of the pipe connecting the two tanks
3. Size of tank B

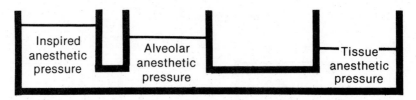

Fig. 4-2. Adaption of a hydraulic model to simulate anesthetic uptake. (After Mapleson, 1961.)

The hydraulic model can be used to represent anesthetic transfer from the lungs to the tissues by blood as shown in Fig. 4-2, where an intermediate tank is placed between the A and B tanks of Fig. 4-1. This new tank represents alveolar anesthetic pressure, and the pipe between it and the original A tank (inspired anesthetic pressure) represents alveolar ventilation. The pipe linking the alveolar pressure tank and the tissue pressure tank (originally tank B) represents the blood flow or perfusion rate for the tissue. The size of the tissue tank is determined by the capacity of the tissue to absorb or dissolve the anesthetic drug (that is, volume × solubility coefficient). From these models it can be seen that increases in ventilation hasten the filling of the alveolar tank. Similarly, increases in tissue perfusion drain the alveolar tank and delay its filling. In this model the inspired pressure tank is kept filled to represent the clinical technique of constant inspired concentrations of anesthetic vapor.

Tissue compartments

The body contains many tissues, which can be classified into compartments according to their differing rates of blood perfusion:
- *Vessel-rich group* (VRG): brain, heart, liver, kidney, gastrointestinal tract, and lungs
- *Lean group* (LG): tissues with intermediate perfusion rates, such as muscle and skin
- *Lipid or fat group*: intermediate perfusion tissue of nonaqueous character
- *Vessel-poor group* (VPG): bone, cartilage, and tendon with very low perfusion

Fig. 4-3 is a redrawing of Fig. 4-2 that divides the tissue tank into these compartments, each with its vascularity represented by the connecting pipe. This model of anesthetic uptake shows that the VRG compartment will fill most quickly. The fat compartment, with a large anesthetic capacity to perfusion ratio, is the slowest filling tank. The VPG, with its negligible perfusion, is usually ignored. The rate of uptake for the various compartments in the case of an inhalation anesthetic of intermediate solubility (in this particular example, halothane) is shown in Fig. 4-4.

It can be seen from these graphs how VRG uptake virtually ceases in 20 minutes while muscle and fat uptake has hardly started. With anesthetics of high blood

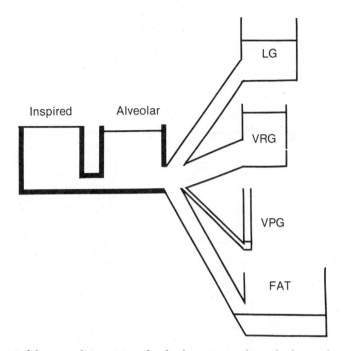

Fig. 4-3. Modification of Fig. 4-2 to divide the tissue tank on the basis of perfusion.

solubility, the rapid uptake by the blood and tissue prevents the alveolar pressure from rising at rates equal to drugs of low or intermediate solubility. Because arterial and alveolar pressures are the same, this delay means tissue pressure is slower to rise. In the case of methoxyflurane, which is highly soluble, the fat compartment does not reach equilibrium with arterial anesthetic pressure for over 2 weeks. Likewise, the bigger the tissue pipes (that is, higher cardiac output), the slower the rate of rise of alveolar pressure. However, the increase of ventilation pipe diameter enables alveolar pressure to rise more rapidly toward inspired anesthetic pressure. Again, the force moving anesthetic into (or out of) the body is the anesthetic pressure gradient between inspired gas and the alveoli. Therefore, by increasing the inspired pressure of an anesthetic, it is "pushed" into the body more quickly. This overpressure technique is used clinically where the anesthetic vaporizer is initially set well above the planned final maintenance level in order to speed induction.

Briefly, the model's simulation of anesthetic uptake reveals that arterial anesthetic pressure rises when ventilation and inspired anesthetic pressure increase and falls when cardiac output and drug solubility increase. Of course, all models like Mapleson's hydraulic model have limitations in mimicking nature. The model is only "one-way" because no depiction is made of venous return (venous anesthetic pressures are equal to the pressure in the tissues drained by the veins). Several other specialized effects that relate to the uptake of large amounts of the weaker

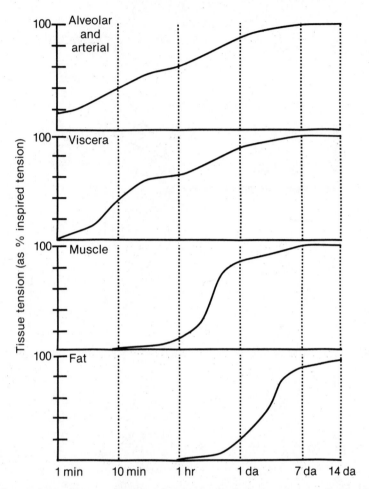

Fig. 4-4. Rates of anesthetic tensions in the various body compartments during the administration of a constant inspired tension of halothane.

anesthetics are not simulated by the hydraulic model. The model can be made to represent anesthetic recovery by removal of the inspired pressure tank (that is, reducing pressure to zero as when an animal breathes room air). This is shown in Fig. 4-5, where the vessel-rich group can drain to the lung more quickly since it has the highest pressure from having had the more rapid uptake. Ventilation and cardiac output are again the limiting factors in recovery.

Until the last decade it was believed that the inhalant anesthetic drugs were inert. However, it has become obvious that the halogenated hydrocarbon anesthetics are all metabolized by the body to greater or lesser extents. This is particularly important if the metabolites are themselves active or toxic. The latter has been shown to be important in humans, where renal toxicity has been caused by the

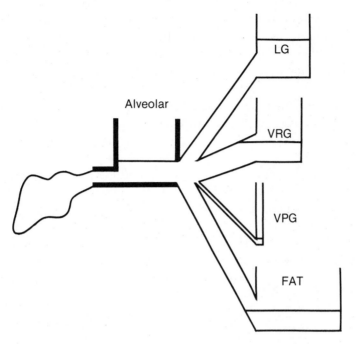

Fig. 4-5. Hydraulic model simulating termination of anesthesia with zero-inspired anesthetic pressure.

release of inorganic fluoride ions in the metabolism of methoxyflurane (most metabolism occurs in the liver). The proportion of the anesthetic drug that is metabolized increases with longer duration of anesthesia, fatness of the patient, and specific drug involved. The nephrotoxicity problem with methoxyflurane has not been shown to occur in normal dogs or cats, but it might be important in animals whose renal function is already compromised.

Clinical significance of anesthetic uptake

Induction

Induction of anesthesia means the process of taking an awake animal through stages I and II of anesthesia to stage III as smoothly and quickly as possible to produce partial pressure in the brain sufficient for anesthesia. Since the brain is a VRG tissue, it will reach anesthetic pressure well before the lean, fat, and VPG tissues have any degree of equilibration with arterial partial pressure. The more soluble the anesthetic drug, the slower the rise of arterial partial pressure. This is most obvious in the contrast between halothane and methoxyflurane (blood/gas λ = 2.4 and 13 respectively), where induction and recovery are much more rapid for halothane. Although induction can usually be hastened by overpressure methoxyflurane is an exception since it has a low saturated vapor pressure (that is, maximal partial pressure possible at room temperature).

There are other limitations to this overpressure technique. Excessively high inspired concentrations can precipitate laryngeal spasm (especially in the cat) or severe respiratory center depression. The less soluble anesthetics reach maintenance levels in the brain most quickly but, unfortunately, they have not to date been shown to be strong or potent drugs (for example, nitrous oxide).

Maintenance

The same factors that affect induction apply to the maintenance of anesthesia. Further, it should be remembered that, as in the hydraulic models, uptake by lean and fat tissues is continuing unabated. The sequel to this continued uptake occurs in recovery when these tissues release the anesthetic drug back into the blood. This creates prolonged low blood concentration, ideal for the liver's metabolizing enzymes to break down the drug. Toxic metabolites can cause delayed toxicity, as classically observed with chloroform, where hepatic and renal damage occurs at 2 or 3 days following anesthesia.

Recovery

During recovery, animals are at low physiologic and metabolic levels. Being cold, hypoventilated, and often in pain, an animal will frequently have a slower recovery than necessary. Increasing ventilation to speed recovery is only practical for agents of intermediate solubility, such as halothane. Nitrous oxide is excreted too rapidly, while methoxyflurane and ether are dissolved in such vast amounts that short-term ventilation is not efficient. When nitrous oxide anesthesia is terminated, the patient should be ventilated with 100% oxygen for 2 to 5 minutes. This is important because when the inspired partial pressure of nitrous oxide becomes zero, the drug flows from the pulmonary blood into the alveoli so rapidly that it results in *diffusion hypoxia*—displacement of oxygen in the lower respiratory tract. Another consideration in keeping recovery short is to allow patients to breathe room air rather than continuing to breath from the anesthetic circuit (unless oxygen

---

Solubility of inhalation anesthetics in rubber (at 20°C)

Nitrous oxide	1.2
Ether	25
Halothane	120
Methoxyflurane	635
Enflurane	74
Isoflurane	62

TABLE 4-3

Effects of three common physical conditions on anesthetic uptake parameters

	Fever	Aging	Shock
Ventilation	↑	↓	↓
Cardiac output	↑	↓	↓
Distribution of cardiac output	(1)	—	(2)
Body composition	—	Less lean, more fat	—
MAC	↑	↓	↑ ↓

(1) Vasodilation of periphery; (2) lean, fat, and viscera less perfused to maintain brain and heart blood flow.

enrichment is indicated). Thus the patient avoids inhaling any anesthetic drug coming out of solution from the circuit's rubber (many anesthetic drugs are extremely soluble in rubber [see p. 186]).

In summary, the effects of anesthetic solubility, alveolar ventilation, and cardiac output on anesthetic uptake and excretion are:

1. *Solubility*. The more soluble in blood a drug, the slower anesthetic induction and recovery will be (see Table 4-4).
2. *Cardiac output*. Increased cardiac output means more drug is taken from the lungs during induction, delaying arterial and VRG partial pressure increases. This delay is less important with the more soluble drugs because the loading of anesthetic drugs into blood passing through the lungs is not a limiting factor.
3. *Ventilation*. Increased ventilation increases anesthetic partial pressure in alveoli and therefore arterial blood. The more soluble drugs benefit from hyperventilation as their uptake into pulmonary blood is usually only slightly less than the anesthetic drug brought into the lungs by ventilation. (That is, the uptake of highly soluble drugs is limited by ventilation.) On the other hand, increased ventilation during recovery aids in elimination of drugs of intermediate solubility.

Pathophysiologic changes in animals affect drug uptake and distribution in complex ways that can only be sorted out by computer studies. In Table 4-3, three common conditions are compared to illustrate the complex interactions that can occur to alter an anesthetic's uptake and distribution.

PHARMACOLOGY OF INHALATION ANESTHETIC DRUGS

Ever since the gas sniffing experiments of the mid-1800s, the search for the ideal anesthetic has continued. An ideal inhalation anesthetic drug must be:

1. Safe with no delayed toxicity (preferably minimal metabolism)
2. Nonflammable
3. Chemically stable and nonreactive with soda lime

TABLE 4-4
Properties of the common inhalation anesthetic drugs

	Nitrous oxide	Ether	Halothane	Methoxyflurane	Enflurane	Isoflurane
Formula	N_2O	$C_2H_5OC_2H_5$	$CF_3CHClBr$	$CH_3OCF_2CHCl_2$	CHF_2OCF_2CHClF	$CF_3CHClOCHF_2$
MAC (%)	188	3.04	0.87	0.23	2.2	1.5
Molecular weight	44	74	197	165	184	184
Boiling point (°C)	−89	35	50.2	104.6	56.5	48.5
Saturated vapor pressure (mm Hg)	800 psi	400	243	22.5	184	261
Flammability levels (%)						
Air	—	1.9 - 48	—	9.0 - 28	—	—
O_2	—	2.0 - 82	—	5.2 - 28	—	—
N_2O	—	1.5 - 24	4.0	4.0	5.8	7.0
First clinical use	1845	1842	1956	1959	1966	1981
Trade name	—	—	Fluothane	Metofane (veterinary use) Penthrane (human use)	Ethrane	Forane
Cost/MAC L (as of Oct. 1981)	1 L pure N_2O = 0.90¢	0.23¢	0.33¢	0.22¢	2.07¢	3.44¢
Solubility (λ)						
Blood	0.47	12.1	2.4	13	1.9	1.4
Oil	1.4	65	224	825	99	60
Rubber	1.2	25	120	635	74	62
Color coding*	Blue	—	Red	Green	Orange	Purple

*Cylinder for N_2O and packaging, vaporizers, etc. for vapors.

4. A potent anesthetic (that is, producing anesthesia at reasonable concentrations)
5. Of low blood solubility for rapid induction and recovery

The major drugs used for inhalation anesthesia today are nitrous oxide, halothane, and methoxyflurane. Diethyl ether is steadily losing favor and probably is not used in any progressive practices today. In Table 4-4 the physical parameters relating to the major drugs are compared. A more detailed description of each drugs' pharmacology in small animals follows.

Nitrous oxide

In animals, nitrous oxide is such a weak anesthetic drug that it cannot produce anesthesia by itself. It is used in concentrations of 50% to 75% to supplement other drugs and, to avoid hypoxia, should always be administered with oxygen. Even at its maximal safe concentration of 75% nitrous oxide requires supplementation with a more potent drug, such as halothane, methoxyflurane, or enflurane, to produce adequate surgical anesthesia. Nitrous oxide can also be used in combination with a narcotic analgesic and a muscle-paralyzing agent for a lighter plane of surgical anesthesia. The enormously high MAC value of 188% for nitrous oxide (see Table 4-4) emphasizes this drug's inadequacy to produce surgical anesthesia alone. An interesting point is that older anesthetic machines have a nitrous oxide flush button designed to rapidly deepen anesthesia, which worked by producing hypoxia!

Nitrous oxide is supplied in compressed gas cylinders of various sizes. The common "E" and "G" tanks hold 1,600 and 13,000 L respectively. When manufactured for medical use, nitrous oxide at room temperature is 90% compressed liquid and 10% gas at a pressure of 750 psig. The international color code for nitrous oxide cylinders is blue.

Properties
- Colorless
- Odorless
- Nonirritating to mucous membranes
- Heavier than air (therefore tends to sink to floor level)
- Nonflammable but, like oxygen, will support combustion

Toxicity

Nitrous oxide is considered relatively nontoxic. However, one must be aware of potential impurities that can occur because of defects in manufacturing the gas. Nitrogen dioxide (NO_2) is of particular concern as it is very irritating and produces profound cyanosis.

When nitrous oxide is used to augment a more potent inhalation agent (for example, halothane or enflurane), the ratio of nitrous oxide to nitrogen dioxide should be between 2:1 or 3:1. This is accomplished by setting the flowmeter for the desired ratio, using a total fresh gas flow of 2 to 3 L. When nitrous oxide is combined with a more potent inhalation anesthetic drug, the concentration for the more potent agent is reduced by 30% to 60% because of nitrous oxide's anesthetic effects. Although a weak anesthetic, nitrous oxide is a powerful analgesic (it is used in childbirth for twilight sleep).

Nitrous oxide does not significantly depress respiration and has only a small depressant effect on the myocardium. So long as it is administered with at least 25% oxygen, nitrous oxide is a safe agent except where there is an enclosed viscus of air. Here there is a risk of increasing the volume or pressure of this air "bubble" since nitrous oxide diffuses into it faster than nitrogen can diffuse out. The most dramatic example is pneumothorax where nitrogen oxide diffusion can double the extent of the pneumothorax in 10 to 15 minutes. This rapid expansion can cause serious complications, such as a ruptured organ, decreased venous return to the heart, or air embolism. Therefore the use of nitrous oxide is contraindicated in the following situations:

- Pneumothorax
- Gastrointestinal obstruction
- Gastric torsion
- Lung cyst
- Diaphragmatic hernia when the stomach is in the thorax

There are two further problems associated with the use of nitrous oxide:

1. Toxic effects on bone marrow with prolonged administration (prolonged meaning days). This was discovered when tetanus patients were kept anesthetized for days at a time with nitrous oxide.
2. Abuse potential. People have died of asphyxia during nitrous oxide parties. Therefore these cylinders should be kept in a secure area.

Diethyl ether

Although first discovered by Valerius Cordus in 1540, ether remained relatively unknown for its anesthetic properties until the 1840s. Since then it has been used extensively in human anesthesia and was the main inhalation anesthetic drug until halothane was introduced in 1956. No single event in history has done more to stimulate and promote the art and science of anesthesiology and surgery than the discovery and use of ether for general anesthesia. Before then patients in need of surgery were manually restrained by several heavy-handed operating room assistants while surgeons boasted more of the speed with which they could perform an operation than the actual procedure involved.

Ether is rarely used in human or veterinary anesthesia today, mainly because of its *highly flammable* properties and its irritation of the respiratory tract mucosa, which stimulates copious amounts of salivary and bronchial secretions. The current primary use of ether in the veterinary profession is for anesthesia of small laboratory rodents in research facilities. Care must always be exercised when using or storing ether due to its explosive nature. One should never smoke, use an open flame, or create a spark in the presence of ether vapors. Even the small spark that can be created by static electricity can lead to an ether fire or explosion.

Ether is supplied as a clear liquid with a pungent odor. The bottle should be kept stoppered and away from strong light to prevent formation of peroxides that are extremely irritating to the respiratory tract. Even though it is very soluble in blood, its highly volatile nature makes a rapid induction possible. Induction, however, is associated with a marked excitatory stage and excessive upper respiratory tract secretions, which can be minimized by atropine premedication. A stable depth of surgical anesthesia, once obtained, is easily maintained. Ether produces good to excellent analgesia and muscle relaxation. Emergence from general anesthesia is slow and often associated with postoperative nausea and vomiting.

Vaporizer location. The vaporizer should be kept outside or inside the patient's breathing circuit. Ether must not be left in vaporizers for more than 2 days if peroxide formation is to be avoided.

Properties
- Colorless
- Pungent odor
- Unpleasant to inhale. Some animals hold their breath during mask or open drop induction. Ether is a potent irritant to respiratory and gastric mucosa, causing copious salivary and bronchial secretions. Postoperative nausea and vomiting are common.
- Heavier than air. Vapor tends to sink to floor level and concentrate into a vapor cloud.
- Highly flammable. Explosions of ether vapor can be caused by small sparks from the bottom of shoes, improperly grounded electric equipment, or electrocautery. If a fire occurs in the vicinity of a patient that is breathing ether, the fire can follow the path of the ether vapor and explode within the patient's lungs.
- Does not tend to corrode metal or react with soda lime

Effect on respiration. Unlike all other inhalation anesthetic drugs discussed, ether at light levels of surgical anesthesia stimulates alveolar ventilation because of its irritant nature and sympathetic stimulation. All other agents depress respiration at any level of anesthesia. However, at deeper planes of anesthesia, ether will depress respiration as do other inhalation anesthetics.

Effect on the cardiovascular system. Ether does not sensitize the myocardium to epinephrine-induced dysrhythmias as does halothane. At typical clinical levels ether maintains blood pressure and cardiac output at near normal levels. In this respect, it allows for a relatively stable cardiovascular system during routine cases. However, should sympathetic blocking drugs be administered, ether can become a potent myocardial depressant.

Toxicity. Ether has an irritating effect on the mucosa of the respiratory and upper digestive tracts. It also stimulates the vomiting center of the brain. Over the years, anesthesia with ether has been associated with the potential for liver toxicity and elevations in blood glucose. It is contraindicated in cases of diabetes mellitus, hepatic dysfunction, and fever (the last because of the risks of ether pyrexial convulsions). Newer anesthetics and derivatives of ether that have been introduced since the late 1950s have almost totally replaced ether in the operating room. Each new agent has been developed in an attempt to eliminate the undesirable aspects of ether and to develop the "ideal" inhalation anesthetic.

Halothane

Halothane is presently the most widely used inhalation anesthetic drug in the world. Its popularity within the veterinary profession rests with its rapid and smooth induction and recovery periods, controllability, and adaptability toward a wide variety of animal species. Halothane provides rapid and smooth induction and recovery periods.

At room temperature halothane can rapidly vaporize up to a concentration of 35% to 40%, which, if inhaled, would be lethal to the patient. Due to its highly volatile nature, halothane should *not* be used to induce anesthesia by the open drop technique. The vaporizer for halothane should be precision calibrated and therefore is a considerably expensive item. Analgesia is fair to good at surgical levels, but muscle relaxation may be poor.

Vaporizer location. The vaporizer should be located outside the patient's breathing circuit.

Properties
- Colorless
- Sweet-smelling
- Not unpleasant to inhale, although cats often hold their breath when a mask induction is attempted. Nonirritating to the mucous membranes of the mouth and respiratory tract. Unassociated with postoperative nausea or vomiting
- Heavier than air
- Nonflammable
- Will corrode brass or aluminum in a moist atmosphere but does not react with soda lime
- Rapid induction and recovery with minimal excitement. Postoperative shivering is common—a significant factor, as shivering can increase the metabolic oxygen requirement dramatically and precipitate hypoxia during recovery.

Effects on respiration. Halothane is a strong respiratory depressant that reduces tidal volume and increases respiratory rate. There is no irritant effect on the respiratory tract.

Effects on the cardiovascular system. Halothane is a potent myocardial depressant, which diminishes contractility in proportion to the depth of anesthesia. In addition to the bradycardia that often occurs, cardiac output and blood pressure are decreased. Bradycardia can be helped by the administration of atropine, but the other parameters respond only marginally to atropine. Halothane relaxes smooth muscle and causes a peripheral vasodilation. It also relaxes the myometrium and should not be used above 0.5% in a cesarean section if the risk of hemorrhage is to be minimized. Cardiac dysrhythmias are common during the use of halothane, especially bigeminy (that is, alternate ventricular systoles), nodal rhythm, and premature ventricular contractions. Hypercapnia (see Chapter 5) increases the incidence of these dysrhythmias. Thus increased ventilation should be one of the first measures taken to counter dysrhythmias. Dysrhythmias are important because they dramatically reduce cardiac output and can precede fatal dysrhythmias such as ventricular fibrillation. Halothane sensitizes the heart to catecholamines that can cause ventricular tachycardia and fibrillation. The highest nondysrhythmogenic dosage of epinephrine that can be given to a dog anesthetized with halothane is 1 to 1.5 μg/ kg over a 20 minute period. Since this dosage was established for healthy dogs, it must act as a guide only in clinical practice.

Toxicity. In addition to its hypotensive effects, the other main criticism of halothane is its role in postoperative hepatitis in humans. There is an incidence of approximately 1 in 10,000 to 100,000 cases, with much shorter odds if halothane anesthesia is repeated within 2 weeks. This hepatitis is simlar to that which occurred after chloroform anesthesia in that it appears 24 to 72 hours postoperatively, producing centrilobular necrosis. Although the mechanism is presently unknown, it is probably related to toxic metabolites. Fortunately, the syndrome has not been reported in either the dog or cat. Overall, considering the amount of halothane administered since 1956, it appears to be one of the safest anesthetic drugs available.

Methoxyflurane

Methoxyflurane is the most potent of the inhalation anesthetic drugs available today but, because of its high solubility and low volatility, has limited use. In veterinary anesthesia, methoxyflurane is often preferred to halothane for orthopedic surgeries for its potency and the fact that its analgesic effects extend well into the postoperative period. In humans, methoxyflurane has lost its popularity because of a dose-related high output renal failure following its use. This nephropathy, however, is caused by fluoride and oxalate metabolites rather than the methoxyflurane per se. There are no well-documented cases in dogs or cats, and all attempts to produce experimental renal failure with methoxyflurane in the dog have failed.

Methoxyflurane is the least volatile of the inhalation anesthetic agents and vaporizes only about 3% at room temperature. Thus it can be administered with relative safety by the open drop method. It may also be placed in a wick-type glass vaporizer within the patient's breathing circuit. Because of methoxyflurane's low volatility, out-of-circle vaporizers are designed to optimize vaporization, which can pose a problem if a methoxyflurane vaporizer is ever mistakenly filled with halo-

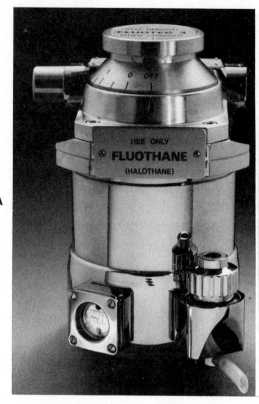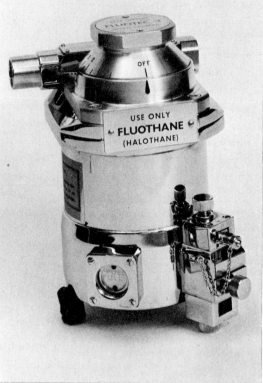

Fig. 4-6. A, Standard filler port on "Tec" vaporizers. **B,** Key Safety Filler System available for "Tec" vaporizers to prevent accidental filling with incorrect drug.

thane. The maximal position of the vaporizer dial, which normally produces 3% methoxyflurane, would now provide 30% halothane to the patient circuit—a rapidly fatal concentration to even the healthiest animal. Such an accident is preventable by the use of safety-filling devices (see Fig. 4-6).

Vaporizer location. The vaporizer is located outside or inside the patient's breathing circuit.

Properties
- Colorless
- Pleasant fruit-like odor
- Nonirritating to mucous membranes, with a low degree of postoperative nausea or vomiting
- Heavier than air
- Nonflammable at clinical concentrations
- Extremely rubber soluble

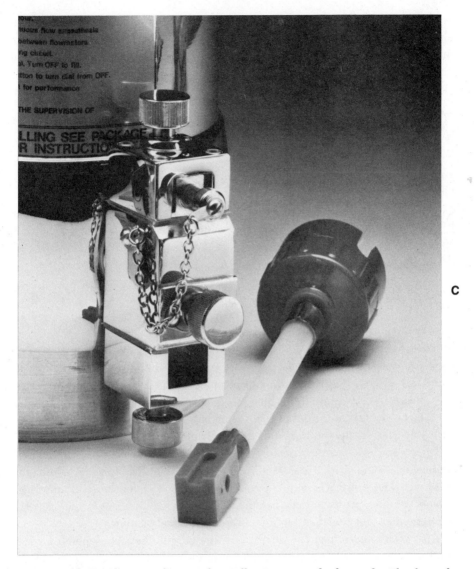

Fig. 4-6, cont'd. C, Close-up of Key Safety Filler System and adapter for Fluothane dispensing bottle. (Courtesy Fraser-Harlake, Inc.)

- Tends not to corrode or react with metals or with soda lime
- Centrally fixed eyes early in stage III—as with ether (in contrast to halothane, where the eyes remain medially rotated until a much deeper plane of anesthesia is reached)

Toxicity. Methoxyflurane sensitizes the myocardium to catecholamine-induced dysrhythmias but to a lesser degree than halothane. Methoxyflurane and halothane are both respiratory depressants at all anesthetic concentrations in that both tidal volume and respiratory rate are decreased, especially with deep levels of anesthesia and/or following premedication with a narcotic. Neither drug is irritating to the mucosa of the respiratory tract, nor does either stimulate salivary or bronchial secretions as would ether. Although sporadic cases of hepatotoxicity after methoxyflurane anesthesia have been reported in humans, none have occurred in animals.

Enflurane

Enflurane is one of the more recent inhalation anesthetic drugs and has become popular in human anesthesia. It induces anesthesia faster than halothane and provides slightly better muscle relaxation and analgesia. Enflurane is supplied as a clear liquid at room temperature and vaporizes to a similar extent as halothane.

Vaporizer location. The vaporizer is located outside the patient's breathing circuit.

Properties
- Colorless
- Ether-like odor, not unpleasant to inhale
- Relatively nonirritating, although postoperative vomiting or nausea can occur. In humans, postoperative headaches are commonly reported.
- Heavier than air
- Nonflammable
- Does not react with soda lime or corrode metal
- Relatively low solubility in blood ($\lambda = 1.9$, compared with 2.4 for halothane), thus providing a more rapid induction and recovery
- May cause hyperventilation or muscle twitching during deep anesthesia

Effects on the cardiovascular system. Enflurane has a dosage-dependent depression of myocardial contractility with resulting hypotension. although the pulse rate does not fall as much as with halothane. At deep levels of anesthesia it is more cardiodepressant than halothane. Less dysrhythmogenic than halothane, enflurane does not sensitize the myocardium to catecholamines.

Effects on respiration. The degree of respiratory depression depends on dosage, but enflurane does not induce the degree of tachypnea associated with halothane. At inspired concentrations of twice MAC, however, apnea occurs in the unstimulated patient.

Toxicity. Compared to halothane and ether, enflurane undergoes the least amount of liver detoxification, as 98% of the agent is eliminated unchanged via the lungs. Enflurane is associated with electroencephalogram (EEG) abnormalities, and seizures can occur with high inspired concentrations and/or hypocapnia. These EEG abnormalities can persist for over a week. Such CNS effects do not occur with its isomer, isoflurane. To date, enflurane appears to be as safe as (if not safer than) halothane in humans. Time will tell of its popularity in the veterinary profession.

Isoflurane

Isoflurane is the newest inhalation anesthetic drug, released for human use early in 1981. It is an isomer of enflurane and shares many of its properies. With a potency between that of halothane and enflurane, it is the least soluble and the most stable of all of the volatile anesthetics.

Vaporizer location. The vaporizer is located outside the patient's breathing circuit.

Properties
- Colorless
- Ether-like odor with slight pungency
- Nonirritating to mucous membranes
- Heavier than air
- Nonflammable
- Does not react with soda lime or metals and has a solubility in rubber similar to that of enflurane (see p. 186)
- Has a lower blood solubility and MAC value than enflurane and therefore is associated with a rapid recovery. The rate of induction is limited by its mild pungency, especially when administered by face mask
- Highly stable and the least metabolized of the volatile anesthetics. No demonstrated toxic effects on either the liver or kidneys
- Does not enhance the dysrhythmogenic effect of epinephrine

Effects on cardiovascular system. At surgical levels of anesthesia isoflurane causes minimal myocardial depression. It does cause hypotension because of decreased peripheral resistance, especially in the muscle vascular bed. Studies indicate that, of the volatile anesthetics, isoflurane has the highest cardiovascular margin of safety. It is also the least dysrhythmogenic inhalation anesthetic drug.

Effects on respiration. There is a dosage related depression of ventilation, which, while slightly greater than that of halothane, is less than enflurane.

Toxicity. Because of its stability, isoflurane has minimal effects on liver and kidney function, even with prolonged anesthesia. It has muscle relaxant properties similar to those of enflurane but greater than halothane. Neither the neurologic side effects of enflurane nor its abnormal EEG patterns are observed with isoflurane. Further, there is no present evidence of isoflurane being a teratogen or carcinogen, which is significant since one pilot study in 1976 suggested that isoflurane might be carcinogenic. Isoflurane is the most expensive anesthetic on the market today, but its future use may ultimately depend on the fact that it is superior to its nearest competitor, enflurane.

OPERATING ROOM POLLUTION

Since 1967 there have been a number of reports of increased spontaneous abortions among operating room (OR) staff. In 1974 a national study reviewed this problem in a retrospective survey of OR personnel. Using pediatricians and non-OR nurses as controls, this study found that there were increased statistical risks of:

1. Spontaneous abortion in pregnant OR personnel (up to twice the risk compared to the controls)
2. Congenital abnormalities in children of OR staff (twice the risk of the control groups)
3. Cancer, especially of the lymphatic system
4. Renal and hepatic disease

This study has been criticized in terms of its design and conclusions, but it has stimulated a more rational approach to the control of anesthetic wastes. It should be stressed that there is *no proof* that any of these risks are directly related to anesthetic wastes, only that one's statistical risks are greater in OR duty. The data could well be attributed to stress or other work-related differences.

Other problems that have been studied include intellectual impairment, immunosuppression, liver enzyme induction, and hypersensitivity reactions. Modern operating rooms include provision for removal of waste anesthetic gases (scavenging), and prospective studies in the future should serve to pinpoint the blame for these health problems (scavenging is dealt with in Chapter 6). Other measures to control anesthetic pollution include:

- Low flow techniques
- Better machine maintenance checks for leaks
- Choice of rebreathing systems
- Conservative anesthetic techniques

It is important that personnel be informed of the potential risks of exposure to anesthetic drugs, and it might be recommended that, until the controversy is resolved, pregnant women not work in the operating room for the first trimester.

The topic of anesthetic pollution is still a controversial subject and presently under federal investigation by the Occupational Safety and Health Administration (OSHA). To date no studies of anesthetic pollution effects have included veterinary personnel. In spite of the present uncertain status of waste gas pollution, OSHA is working on a document for release in the near future that may set specific limits on the levels of waste anesthetic gases permitted in human operating rooms, dental offices, and veterinary hospitals.

REFERENCE

1. Mapleson, W.W.: Simple analogue for the distribution of inhaled anaesthetics about the body, abstracts of contributed papers, Stockholm, 1961, International Biophysics Congress, p. 81.

ADDITIONAL READINGS

Eger, E.I., II: Anesthetic uptake and action, Baltimore, 1981, The Williams & Wilkins Co.
Lichtiger, M., and Moya, F.: Introduction to the practice of anesthesia, New York, 1978, Harper & Row, Publishers, Inc., Chapter 12.
Sawyer, D.C., Evans, A.T., and DeJoung, D.J.: Anesthetic principles and techniques, East Lansing, 1977, Michigan State University Press.

5

Practice of inhalation anesthesia

PERFORMANCE OBJECTIVES

After completion of this chapter, the student will:

- List the advantages of endotracheal intubation
- Discuss the complications associated with intubation of the trachea in dogs and cats
- List and discuss the four primary functions of the anesthesia machine
- Differentiate between "E" and "H" size compressed gas cylinders for oxygen and nitrous oxide in terms of color coding, physical state, filling volume, pressure, and pin-indexing
- Discuss the two major purposes of the patient breathing circuit
- List the clinical signs and physiologic complications associated with hypercapnia in an anesthetized animal
- Differentiate between semiopen and circle breathing circuits as they pertain to carbon dioxide elimination, the presence of one or more valves, the use of a reservoir bag, and acceptability relative to the size of the animal
- List the components of a circle breathing system and differentiate between a semiclosed and closed circle system
- List the major disadvantages associated with the use of semiopen breathing circuits for small animals
- Explain the purpose and technique for denitrogenation of the patient's lungs during the induction phase of inhalation anesthesia

ENDOTRACHEAL INTUBATION

A major prerequisite to proper administration of inhalation anesthesia is the placement in the trachea of a specially designed tube called an endotracheal tube. Although inhalation anesthesia can be accomplished by the use of a face mask, it is not desirable for long-term administration because of its disadvantages. A face mask adds considerably to mechanical dead space; it often leaks to room air, adding unnecessarily to pollution from anesthetic gases; it permits rebreathing of exhaled carbon dioxide and dilution of the delivered anesthetic concentration with room air and exhaled gases; and it does not allow the anesthetist to assist or control the animal's ventilation. Thus the advantages of endotracheal intubation in the anesthetized animal significantly outweigh its disadvantages.

Advantages

- Endotracheal intubation ensures an open (patent) airway.
- It can be lifesaving in the event of respiratory and/or cardiac arrest by allowing for immediate ventilation.
- It reduces anatomic dead space and allows for more efficient ventilation.
- It provides a means of preventing aspiration pneumonitis when an inflatable cuff is used.
- It allows for better suctioning of the trachea and bronchi should aspiration occur.
- It facilitates administration of oxygen and inhalation anesthetic drugs.
- It allows for better control of the animal's ventilation by providing a means for positive pressure ventilation.
- It allows for improved oxygenation of arterial blood.
- It prevents atelectasis of lung alveoli by providing a means for intermittent sighs during lengthy procedures.
- It protects the airway of an unconscious or comatose animal.
- It allows for control of lung ventilation during open-chest surgery.
- It ensures an unobstructed airway during the anesthetic and postanesthetic periods in brachycephalic breeds of dogs or cats.
- It decreases the chance for airway obstruction during surgical, diagnostic, or dental procedures involving the head and neck, especially when the head must be placed in a twisted or flexed position.
- It encourages visual inspection of the animal's mouth, pharynx, and larynx during intubation. Trauma, inflammation, or swellings that may have gone unnoticed can be indicated on the animal's record and may serve as a warning, should the animal have difficulty breathing during the recovery period.
- It provides a means for administering such special respiratory care as positive end expiratory pressure (PEEP), oxygen therapy, nebulization, humidification, and bronchoscopy.

Endotracheal intubation is a simple manipulative skill that is easily learned with practice, even with cats. It should be a routine procedure whenever an animal undergoes general anesthesia, no matter what drug is used or the length of the procedure.

Complications

The complications associated with endotracheal intubation are rare and most often due to an error in technique. Complications, however, are potentially dangerous both to the health of the animal and to the reputation of the veterinarian. They can occur at the time of intubation, during anesthesia, during the recovery period, or, in some cases, days later.

Misplacement of the tube

A common error in learning how to intubate is to place the tube into the esophagus instead of the trachea. This occurs most often with cats due to their narrow glottis and tendency toward laryngospasm. A misplaced tube will not provide anesthesia, and the animal will begin to show signs of awakening within 5 to 10 minutes. Airway obstruction can occur with subsequent hypoxia if the tube occludes the opening into the trachea. Gastric distention can also develop, leading to vomiting and/or impaired ventilation as a result of compression of the diaphragm. These complications can be avoided if one directly observes the passage of the tube into the trachea with the aid of a laryngoscope. Once in place the endotracheal tube should be secured to prevent accidental dislodgement. Confirming that the tube is in the trachea is important before proceeding further.

Trauma

Physical damage to the teeth or mucous membranes of the mouth, soft palate, pharynx, larynx, or trachea can result from repeated or overzealous attempts to intubate with a tube that is either too large, too stiff, or too dry. Hemorrhage can result, leading to aspiration and problems after extubation. A certain degree of mechanical irritation is associated with the presence of a foreign body in the trachea, and drying of the tracheal mucosa can occur due to inhalation of dry gases over a long period—resulting in a mild tracheitis for a short period after extubation (up to 3 days). Necrosis of the tracheal mucosa can occur if too large a tube is left in place for longer than 30 minutes or if the cuff on the endotracheal tube is overinflated. This can lead to a serious scarring and narrowing (stenosis) of the trachea because of pressure necrosis. In addition, atropine may cause a drying and thickening of tracheal secretions that may require additional postoperative effort by the animal to remove the secretions. Trauma to the lips or gums can result from a tube that is secured too tightly with gauze or rubber bands.

Endobronchial intubation

If the endotracheal tube is advanced too deeply, it may enter a mainstem bronchus (see Fig. 5-1), usually the right side. This can lead to a serious ventilation-to-perfusion inequality since one entire lung field would receive no ventilation. Hypoxia and hypercapnia would develop if the error went unnoticed. Anesthetic depth would be difficult to control, and induction time would be much longer than expected. The unventilated lung field would tend to collapse and become atelectatic. This situation is more apt to occur in cats and short-necked dogs with the use of a tube that is too long (see Fig. 5-2).

It is best to premeasure the length of the tube against the animal's neck prior to insertion. Ideally, the endotracheal tube should be placed with the tip midway between the larynx and thoracic inlet, with the adapter end extending just beyond the incisor teeth. Since most endotracheal tubes are made for humans, it is often necessary to shorten some sizes for use on short-necked animals. Once the tube is placed in the trachea it should be checked for correct position by auscultating both sides of the chest for breath sounds. Applying positive pressure to the reservoir bag while observing for bilateral chest expansion will also help ensure correct tube placement. If there is still any doubt, the tube should be retracted a short distance and the process repeated. Signs of incorrect endobronchial intubation are an animal taking longer than normal to respond to changing anesthetic concentrations and showing symptoms of inadequate ventilation.

Laryngospasm

Directly touching the vocal cords of a lightly anesthetized animal can cause a reflex closure of the vocal cords. The cords may reopen if the stimulus is removed, or the cords may go into spasm and cause obstruction to the airway (see Fig. 5-3). Cats are highly prone to laryngospasm, and care must be taken not to touch the vocal cords with the laryngoscope blade or the tip of the endotracheal tube. Spraying or painting the larynx of cats with lidocaine helps to prevent laryngospasm during intubation. If severe laryngospasms occur, the animal can be ventilated with 100% oxygen through a face mask. If laryngospasms do not subside within 1 minute and the animal cannot be intubated, the use of a muscle paralyzer such as succinylcholine may be necessary to break the spasms before hypoxia and cyanosis occur. Laryngospasms can also occur after the tube has been placed. If the endotracheal tube is too large, damage to the vocal cords may result, in which case the animal may exhibit hoarseness or difficulty swallowing following recovery.

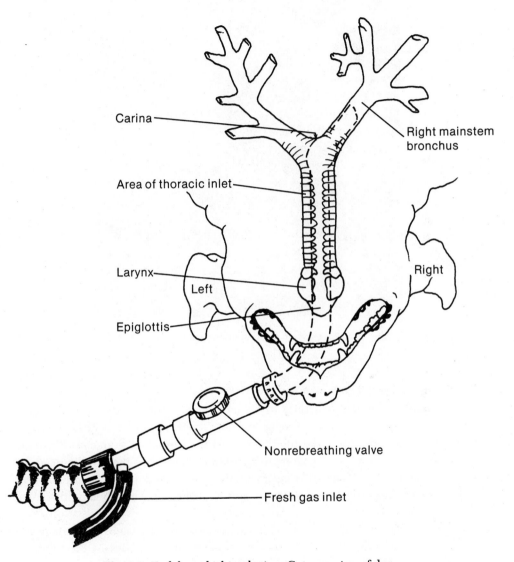

Carina

Right mainstem bronchus

Area of thoracic inlet

Larynx

Left

Right

Epiglottis

Nonrebreathing valve

Fresh gas inlet

Fig. 5-1. Endobronchial intubation. Cutaway view of dog.

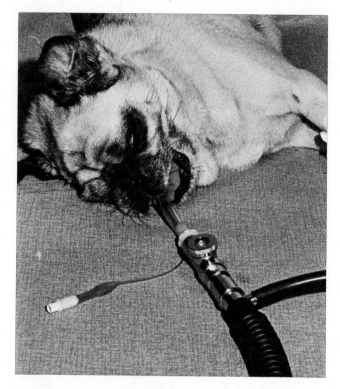

Fig. 5-2. Excessively long endotracheal tube in pug dog.

Obstructed endotracheal tube

Partial or complete obstructions to the endotracheal tube can occur at any time (see Chapter 2 for a discussion of signs of obstruction) and from a variety of causes:

- Occlusion of the tip of the tube (1) against the carina of the trachea (this may result in "bucking" or coughing in an attempt to displace the tube; it may also cause apnea if the animal is insufficiently anesthetized) or (2) against the wall of the trachea especially if the tube does not have a side hole behind the bevel (see Fig. 5-4).
- Occlusion of the tube due to overly tight gauze, rubber bands used for securing tube in position, or the animal biting down and compressiog the tube.
- Occlusion of the tube lumen by blood, saliva, or mucus
- Overinflation of the cuff, causing compression of the tube diameter or migration of the cuff over the tip of the tube. A general rule is that no more than 5 cc of air should be used to inflate the cuff. If it requires more than 5 cc to provide a tracheal seal, a larger tube should be inserted. Low pressure cuffs are available to help prevent this complication.
- Compression of the tube due to a surgical retractor or gauze pads

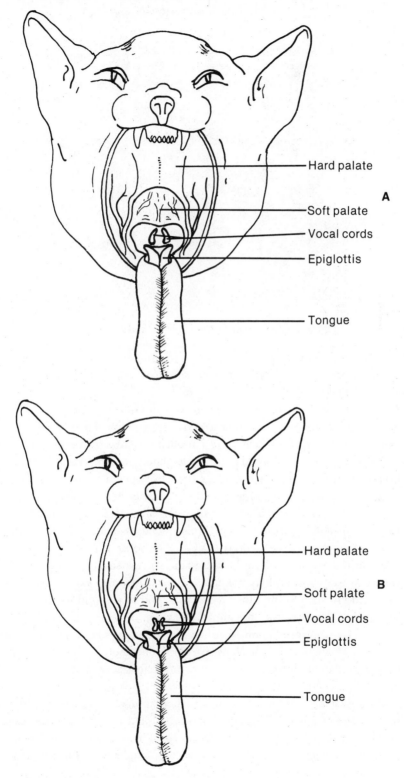

Hard palate

Soft palate

A

Vocal cords

Epiglottis

Tongue

Hard palate

B

Soft palate

Vocal cords

Epiglottis

Tongue

Fig. 5-3. Cat larynx showing **A,** open vocal cords and **B,** laryngospasm.

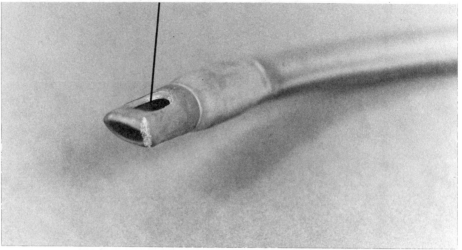

Fig. 5-4. Close-up of Murphy eye on endotracheal tube.

- Kinking of the tube due to overflexion of the head or neck or incorrect positioning of the tube distal to the incisor teeth. Use of a special coiled tube prevents kinking (see Figs. 2-20 and 5-5).
- Tube aspiration. If allowed to regain its reflexes while the endotracheal tube is still tied in place, the animal could bite through the tube and inhale the distal portion into the trachea or a bronchus. This can be avoided if careful attention is paid to the animal during its emergence from anesthesia.
- Cardiovascular complications. Dogs tend to respond to intubation of the trachea with an increase in parasympathetic activity because of stimulation of the vagus nerve. Bradycardia and hypotension are commonly associated with intubation in dogs. Cardiac dysrhythmias, such as bigeminal rhythm and premature ventricular contractions (PVCs), can occur. Cardiac arrest during intubation is seen more often in dogs than cats, especially in cases of cardiovascular disease, hypoxia, hypercapnia, or shock. Atropine can be used to counter the vagal effects. On the other hand, cats tend to respond to intubation of the trachea with an increase in sympathetic tone. Tachycardia and laryngospasm often accompany intubation. Cardiac dysrhythmias may also occur, although with less frequency than in dogs. Atropine does not counteract laryngospasm (although it does decrease the stimulatory effect secretions may have on the larynx).

The cardiovascular responses to endotracheal intubation can be modified or accentuated by preanesthetic drugs and anesthetics. Thiamylal, for instance, tends to increase the incidence of cardiac dysrhythmias. Phenothiazines, however, have a protective influence on the heart's response to epinephrine-induced dysrhythmias.

Hypotensive drugs, especially narcotics, tend to accentuate hypotension and bradycardia.

Intubation of the trachea coupled with anesthetic induction is one of the most dangerous periods of anesthesia. Careful monitoring and close attention to detail are essential if serious anesthetic emergencies are to be avoided.

Anesthesia for endotracheal intubation

Before an endotracheal tube can be passed through the larynx into the trachea, the animal must be anesthetized. Tracheal reflexes would cause the animal to expel the tube by forceful coughing, gagging, or biting. Passing an object of any dimension through the vocal cords of an awake or insufficiently anesthetized animal causes severe spasms of the vocal cords. Muscle-paralyzing drugs should not be used for intubation unless the animal is first rendered unconscious with a general anesthetic drug.

Three methods that can be used with veterinary patients to induce anesthesia before intubating the trachea are:

1. Intravenous injection of an ultrashort-acting anesthetic drug as either a rapid or slow induction sequence
2. Mask (or chamber) inhalation of halothane in oxygen or oxygen plus nitrous oxide
3. Intravenous injection of ultrashort-acting barbiturate followed by a low dose of a muscle-paralyzing drug such as succinycholine

The first method is the one most often practiced for inducing anesthesia in the dog and adult cat. Mask induction without a sleep-inducing dose of barbiturate is not practical in healthy animals weighing more than 10 to 15 kg due to problems of restraint and the requirement of extremely high fresh gas flows. The last method is not commonly used with dogs and cats because of the additional risks associated with muscle paralyzers and the essential requirement for artificial ventilation during the period of muscle paralysis. In methods 1 or 2 the larynx may also be coated or sprayed with a local analgesic drug to lessen the chance for laryngospasm. Slow barbiturate and/or mask inductions should not be attempted when rapid control of the airway is necessary (for example, in brachycephalic dogs or those with a full stomach or diaphragmatic hernia).

The trachea is intubated when the jaw muscles are sufficiently relaxed to allow the mouth to be opened wide with minimal resistance. In addition, the pharyngeal and laryngeal reflexes must be adequately obtunded to permit inserting the endotracheal tube into the trachea without violent coughing or laryngospasm.

Equipment for intubation

Endotracheal tubes

Two basic types of tubes are used for endotracheal intubation: soft and spiral. Soft endotracheal tubes are made out of soft plastics or rubber, but they tend to kink when flexed, especially the red rubber variety. Spiral tubes, also known as anode or Tovell tubes, contain a coil of metal or nylon embedded in latex rubber. They have the advantage of being more resistant to kinking or collapse from externally applied pressure, thereby decreasing the likelihood of airway obstruction while the animal is under anesthesia. Spiral tubes are quite flexible and can even be tied into a knot without collapsing (see Fig. 5-5). Due to their flexible nature, a stylet may be required to add rigidity during intubation of the trachea. Spiral tubes come in a variety of sizes and usually have an inflatable cuff on the patient end. Since these tubes are more expensive than soft tubes, they should be reserved for procedures involving the eye, head, or neck, where surgical draping makes it difficult to observe the animal's endotracheal tube for kinking. A spiral tube composed of a nylon inner spiral should be used for radiographs of the head or neck as stainless steel will interfere with radiographic interpretation. Although spiral tubes were developed to prevent collapse or kinking of the airway during anesthesia, they are not totally infallible. Since the inner coil of metal or nylon does not extend the entire length of the tube, it is possible for a kink to occur when either end of the tube is put into an extremely flexed position, especially if the endotracheal tube

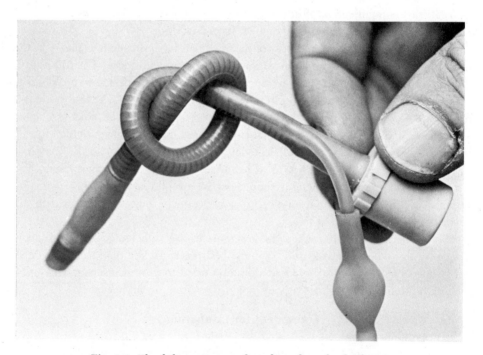

Fig. 5-5. Flexibility extreme of anode endotracheal tubes.

adapter is not seated well into the spiral or if the unspiraled patient end is pressed against the wall of the trachea in such a way that it kinks or invaginates.

Soft endotracheal tubes are made of rubber, vinyl plastic, or silicone. Red rubber tubes, extremely flexible at diameters under 6 mm, are relatively rigid in larger sizes. When using a small diameter rubber tube to intubate a cat, it may be necessary to introduce a metal stylet to add rigidity and form to the tube before attempting to pass it through the larynx. Rubber tubes are porous and tend to absorb anesthetic vapors or germicidal solutions, which can then act as tracheal irritants. With age, the red rubber tends to dry and crack especially where the adapter fits into the proximal end of the tube. Plastic tubes tend to be harder and stiffen more with age than the red rubber tubes. They are also inclined to soften once they reach body temperature and mold to the shape of the animal's airway. Recently, a synthetic type of medical grade rubber has become available for the manufacture of silicone tubes. Popular because of its lack of tissue-irritating properties, silicone rubber is smooth, nonporous, relatively frictionless, and easily repaired. It does not deteriorate, and it is not broken down by body fluids.

There are at least five different systems to classify the size of endotracheal

TABLE 5-1

A comparison of three commonly used systems for classifying
endotracheal tubes by size

Magill scale	French scale	Internal diameter scale (mm)
00	13	4
0	16	5
	18	
1	20	5
2	22	6
3	24	7
4	26	8
5	28	8
6	28	9
7	30	10
8	32	11
9	34	12
10	36	
	38	
	40	
	42	
	44	
	46	
	48	

TABLE 5-2

Guide for a selection of veterinary endotracheal tubes according to body weight

Body weight (kg)	Magill scale	Internal diameter (mm)
Cats		
1.0	00	3
2.0	0	4
4.0	1	4.5
Dogs		
2.2	2	5
4.0	4-5	6
7.0	6-7	7
9.0	8	7-8
12.0	9-10	8
14.0	9-10	9-10
16.0	10-11	10-11
18.0	11-12	11-12
20.0	11-12	12

tubes, which leads to considerable confusion in selecting or ordering tubes from various supply companies. The American Society of Anesthesiologists (ASA) has adopted the internal diameter (ID) system as a standard means for designating endotracheal tube sizes (see Table 5-1).

For the most part endotracheal tubes for small animals are the same as those used in human anesthesia. An orotracheal tube for humans is normally used for intubating dogs (see Fig. 5-6). Tubes for human infants and neonates are used for intubating cats or small dogs. Once a tube size has been selected, it should be premeasured against the length of the animal's neck. If necessary the adapter end should be shortened to prevent the chance of endobronchial intubation. The patient end of the tube should rest about midway between the larynx and first rib. The proximal end of the tube should protrude 1 to 2 cm beyond the incisor teeth so that it can be secured to prevent accidental swallowing or aspiration. If the tube protrudes too far beyond the incisor teeth, it increases dead space and is more susceptible to kinking or dislodgement.

The size of most endotracheal tubes is marked on the side of the tube along with several other reference markings (see Fig. 5-7). The information included on the tube varies according to the manufacturer and usually consists of:
- The manufacturer's brand name or symbol
- The word "oral" or "nasal" designating its intended route of passage in humans
- The internal diameter (ID) in millimeters
- The outside diameter (OD) in millimeters (or some other number system such as French or Magill)

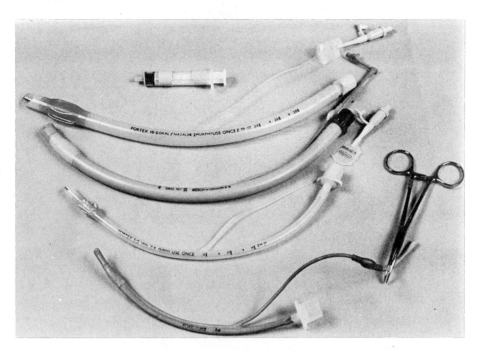

Fig. 5-6. Four different types and sizes of endotracheal tubes. From top to bottom: 5 ml cuff syringe; 10.5 mm plastic low pressure cuff; 9 mm red rubber, high-pressure cuff; 5.5 mm plastic low pressure cuff; 16 French red rubber high pressure cuff.

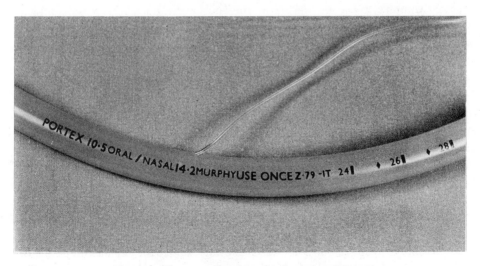

Fig. 5-7. Close-up of endotracheal tube markings.

- The letters "IT" (implantation tested), meaning the material used in manufacture of the tube has been implanted in rabbits to test for tissue reactivity. Some tubes have the symbol "Z-79" (representing the Z-79 Committee of the American National Standards Institute), which means the tube has passed various tests during manufacture.
- The words "Use once" meaning it should be discarded after use and not sterilized for reuse in humans
  - The length of the tube (in centimeters) as measured from the patient end, which serves as a guide when positioning the tube in the trachea

Endotracheal tube markings are placed on the beveled side and read from the patient end of the tube to the machine end. It is possible, therefore, to determine the position of the bevel within the animal's trachea should this become necessary.

Inflatable cuffs

In order to provide an airtight seal between the outside wall of the endotracheal tube and the inside of the trachea, many tubes come supplied with balloon-like cuffs on the patient end. When inflated with air, the cuff prevents leakage of gas around the tube and fluids from coursing their way into the lungs. A good tracheal seal also prevents dilution of inspired anesthetic gases with room air, which is necessary when giving positive pressure ventilation. In addition, it prevents leakage of anesthetic gases into the room air and positions the tube in the center of the trachea so the tip does not traumatize the tracheal mucosa.

A variety of inflatable cuffs is available. Slide-on cuffs can be used for tubes that are supplied without a permanently bonded cuff. The cuff material is usually manufactured from the same rubber or plastic as the tube.

The amount of pressure exerted by the cuff on the tracheal mucosa is a major concern, especially during long procedures and/or when using positive pressure ventilation. Thre basic types of cuffs are available on endotracheal tubes: high pressure cuffs, low pressure cuffs, and sponge cuffs.

High pressure cuffs have rigid walls and require considerable air pressure for inflation. The residual volume of air contained within the balloon cuff is less than in the newer, low pressure cuffs. When inflated to form an airtight seal, high pressure cuffs can exert excessive tension on a small area of the tracheal wall. Distortion of the trachea, tracheal necrosis, and/or compression of the tube can occur if volumes of air above the minimal amount needed to prevent leaks are injected into the cuff. The least amount of volume needed to form a minimal seal should be used when injecting air into high pressure cuffs. This is best accomplished by applying positive pressure to the reservoir bag while simultaneously injecting air into the pilot tube. When air is no longer heard escaping around the endotracheal tube, the injection is stopped and the cuff sealed. When administering a sigh to the animal's lungs, it is desirable to have a slight leak. Generally, if it requires more than 5 cc of air to attain a seal, the tube should be replaced with one of a larger diameter. High-pressure cuffed endotracheal tubes should not be used for long procedures or when positive pressure ventilation is to be used for an extended period.

Low pressure cuffs contain a greater volume of residual air than high pressure cuffs. They are prestretched and distribute their pressure over a larger surface area on the tracheal wall. Therefore, less pressure is required to produce an airtight seal. If the cuff is overinflated, a portion of it could herniate over the end of the tube, causing partial or total airway obstruction. Only that volume necessary to prevent a leak (as described in the preceding paragraph) should be injected when inflating the cuff with air. Low pressure cuffs should be used during long procedures or when administering positive pressure ventilation. Complete evacuation of the low pressure cuff is essential before insertion or extubation.

Sponge cuffs are made of polyurethane foam bonded to the endotracheal tube. The foam expands once it is inserted into the trachea and molds to it, forming an effective seal. The selection of tube size is critical since too small of a tube could result in an incomplete seal. If too large a tube is inserted, excessive tracheal pressure may result once the foam expands. Therefore, sponge cuffs are not used extensively with small animals.

All inflatable cuffs have inflating tubes that connect to the cuff for inflation once the tube is inserted in the trachea (see Fig. 5-6). A small pilot balloon at the inflating end of the tube indicates whether or not the cuff is inflated. The free end of the inflating tube is designed to accept a syringe for inflation and may be adapted with a one-way valve to prevent escape of air once it is injected. Care must be taken when inserting the endotracheal tube not to tear the cuff or inflating tube on the animal's teeth or laryngoscope blade. When the tube is secured in place, the inflating tube or pilot balloon should not be obstructed. Further, the functioning of the cuff and pilot balloon should always be checked before the animal is anesthetized for tracheal intubation, and care must be taken to avoid contaminating the patient end of the tube before its insertion into the trachea.

Care of endotracheal tubes. In most veterinary hospitals, endotracheal tubes are reused unless they become damaged or contaminated during an infectious case. After they are used, all endotracheal tubes should be scrubbed inside and out with soapy water, with care taken not to damage the inflatable cuff apparatus. If the tube cannot be scrubbed immediately after use, it should be immersed in a bucket of soapy water until it can be scrubbed and rinsed thoroughly. Then it can be immersed in an acceptable disinfectant solution (see Chapter 6). After adequate disinfection time, the tubes should be thoroughly rinsed in clean water and allowed to dry before they are repackaged for future use. When tubes have been used for an animal with a contagious respiratory infection, they should be sterilized by gas or gluteraldehyde or disposed of through incineration. Autoclaving is not recommended as it may destroy the plastic and/or shorten the life of the tube.

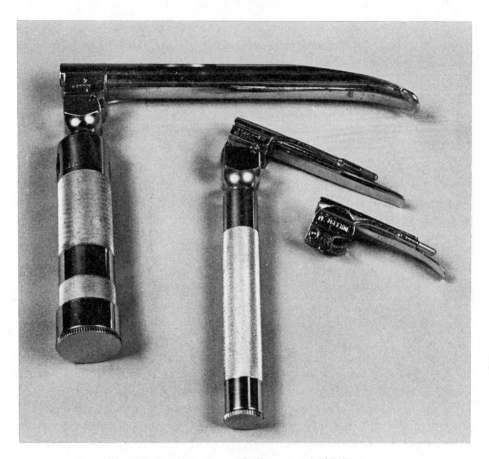

Fig. 5-8. Laryngoscope with three straight-blade sizes.

Laryngoscopes

A laryngoscope is a handheld device used for visualizing the larynx and nearby tissues. It is most often used to facilitate endotracheal intubation. Situations will occur when a laryngoscope cannot be used for intubation—for example, when an animal has a severe fracture of the mandible or a large oral tumor. It should be remembered that a laryngoscope is capable of breaking teeth or traumatizing the delicate tissues of the mouth and pharynx.

The basic parts of a laryngoscope are the handle and the blade (see Fig. 5-8). The blade, either curved or straight, is usually made of stainless steel and is detachable for purposes of cleaning and disinfection. A small lamp or fiberoptic point is recessed near the end of the blade to illuminate the laryngeal area. The bulb is powered from the handle through an electric contact that forms a circuit when the blade is in position for use. The blade should not be left in the "on" position when not in active use. Disposable or rechargeable batteries are used as the power source. Plastic disposable laryngoscopes are also available but are designed more for human use.

There are numerous laryngoscope blades available commercially—most of them designed for human use and named after their inventors. Of these only three or four are used routinely for dog and cat intubation, and their selection becomes a matter of individual preference. Most blades are variations on one another and reflect subtle differences in the shape and curve of the blade or in the position of the built-in light source. The majority of laryngoscope blades are designed for right-handed human anesthetists and contain a flange along one edge of the blade. The flange serves to deflect surrounding soft tissue and guide the tube down the blade and through the larynx. Unfortunately for right-handed veterinary anesthetists, this flange is in the way since animals are usually intubated in sternal recumbency while humans are intubated in dorsal recumbency. Ideally, veterinary anesthetists—to avoid having to pass the endotracheal tube over and across this flange—should seek a laryngoscope either without a flange blade or one designed for a left-handed human anesthetist (see Fig. 5-9).

When a *curved* laryngoscope blade is used, the tip should be placed in the vallecula (furrow) between the epiglottis and the base of the tongue (see Fig. 5-10). Pulling the tongue forward helps the anesthetist to check for correct placement of the laryngoscope blade. The blade is then used to depress the tongue and epiglottis, which pulls the epiglottis forward and exposes the larynx. The blade and handle are never to be used as a lever as this can cause trauma to teeth and soft tissue. When a *straight* laryngoscope blade is used, the tip of the blade depresses the tip of the epiglottis in order to expose the larynx, vocal cords, and glottis. Straight blades, when used to depress the epiglottis of a cat, may stimulate laryngospasm if advanced too far over the epiglottis.

Laryngoscopes are preferred over digital or blind intubation because they (1) allow direct visualization of the larynx and surrounding anatomic structures and (2) decrease the chance of inadvertent trauma to the pharynx and larynx caused by blind endotracheal intubation.

Techniques for endotracheal intubation

Techniques for intubating dogs and cats vary according to the species and individual preference of the anesthetist. Generally, one of three different methods is used:

1. Direct visualization of the tracheal opening (glottis) with a laryngoscope
2. Tactile intubation where the index finger of one hand is used to depress the epiglottis and guide the tube into the trachea. This method is of little use in cats, but it does allow some direct vision of the larynx in larger dogs.
3. Blind intubation, where the tube is passed through the mouth and manipu-

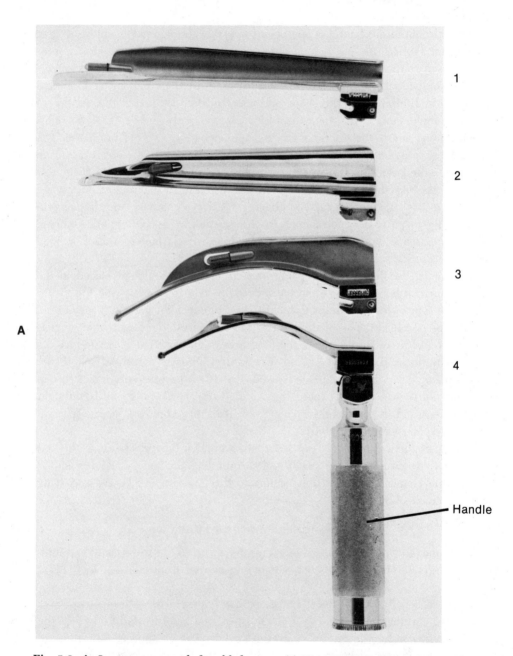

Fig. 5-9. A, Laryngoscope with four blade sizes: (1) Wis-Foregger, (2) MacIntosh straight, (3) MacIntosh curved, (4) Bizarri-Guiffrida.

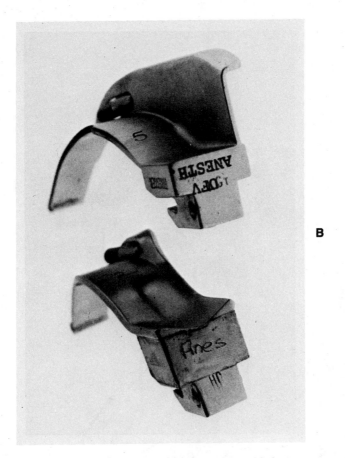

B

Fig. 5-9, cont'd. B, End-on view of two curved blades. Bottom blade (Bizarri-Guiffrida) has a minimal flange.

lated over the epiglottis and into the trachea. If the tube is being controlled with the right hand, the left is used to open the mouth and extend the tongue (see Figs. 5-11 and 5-12). The tube is then guided along the roof of the mouth and over the epiglottis, using the curve of the tube to direct the tip down through the vocal cords into the trachea. This method requires considerable dexterity and a knowledge of the local anatomy to avoid traumatizing the pharynx or larynx. Since there is a tendency to pass the tube into the esophagus or stimulate laryngospasm during a blind intubation, this technique is not recommended as a routine procedure. However, it may be the only means available when intubating a dog (or cat) without assistance or when the mouth cannot be opened wide enough to allow visualization of the larynx. *Text continued on p. 221.*

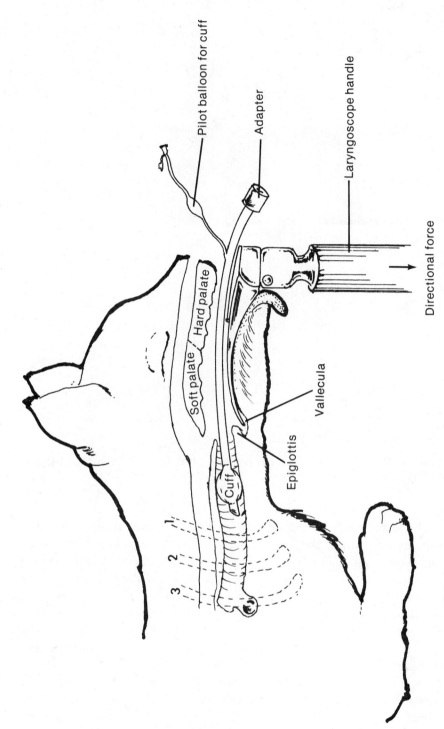

Fig. 5-10. Schematic cutaway view of cat showing correct position for curved laryngoscope blade.

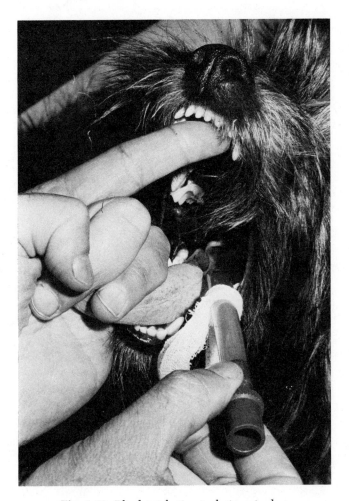

Fig. 5-11. Blind intubation technique in dog.

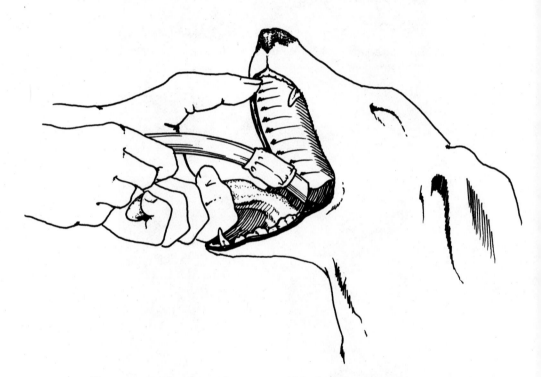

Fig. 5-12. Hand positions for unassisted blind intubation of dog trachea.

Each of these techniques requires extending the tongue and head so that the mouth and larynx are in a nearly straight line.

Dog intubation

Dogs are generally easier to intubate than cats. The mouth opens wide and the larynx has a large glottis that lies in a relatively easy position to visualize (see Fig. 5-13). Brachycephalic breeds are more difficult to intubate due to a large tongue and overly long soft palate. In addition, the smaller brachycephalic breeds have a short neck, and care must be taken not to pass the tube too far into a mainstem bronchus. Intubation is easiest when the dog is placed in sternal recumbency; however, intubation is also possible in lateral or dorsal recumbency.

Preparation for intubation. Before inducing anesthesia in a dog or cat, it is best to assemble and check all supplies and equipment necessary for endotracheal intubation, selecting at least two different tube sizes in case the first one turns out to be too large or too small. Supplies that are generally needed for or during intubation include:

Anesthesia form
Syringe and needle for the thiobarbiturate
Alcohol and cotton
Gauze for securing the tube in place
Laryngoscope
Endotracheal tubes with adapters
Electric clipper
Intravenous catheter
Intravenous fluid setup
Three strips of 1 inch adhesive tape for securing the intravenous catheter or syringe
Water soluble lubricating jelly
Small cuff-inflating syringe
Bland ophthalmic ointment
Esophageal stethoscope
Inhalation anesthesia machine
Face mask
Ambu bag
Emergency drugs
Any other preferred items

Obviously all these supplies cannot be placed on the same table as the animal. However, anesthesia should not be induced until all necessary equipment is immediately available. Anesthetic induction is a high risk period for the animal, and intubation must proceed smoothly and without unnecessary delays.

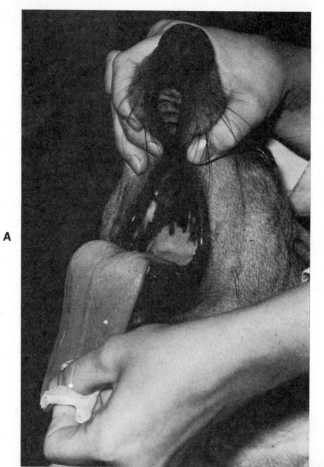

A

Fig. 5-13, A and B. For legend see opposite page.

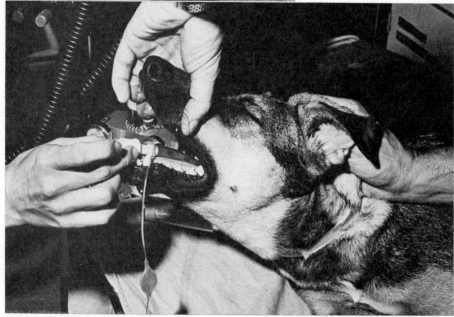

B

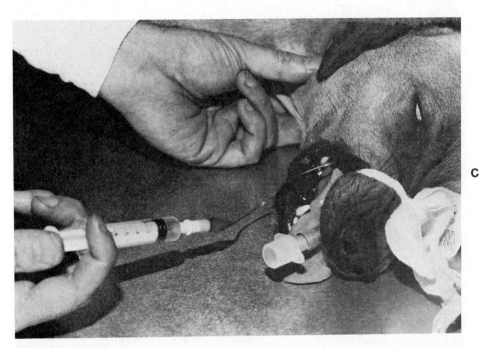

Fig. 5-13. A, Assistant restrains dog's head and tongue before endotracheal intubation. Head and neck should form a straight line while gentle traction on the tongue pulls the larynx anteriorly. **B,** Endotracheal tube is placed into the lumen of the trachea so that the adapter protrudes just beyond the lower incisor teeth, and the curvature of the tube matches that of the dog's head and neck. **C,** Endotracheal tube is secured to the dog's upper jaw with a soft gauze tie. The cuff is inflated while the tracheal-laryngeal region is palpated for correct placement and air leakage around the outside diameter of the tube. If inhalation anesthesia is being used, the endotracheal tube should be connected to the breathing circuit of the anesthesia machine at this stage. Once connected to the machine, oxygen and anesthetic vapor are allowed to flow.   *Continued.*

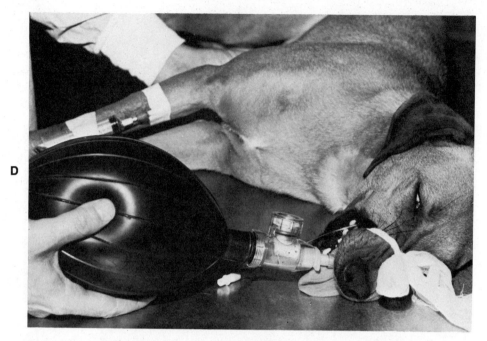

Fig. 5-13, cont'd. D, Emergency ventilation. An Ambu bag connected to the endotracheal tube may be used to artificially ventilate an animal with room air should apnea occur. A source of 100% oxygen can be connected to the open end of the Ambu bag, allowing for a higher inspired oxygen tension. Connecting the patient to the breathing circuit of the anesthesia machine also provides a means to support ventilation with 100% oxygen. The nonrebreathing valve (foreground) on the Ambu bag permits single-handed ventilation while the other hand is free for palpating the apex beat (background) or femoral pulse. Note that the right eyeball is rotated ventrally and medially so that the iris is hidden behind the prolapsed third eyelid.

Procedure. Following is a stepwise description for a normal dog intubation performed with technical assistance:

1. Assemble all necessary supplies and equipment, and verify all are in working order.
2. Induce general anesthesia.
3. Place dog in sternal recumbency.
4. Lubricate patient end of tube with a sterile, water soluble lubricant. If a stylet is to be used, it should also be lubricated before being placed inside the tube.

5. Have assistant hold the mouth open and align the head and neck by grasping the upper lips in one hand and extending the tongue with the other hand. Proper position allows an easier intubation. The assistant must also restrain the dog to prevent twisting of the neck or loss of the sternal position.

6. Place laryngoscope blade in its correct position to visualize the arytenoid cartilages (vocal cords).

7. Under direct visualization pass the lubricated end of the tube through the tracheal opening (glottis).* The tip of the tube should be about halfway between the larynx and first rib. The adapter end should not extend more than 2 to 3 cm beyond the incisor teeth. Turn laryngoscope off.

8. Secure the tube with a gauze half-knot, then tie the gauze around the upper or lower jaw behind the canine teeth or, on small dogs, in back of the ears. A quick release knot is used in case the tube has to be removed quickly. Test the setup by lightly pulling on the tube. It should not slip through the half-knot or dislodge from the jaw.

9. Connect the adapter of the endotracheal tube to the anesthesia machine as soon as possible. Do not allow the breathing hoses of the anesthesia circuit to add drag on the tube, as it may dislodge from the trachea.

10. Inflate the cuff of the endotracheal tube with just enough air to form a seal between tube and trachea. This is best accomplished by closing the pop off valve on the anesthesia machine and applying 10 to 15 cm H_2O positive pressure to the reservoir bag. If a leak is heard around the tube, inject air into the cuff until the leak is very slight or heard only when administering a sigh.

11. Before proceeding, check to be sure there are no kinks or occlusions of the endotracheal tube or breathing circuit. Support the dog's head and breathing tubes to minimize drag on the endotracheal tube. Premeasure and insert an esophageal stethoscope and/or attach other monitoring devices.

*The opening into the trachea is centrally located. The opening into the esophagus is to the left and dorsal to the glottis. The endotracheal tube should be passed with the curve matching the normal curvature of the dog's head and neck. To make sure that the tube is in the trachea, it may be necessary to palpate the esophagus along the left side of the neck. If two tubular structures are felt, it means the endotracheal tube has been misplaced. In addition, the adapter end of the tube should be felt for exhaled air. If the tube is correctly positioned, the air will exit the tube with discernible force. Placing a mirror or shiny metal object in front of the adapter end is also helpful in assuring correct placement of the tube. If the tube is in the trachea, exhaled water vapor can be observed on the mirror or metal surface. If the dog is lightly anesthetized, it often elicits a cough or two as the tube enters the trachea. The animal cannot vocalize if the tube is correctly positioned through the larynx into the trachea.

Cat intubation

A cat is more difficult to intubate because of its small mouth and sensitive larynx. Although the tongue is relatively small, the oral cavity is also reduced in size. The dome-shaped vocal cords tend to direct the tube to either side, usually into the esophagus. The jaws of a cat do not open as widely as a dog, leaving little room for the assistant's fingers or a laryngoscope blade. Since the reflex causing laryngospasm persists even into deeper planes of anesthesia, the use of a local analgesic spray on the larynx is advocated to lessen the chance of laryngospasm, which can occur both during and after tube insertion. However, cats can be intubated without the use of a local analgesic if one is careful not to touch the vocal cords or adjacent tissue with the tube or laryngoscope. But if the larynx does enter into spasm, it is best not to proceed until the cords have relaxed or the anesthesia is deepened. When inhalation anesthesia by face mask is used, it is important to make certain the cat is sufficiently anesthetized to allow tracheal intubation. Jaw tone, eye position, and reflexes should be assessed before removing the face mask (see Fig. 5-14). Healthy cats recover from the effects of halothane very rapidly. Thus if too much time is spent in preparation, the cat may awaken and/or laryngospasm may occur.

Cats should be intubated by direct visualization of the larynx. When assistance is available, it is easiest to place the cat in a sternal position. Unassisted cat intubation can be accomplished with practice and is best achieved with the cat in dorsal recumbency. Blind intubation is not recommended because of the sensitive nature of the cat's pharyngeal and laryngeal reflexes. A cuffed or uncuffed endotracheal tube can be used (see Fig. 5-15), ranging usually from 2.5 to 4.5 mm (ID) in size. A soft metal stylet may be useful in directing the small tube through the larynx. A small curved pediatric size laryngoscope blade (75 to 85 mm) can be used to illuminate the delicate tissues of the larynx. The vocal cords should not, of course, be touched with the laryngoscope or endotracheal tube.

Procedure (see Fig. 5-16). When passing the endotracheal tube it is best to hold the tip so it is anterior to the vocal cords, which will allow observation of the movement of the cords (see Fig. 5-3). When the cat exhales, the cords open to their greatest width so that passage of the tube through the glottis is easiest toward the end of exhalation. The endotracheal tube should never be forced through the vocal cords if the tube is too large or the cords are in spasm. Inspection of the cat's mouth and laryngeal area should be a routine step during the intubation procedure. When positioning for intubation, the assistant should not place his or her fingers in the cat's mouth (a gauze tie along the upper and lower jaw can be used to hold the mouth open without obstructing the anesthetist's view [see Fig. 5-17]). If lidocaine is used on the larynx 15 to 30 seconds should be allowed for effect before intubation is attempted. If a cuffed endotracheal tube is used it is important not to inject more than a total of 1 to 2 cc of air when the cuff is inflated (a tube should never be passed into or out of the larynx when the cuff is inflated). *Text continued on p. 231.*

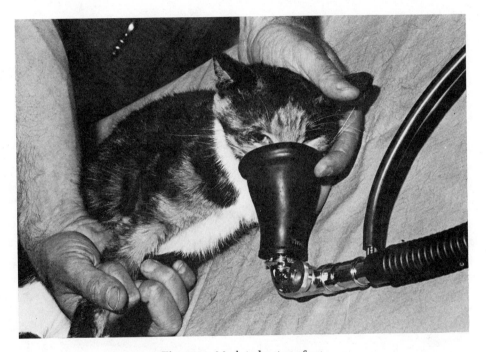

Fig. 5-14. Mask induction of cat.

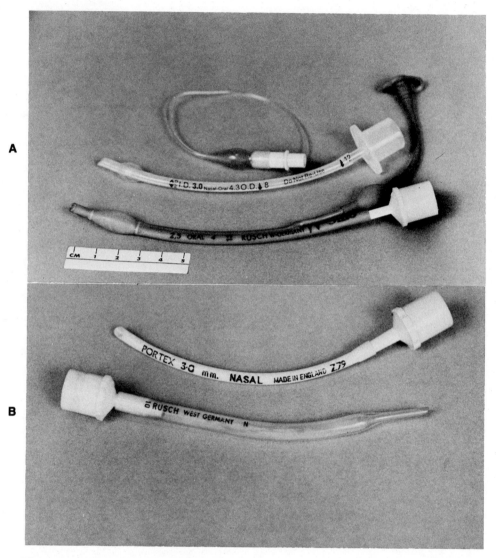

Fig. 5-15. A, Cuffed and **B,** uncuffed endotracheal tubes for cats or small dogs. The tapered tube at the bottom is designed to prevent endobronchial intubation.

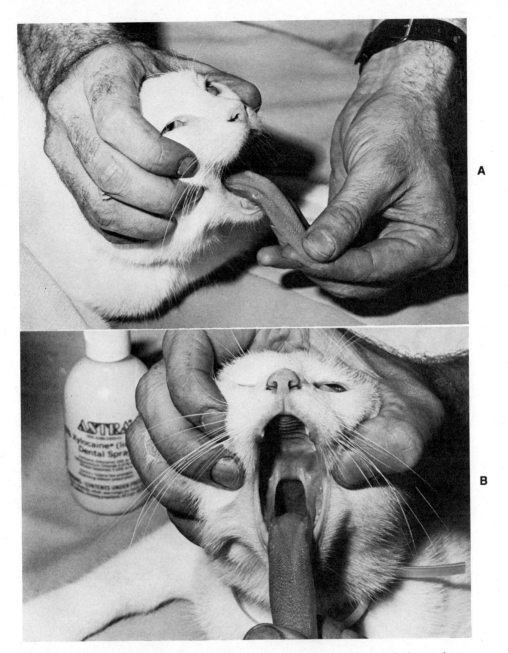

Fig. 5-16. Cat intubation sequence. **A,** When cat is anesthetized adequately for intubation, the jaw is relaxed and the tongue can be pulled anteriorly to expose the posterior pharynx and larynx. The assistant places the cat in sternal recumbency. One hand grasps the cat's head and raises it by lifting on the posterior maxilla. **B,** Anterior view of anesthetized cat's oral cavity. By lifting the cat's head, the lower jaw hinges open, and the tongue can be pulled forward to expose the larynx. Care must be taken not to overextend the tongue or puncture the ventral aspect of the tongue with the lower canine teeth. The tongue is purposely overextended in these photographs to better demonstrate the anatomy of the posterior oral cavity. Note that even with overextension of the tongue, the epiglottis and larynx remain hidden from view. *Continued.*

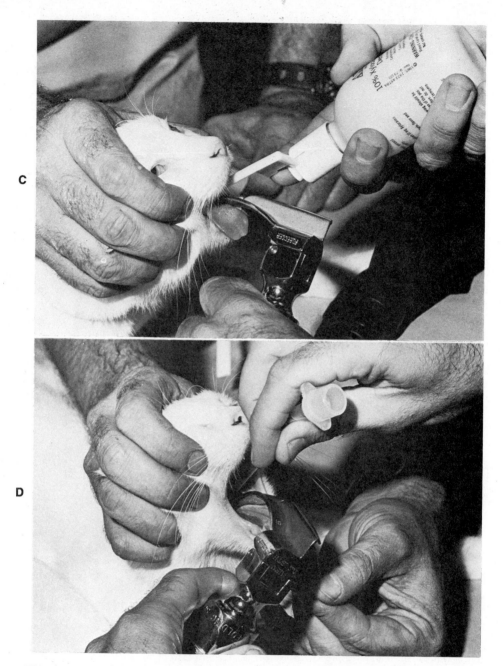

Fig. 5-16, cont'd. C, The assistant releases the tongue while the anesthetist exposes the larynx with a laryngoscope and desensitizes the area with lidocaine spray before insertion of the endotracheal tube. **D,** The assistant holds the cat to expose the larynx while the anesthetist gently passes the endotracheal tube through an open glottis. Care must be taken not to touch the larynx with the laryngoscope blade or endotracheal tube as laryngospasm can be precipitated.

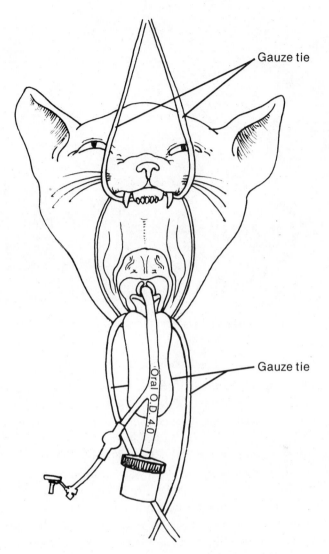

Fig. 5-17. Use of a gauze tie for opening cat's mouth.

When the endotracheal tube is in place (see Fig. 5-18), gauze is tied around the tube and the lower jaw posterior to the canine teeth or behind the ears to prevent dislodgement. Care should be taken to avoid incorporating the cat's tongue in the tie or compressing the endotracheal tube. Once the tube is secured, an esophageal stethoscope may be passed to monitor heart sounds and respiration. Kinking or twisting of the endotracheal tube is more often a complication with cats than with dogs, especially if the tube extends too far out of the mouth.

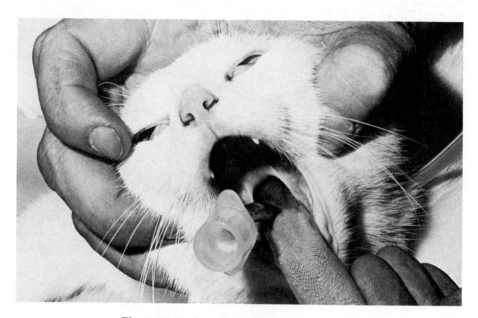

Fig. 5-18. Endotracheal tube in place in a cat.

Extubation

The endotracheal tube is generally left in place until the animal begins to swallow, cough, or chew on the tube. Brachycephalic breeds require special attention during this period. Removal of the tube in these animals must not take place until they are more fully conscious and able to maintain a free airway.

Vomiting may occur during the early stages of the recovery period before the animal has regained its reflexes. Since blood, saliva, or regurgitated fluid may have collected in the pharynx or upper trachea during the anesthetic period, suctioning of these regions through the endotracheal tube may be necessary before the tube is removed. However, sustained and excessive suction within the trachea should be avoided since it can collapse the lungs and deplete them of oxygen. The suction catheter is introduced into the tube, but suction is applied only while withdrawing the catheter. The animal is then ventilated with 100% oxygen before attempting any additional suction. It is usually unnecessary to suction more than once or twice to clear an endotracheal tube. Allowing the animal to regain its swallowing reflex before extubation will lessen the chances for aspiration of collected fluid into the lungs.

The cuff should always be deflated before the tube is removed from the trachea. The pilot balloon should also be checked to verify that the cuff is deflated. Pulling a tube out of the trachea with its cuff fully inflated can cause unnecessary trauma to the larynx and/or laryngospasm. Before the tube is removed, the animal should be allowed to breath 100% oxygen for 3 to 5 minutes after discontinuing anesthesia.

In addition, the gauze tie should be loosened and the cuff deflated in anticipation of the possible need for a rapid extubation, should the animal regain its reflexes sooner than anticipated. Whenever possible the tube should be removed at the peak of inhalation, just as exhalation begins.

During emergence from anesthesia, the animal should be positioned so that its head, neck, and tongue are extended. After the tube has been removed, it should be inspected for blood or mucus and checked for cuff leaks before cleaning and disinfection.

THE INHALATION ANESTHESIA MACHINE

For many years inhalation anesthesia was practiced without the convenience of an anesthesia machine, using only a mask and ether (or chloroform) by open drop technique. Anesthesia machines were developed to enable the anesthetist to accurately measure and administer anesthetic gases to the patient. The use and acceptance of these machines—manufactured by a number of different companies—have greatly increased the safety and ease of administering general anesthesia to veterinary patients. In spite of differences in their outward appearance, all inhalation anesthesia machines contain two basic components:

1. A system for delivering compressed oxygen gas mixed with anesthetic vapor. In addition, there may be a system for compressed nitrous oxide and cyclopropane gases.
2. A patient breathing circuit (see Fig. 5-19)

Safety in anesthesia dictates that those who are to administer inhalation anesthesia have both a working knowledge of the gas anesthesia machine and the principles of its design and construction. The student is urged to read further on the design and functioning of these machines, especially about complications that may result from their incorrect use. Machines are, of course, subject to malfunction, and an anesthesia machine incorrectly used can become a lethal instrument. Some potentially dangerous situations to watch for are:

- Depletion of compressed oxygen supply during a procedure. The animal rapidly becomes hypoxic, especially if allowed to breath 100% nitrous oxide.
- Anesthetic vaporizer filled with the wrong anesthetic drug, causing an irregular anesthetic state or an overdosage
- Anesthetic vaporizer inadvertently set at a high concentration, resulting in anesthetic overdosage
- Depletion of anesthetic liquid during a procedure, with the animal emerging from anesthesia
- Compressed nitrous oxide cylinder connected to the oxygen yoke (or vice versa) so that the animal receives an incorrect gas mixture and asphyxiates or has an irregular anesthesia period
- Carbon dioxide absorber becomes exhausted, with animal rebreathing its exhaled carbon dioxide, leading to hypercapnia and respiratory acidosis

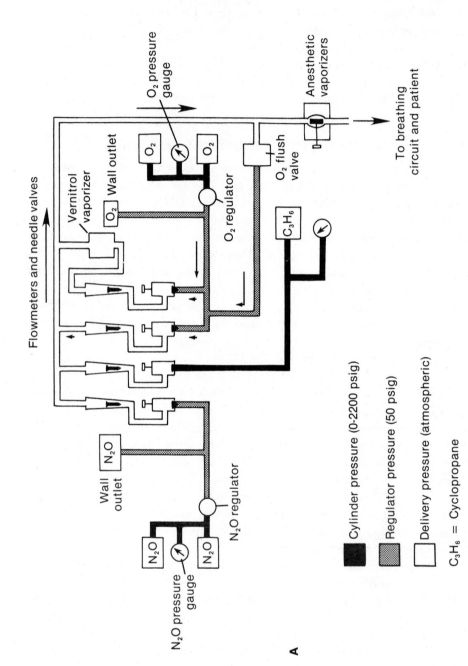

Fig. 5-19, A. For legend see opposite page.

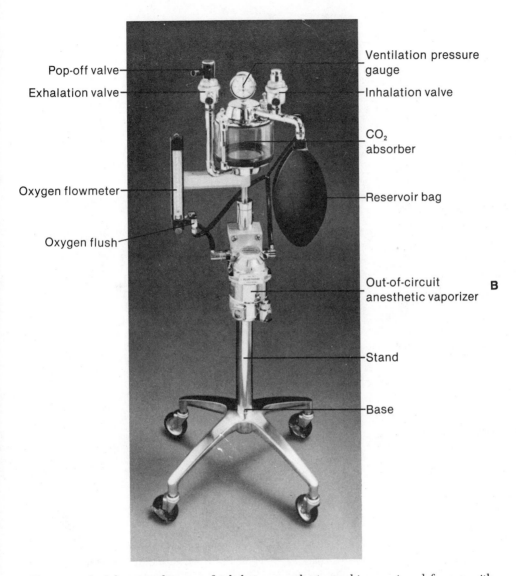

Pop-off valve

Exhalation valve

Oxygen flowmeter

Oxygen flush

Ventilation pressure gauge

Inhalation valve

CO_2 absorber

Reservoir bag

Out-of-circuit anesthetic vaporizer

Stand

Base

B

Fig. 5-19. A, Schematic diagram of inhalation anesthesia machine equipped for use with three compressed gases (nitrous oxide, oxygen, and cyclopropane [$C_3 H_6$]) in addition to a Vernitrol vaporizer and one or more direct-reading calibrated anesthetic vaporizers, all of which are located outside the patient breathing circuit. Nitrous oxide and oxygen gases can be delivered from pipeline wall outlets or from two compressed "E" cylinders attached to the machine, whereas cyclopropane is delivered only from a single "E" cylinder attached to the machine. Arrows indicate direction of oxygen flow. **B,** Basic inhalation anesthesia machine. Single oxygen flowmeter connects to pipeline system. Breathing tubes and Y-piece are not shown.

Continued.

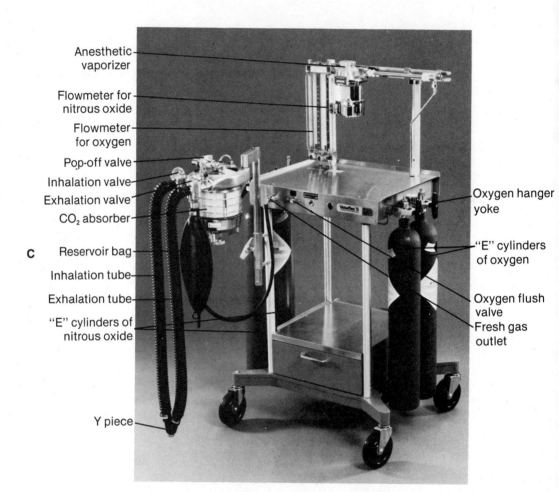

Anesthetic vaporizer

Flowmeter for nitrous oxide

Flowmeter for oxygen

Pop-off valve

Inhalation valve

Exhalation valve

CO_2 absorber

Reservoir bag

Inhalation tube

Exhalation tube

"E" cylinders of nitrous oxide

Y piece

C

Oxygen hanger yoke

"E" cylinders of oxygen

Oxygen flush valve

Fresh gas outlet

Fig. 5-19, cont'd. C, Two-gas inhalation anesthesia machine with out-of-circuit vaporizer for methoxyflurane. There are two yokes for oxygen and two for nitrous oxide. The line leading from the fresh gas outlet can be directed into a circle system (as shown) or a nonrebreathing circuit. (**A,** Redrawn with permission from Lichtiger, M., and Moya, F.: Introduction to the practice of anesthesia, ed. 2, New York, 1978, Harper & Row Publishers, Inc., p. 104; **B,** courtesy Fraser-Harlake, Inc.; **C,** courtesy Pitman-Moore, Inc.)

Although certain safety systems have been designed into anesthesia machines to prevent some of these complications, it is still possible for the safety system to fail. A thorough check of the machine should be performed to ensure safe and proper functioning before its use on an animal.

An inhalation anesthesia machine can be used for:

1. Administering general anesthesia for short-term or long-term procedures
2. Providing supplemental oxygen and/or a light level of anesthesia for animals undergoing a local or epidural block
3. Providing a source of 100% oxygen for emergency resuscitation or during cardiac arrest. Because of its oxygen delivery system and reservoir bag, the anesthesia machine can be used to sustain an animal's ventilation by providing a means for positive pressure breathing

Basic functions

Anesthesia machines have four primary purposes related to their anesthesia function:

1. Storing compressed oxygen, nitrous oxide, and anesthetic liquid(s)
2. Calibrating compressed gases and anesthetic vapor
3. Mixing oxygen and nitrous oxide with anesthetic vapor into a desired proportion
4. Delivering anesthetic vapor and fresh gas(es) to the patient

In addition, anesthetic machines should function to:

• Remove the patient's exhaled carbon dioxide by means of absorption or evacuation from the breathing circuit
• Scavenge waste anesthetic gases (including nitrous oxide) from the breathing circuit to prevent unnecessary inhalation by the anesthetist and other operating room personnel

A discussion of these primary functions of inhalation anesthesia machines follows. Although considered separately, each component has a crucial role in the overall performance of the machine in delivering anesthetic gases safely and efficiently to the patient. Errors or malfunctions in one component will surely affect the total purpose of the anesthesia machine—to deliver anesthesia while simultaneously maintaining the patient's metabolic requirements for oxygen supply and carbon dioxide elimination.

Storage of compressed gases and anesthetic liquids

Oxygen and nitrous oxide. The compressed gases generally used for anesthesia with dogs and cats are 100% oxygen (O_2) and 100% nitrous oxide (N_2O). Medical grade oxygen is supplied as a compressed gas in metal cylinders under pressure (2,000 psig)*. Storage of the larger "G" or "H" size cylinders must be in accordance

*See Appendix B for other pressure values.

with specific guidelines determined by the National Fire Protection Agency (NFPA) as well as state and local fire authorities. The pressure within the oxygen cylinder begins decreasing from 2,000 psig as soon as the tank is opened and allowed to flow. When the cylinder pressure gauge on an oxygen cylinder reads less than 100 psig, the cylinder should be replaced with a full one. The anesthesia machine should also be adapted with at least one yoke for a smaller "E" size compressed oxygen tank in the event the central supply fails or the machine is to be used in an area without pipeline oxygen. An inhalation anesthesia machine cannot function until a source of oxygen is either attached directly to the machine yoke or piped in from a central oxygen supply. Some large veterinary hospitals have a special storage room to function as the central supply source for oxygen. Incorporation of a central oxygen storage area into the design of a busy veterinary hospital allows for a more economical use of compressed oxygen and nitrous oxide.

Medical grade nitrous oxide is supplied as a mixture of compressed liquid and gas in metal cylinders under a pressure of approximately 750 psig at room temperature. If a nitrous oxide tank is allowed to heat up, the pressure within the tank will increase. Since the pressure within a nitrous oxide tank does not begin to decrease until all of the compressed liquid has been vaporized, the pressure remains at about 750 psig until it is about 80% empty. The only reliable method for determining the amount of gas remaining in a nitrous oxide cylinder is to weigh the cylinder. It is important to pay close attention to the cylinder pressure gauge of a nitrous oxide tank in order to avoid exhaustion of the gas during a procedure. When the pressure gauge begins to drop below 500 psig, the cylinder should be considered virtually empty and replaced with a full cylinder. The student should become familiar with the color coding, pressure, volume, and relative cost for the commonly used compressed gas cylinders (see Tables 5-3 and 5-4).

When compressed oxygen and nitrous oxide are stored centrally, the area should be located away from flammable materials, including gasoline, grease, or oil. Ideally, the storage room should be located outside the hospital building and away from air conditioning, heating, or ventilation units. It should have a single entry door and be constructed in accordance with all fire protection codes pertaining to storage of combustible gases under pressure. The large oxygen and nitrous oxide cylinders should be chained in the upright position to prevent accidental displacement or damage to the cylinder valve. Cylinders not in active use should have the outlet port of the cylinder head capped to prevent contamination by dust or oil. Should dust particles or dirt accidentally enter the compressed gas circuit of the anesthesia machine, a fire or explosion could result when the foreign material comes in contact with oxygen under high pressure. It is common practice to open the outlet valve of an oxygen or nitrous oxide tank before attaching it to the anesthesia machine in order to blow out any dust or debris that may have collected within the outlet port (this process is known as "cracking" the cylinder head). When

TABLE 5-3
Cylinder characteristics for some common medical gases

Cylinder dimensions	Weight (empty)	Capacity	Carbon dioxide	Cyclopropane	Nitrous oxide	Oxygen
E (4¼" od × 26")	5.9 kg (13 lb)	Pounds	6.6	5.5	6.4	1.9
		Liters	1,590.0	1,438.0	1,590.0	659.0
		Gallons	420.0	380.0	420	174.0
M (7" od × 43")	31.8 kg (70 lb)	Pounds	30.6		30.6	8.8
		Liters	7,570.0		7,570.0	3,000.0
		Gallons	2,000.0		2,000.0	800.0
G (8½" od × 51")	50 kg (110 lb)	Pounds	50.0		56.0	15.5
		Liters	12,358.0		13,836.0	5,331.0
		Gallons	3,260.0		3,655.0	1,408.0
H and K (9¼" od × 51")	59 kg (130 lb)	Pounds			64.3	16.0-22.0
		Liters			15,899.0	5,570-7,500
		Gallons			4,200.0	1,470-2,000

Adapted in part from Dorsch, J.A., and Dorsch, S.E.: Understanding anesthesia equipment: construction, care and complications, Baltimore, 1975, The Williams & Wilkins Co., p. 2.

TABLE 5-4

Color codes and properties of compressed medical gas cylinders

Gas	Formula	United States	International	$21°C$ service pressure (psig)	State in cylinder	Filling density
Oxygen	O_2	Green	White	1800-2400*	Gas	
Carbon dioxide	CO_2	Gray	Gray	838	Liquid<88°	68%
Nitrous oxide	N_2O	Blue	Blue	745	Liquid<98°	68%
Cyclopropane	C_3H_6	Orange	Orange	75	Liquid	55%
Ethylene	C_2H_4	Red	Violet	1200	Liquid<50°	31%-35%
Helium	He	Brown	Brown	1600-2000*	Gas	
Nitrogen	N_2	Black	Black	1800-2200*	Gas	
Air		Yellow	White and black	1800	Gas	

From Dorsch, J.A., and Dorsch, S.E.: Understanding anesthesia equipment: construction, care and complications, Baltimore, 1975, The Williams & Wilkins Co., p. 4.

*Depending on type of cylinder.

the outlet valve on the top of a compressed gas cylinder is opened, it should be turned in a counter clockwise direction between 180 to 360 degrees. Turning the valve more than one full revolution does not open the cylinder any further. Caution must be exercised when opening the stem valve on "E" cylinders. Overzealous attempts to turn a closed stem valve in a clockwise direction could result in rupture of the valve. When transporting full cylinders, care must be taken not to drop the cylinder. If the stem valve is broken by a blow or a fall, the compressed gas exiting from the cylinder could cause serious injury. In the case of a full "G" or "H" cylinder of oxygen, the force of propulsion is capable of projecting the cylinder through doors, windows, or even a cinder block wall!

Although oxygen and nitrous oxide are nonflammable gases, they will support combustion in the presence of a flame or ember—acting as fuel for any fire. For this reason oil or grease must never be used on any part of the anesthesia machine or breathing circuit.

Pin-Index Safety System. To prevent the accidental mismatching of oxygen with nitrous oxide (or other compressed gases) all "E" size cylinders and cylinder yokes are pin-indexed. The yoke on the anesthesia machine has two pins that match two holes in the neck of the appropriate cylinder valve head (see Fig. 5-20). Unless the yoke pins are broken off, it is physically impossible to attach a cylinder to an incorrect yoke, which prevents a gas from entering the machine through the wrong flowmeter. When compressed gases are piped into the operating area from a central supply, each gas has a special coupling system to take the place of the pin-index system and is called the Diameter-Index Safety System.

Anesthetic liquids. Most inhalation anesthetic drugs are liquid at room temperature. They are stored in special vaporizers designed to transform the liquid into a vapor by passing oxygen and/or nitrous oxide over or through the liquid. As the anesthetic molecules vaporize, they are carried out of the vaporizer along with the oxygen and led into the patient breathing circuit.

Before oxygen (with or without nitrous oxide) from the compressed gas cylinder is allowed to flow through the anesthetic vaporizer, its pressure must first be reduced to slightly above atmospheric pressure. To accomplish this, the gas leaving the cylinder goes through a pressure regulator that reduces the pressure to about 50 psig. Flowmeter controls further reduce the pressure of oxygen and nitrous oxide to just above that of the atmosphere (15 psig). From the flowmeter the gases are directed into or through the anesthetic vaporizer and then to the patient breathing circuit (see Fig. 5-20, A).

Several different types of anesthetic vaporizers are available commercially. The location of the anesthetic vaporizer *outside* or *inside* of the patient breathing circuit depends on the particular anesthetic drug and the type of breathing circuit used (see Fig. 5-21). All present inhalation anesthetic liquids (except ether and methoxyflurane) require a precision vaporizer that is located outside of the patient breath-

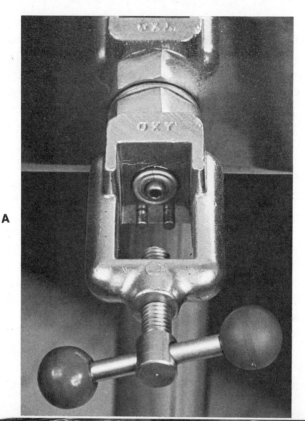

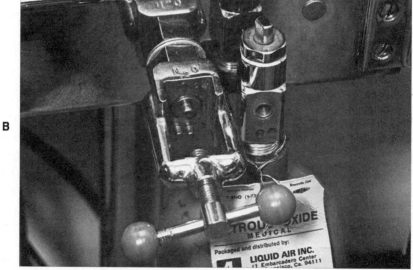

Fig. 5-20. Pin-Index Safety System for **A,** oxygen yoke on anesthesia machine and **B,** nitrous oxide yoke and "E" cylinder.

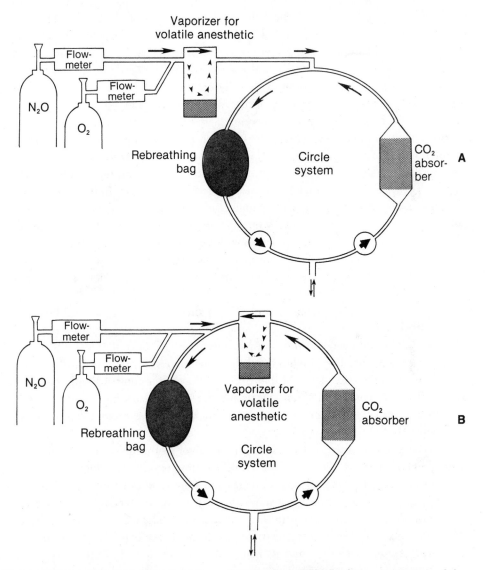

Fig. 5-21. Schematic representation of anesthetic system with **A,** the vaporizer out of the circle (VOC) and **B,** the vaporizer inside the circle (VIC). (Redrawn with permission from Soma, L.R., and Klide, A.M.: Techniques and equipment for inhalation anesthesia in small animals, Journal of the American Veterinary Medical Association **152:**957, 1968.)

ing circuit. By definition any non-rebreathing system employs an anesthetic vaporizer located out of the breathing circuit.

Calibration of compressed gases and anesthetic vapor

Compressed gases. Before compressed oxygen and nitrous oxide can be used for vaporization of the anesthetic liquid and inhalation by the patient, their cylinder pressures must be reduced. When the outlet valve of a full oxygen cylinder is turned on, the pressure within the tank is measured by the *cylinder pressure gauge*. When a central gas supply is used, the pressure gauges are located in the supply room and/or on a control panel located within the working area of the hospital. When "E" cylinders are used directly on the anesthesia machine, the pressure gauge is located in the vicinity of the yoke attachment for easy viewing. When the compressed gas cylinder valve is opened the *pressure regulator* (pressure reduction valve) immediately steps the cylinder pressure down to 50 psig before channeling the oxygen or nitrous oxide to the *flowmeter control*.

Anesthesia machines will not function accurately when compressed gas cylinders contain less than 50 psig. In general, a compressed oxygen cylinder of any size is considered empty when its pressure gauge reads 100 psig or less. Anesthesia should never begin with an empty or nearly empty compressed oxygen cylinder, especially when using nitrous oxide in combination with oxygen. When the flowmeter controls are in the "off" position and the compressed gas cylinders are open, pressure will remain within the compressed gas circuitry between the cylinder and the flowmeter.

When an anesthesia machine is not in use, this line pressure should be evacuated to prevent unnecessary compression of the pressure gauge, pressure regulator, and gas pipings. To evacuate the line pressure, the "E" tank should be turned off (or disconnected from the pipeline) and the flowmeter(s) turned on until the cylinder pressure gauge reads zero. At that time the flowmeter control should be turned back to the "off" position. (When evacuating the line pressure for oxygen, it is not necessary to turn the oxygen flowmeter on if the anesthesia machine has an oxygen flush valve.)

Once oxygen or nitrous oxide reaches the level of the flowmeter control, it is subsequently measured in liters (or cubic centimeters) of gas flow *per minute*. Flowmeters are calibrated for a specific gas and cannot be interchanged. They consist of a tapered glass tube enclosed within an outer protective glass or plastic casing. Inside the tapered glass tube is a float that is shaped like a ball or a bobbin (see Fig. 5-22), and alongside the tube a calibrated scale reads the desired gas flow. The tapered glass tube and its float come as a single unit. If the tube should break the entire unit requires replacement. Some flowmeters measure gas flows according to the center of the floating ball while bobbin-type flowmeters use the upper end of the bobbin as a gauge.

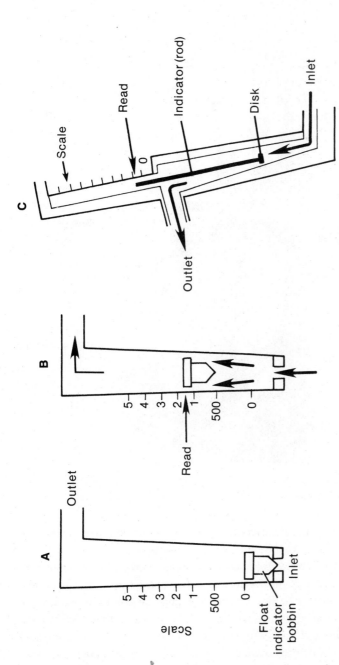

Fig. 5-22. A and **B**, Variable orifice flowmeter. Gas enters at the base and flows through the tube, causing the float to rise. The gas passes through the annular opening around the float. The area of this annular space increases with the height of the indicator. Thus the height of the indicator is a measure of gas flow. **C,** Disk indicator flowmeter. Gas enters at the base of the flowmeter and passes to the outlet, causing the stem and disk to rise. As the disk rises, the indicator passes upward, indicating gas flow. Since the tube through which the disk passes is tapered, this is a variable orifice flowmeter. (Redrawn from a diagram provided by Pitman-Moore, Inc.)

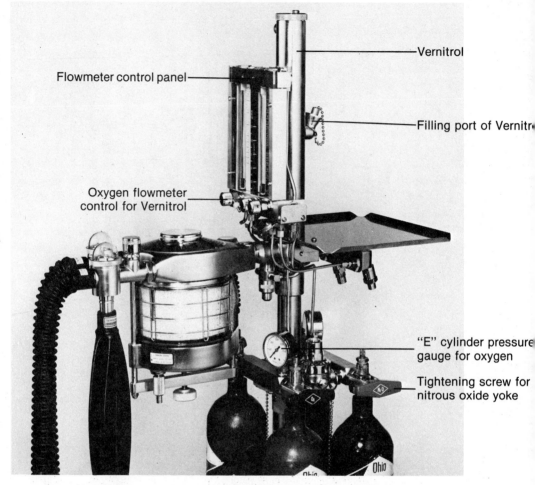

A

Flowmeter control panel—

Oxygen flowmeter
control for Vernitrol

Vernitrol

Filling port of Vernitr

"E" cylinder pressure
gauge for oxygen

Tightening screw for
nitrous oxide yoke

Fig. 5-23. A, Side view of anesthesia machine containing Vernitrol vaporizer for methoxy-flurane. Vaporizer is located outside the patient breathing circuit (circle system).

Anesthetic vapor. Anesthetic vaporizers provide a measurement of vapor concentration by one of two methods: indirect or direct calculation.

Indirect calculation. Vaporizers such as the Copper Kettle or Vernitrol have separate flowmenters for oxygen that are used to vaporize the liquid anesthetic drug and mix it with the main gas flow before directing the combined mixture to the patient breathing circuit (see Fig. 5-23). Such vaporizers are, therefore, located outside the patient breathing circuit. The percentage (concentration) of anesthetic vapor to reach the patient must be calculated by the anesthetist, and it varies according to the oxygen flow through the vaporizer and the total gas flow (oxygen plus nitrous oxide) being delivered from the flowmeter(s). These vaporizers are not popular due to the need for additional calculations involving the vapor pressure of

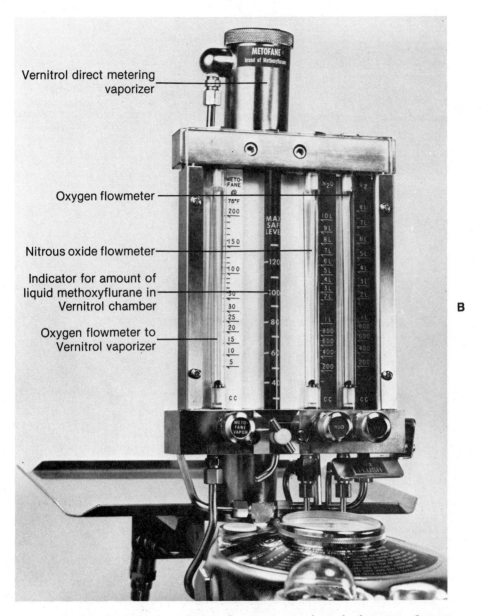

Fig. 5-23, cont'd. B, Same machine showing flowmeter control panel. The oxygen flowmeter on the left controls the flow of oxygen into the Vernitrol vaporizer for vaporization purposes. Readings are for the volume (in cubic centimeters) of methoxyflurane being vaporized and then mixed with the total fresh gas flow (shown on the right half of the panel).   *Continued.*

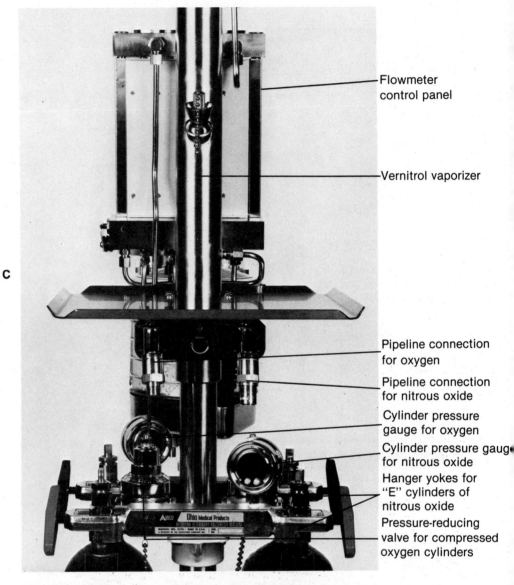

C

Flowmeter control panel

Vernitrol vaporizer

Pipeline connection for oxygen

Pipeline connection for nitrous oxide

Cylinder pressure gauge for oxygen

Cylinder pressure gauge for nitrous oxide

Hanger yokes for "E" cylinders of nitrous oxide

Pressure-reducing valve for compressed oxygen cylinders

Fig. 5-23, cont'd. C, Rear view of anesthesia machine with Vernitrol vaporizer. (Courtesy Pitman-Moore, Inc.)

the particular anesthetic liquid, its temperature, and the oxygen flow through the vaporizer relative to the total gas flow. The Copper Kettle or Vernitrol vaporizers can be used to vaporize any liquid anesthetic drug, given the information required to calculate the concentration to be delivered. The Vernitrol vaporizer is commonly used for vaporizing methoxyflurane.

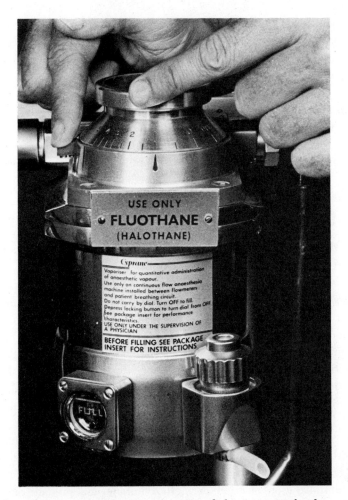

Fig. 5-24. Fluotec vaporizer turn-on. Concentration dial is set at 1% by depressing the lock on the left side and rotating the dial.

Direct calculation. Anesthetic liquids, such as halothane, enflurane, and isoflurane, are potent and tend to vaporize at room temperature in extremely high concentrations. These anesthetic drugs require specially designed vaporizers located outside the patient breathing circuit, which compensate for changes in temperature and gas flows. Direct calculating vaporizers accept the total fresh gas flow as it emerges from the flowmeter(s). Most modern vaporizers have a switch mechanism to lock the vaporizer dial in the "off" position. This lock must be manually overridden in order to turn on the vaporizer (see Fig. 5-24). The desired anesthetic concentration is obtained by setting the dial on the top of the vaporizer. The vaporizer automatically compensates for changes in total gas flow (oxygen or oxygen plus nitrous oxide) and temperature. Direct reading vaporizers are relatively expensive but considered safer because they eliminate human error in calculating vapor concentrations for varying temperatures. Due to their delicate inner mechanisms these vaporizers need servicing and recalibration on the average of once every 2 years.

Modern direct reading vaporizers are accurate over a wide range of total gas flow rates. Older model vaporizers require compensation when the total gas flows are less than 800 ml/minute or greater than 3 L/minute. Direct reading vaporizers are calibrated specifically for a single anesthetic liquid. Inaccurate concentrations will result if the incorrect anesthetic drug is placed in the vaporizer. Thus care must be taken in filling these vaporizers. Should the wrong anesthetic liquid be placed in the vaporizer it must be drained immediately and oxygen flushed through the empty vaporizer for at least 15 to 20 minutes (it is preferable to allow the vaporizer to air overnight). When the concentration dial of a direct reading vaporizer is in the "off" position and the flowmeter(s) are on, the entire fresh gas flow will bypass the vaporization chamber and can then be directed to the patient breathing circuit. In this way the patient can be ventilated with 100% oxygen (or a mixture of oxygen and nitrous oxide) without anesthetic vapor.

Most direct reading vaporizers are made with a thick casing of copper to prevent rapid temperature fluctuations from taking place within the anesthetic liquid. An indicator window at the bottom of the vaporizer permits inspection of the liquid level remaining in the vaporization chamber. When filling (or emptying) a vaporizer with anesthetic liquid while the flowmeter is on, the concentration dial must be in the "off" position; otherwise anesthetic vapor and liquid will be expelled into the room air. Care must also be taken to close the filling port securely to avoid spillage of anesthetic liquid before turning on the vaporizer.

In-circuit vaporization. Older anesthesia machines made use of a glass jar-type vaporizer with string wicks, which was usually positioned on the inhalation arm of the patient breathing circuit (see Fig. 5-25). These vaporizers were originally designed for administration of ether or methoxyflurane and predate direct reading vaporizers. The Ohio No. 8 (see Fig. 5-26) is an example of a vaporizer in-circuit (VIC). All the other vaporizers discussed are examples of vaporizers out-of-circuit (VOC). In-circuit vaporizers make use of the gas flows within the circle breathing system to vaporize the liquid anesthetic drug. When the total fresh gas flow to the circle is high, the anesthetic concentration inhaled by the animal decreases due to cooling of the liquid. Conversely, at a given dial setting the anesthetic concentration increases as the total fresh gas flow decreases. With the Ohio No. 8 vaporizer the concentration dial on top of the glass jar consists of settings ranging from "off" to "full open" with nine arbitrary positions in between. In the "off" position the total gas flow going through the circle bypasses the vaporization chamber and goes directly to the patient. In the "full open" position the entire gas flow is diverted into the vaporization chamber, thereby allowing for maximal vaporization of the liquid anesthetic drug at room temperature—approximately 3% for methoxyflurane and nearly 33% for halothane. Thus, should halothane be mistakenly placed in this

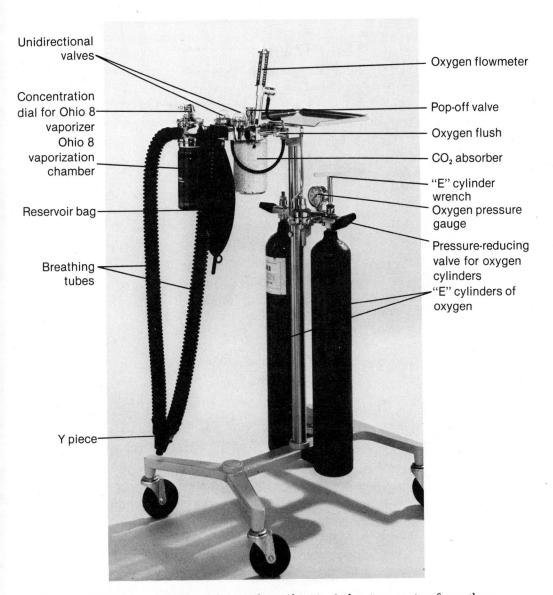

Unidirectional valves

Concentration dial for Ohio 8 vaporizer

Ohio 8 vaporization chamber

Reservoir bag

Breathing tubes

Y piece

Oxygen flowmeter

Pop-off valve

Oxygen flush

CO_2 absorber

"E" cylinder wrench

Oxygen pressure gauge

Pressure-reducing valve for oxygen cylinders

"E" cylinders of oxygen

Fig. 5-25. Inhalation anesthesia machine with an Ohio No. 8 glass jar vaporizer for methoxyflurane. The vaporizer is located inside the patient breathing circuit. Two yokes are present for attaching two "E" cylinders of compressed oxygen. (Courtesy Pitman-Moore, Inc.)

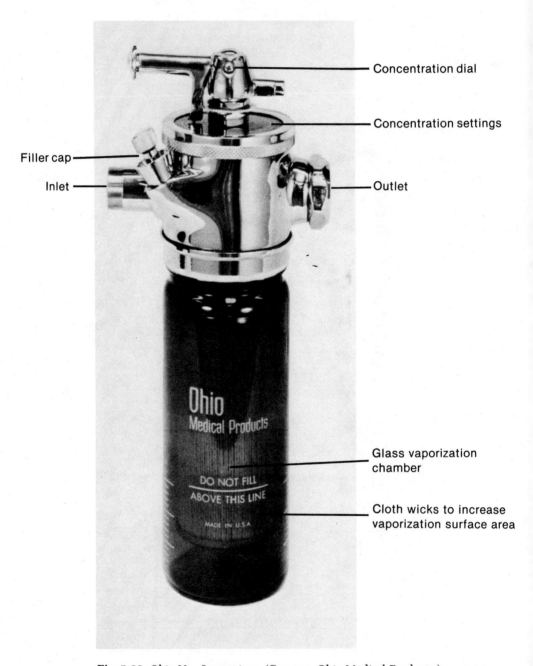

Concentration dial

Concentration settings

Filler cap

Inlet

Outlet

Glass vaporization chamber

Cloth wicks to increase vaporization surface area

Fig. 5-26. Ohio No. 8 vaporizer. (Courtesy Ohio Medical Products.)

type of vaporizer and the animal allowed to breathe a concentration of this quantity, cardiac arrest could occur within minutes. Consequently, the only anesthetic drug presently recommended for use in a VIC vaporizer is methoxyflurane. It is important that the level of anesthetic liquid be neither too low nor too high since maximal efficiency depends on proper wick saturation and air space within the vaporization chamber.

In-circuit vaporizers are considered less accurate and potentially more dangerous than calibrated, direct reading, out-of-circuit vaporizers.

ADVANTAGES OF IN-CIRCUIT VAPORIZERS

- They are inexpensive.
- The animal tends to regulate its own depth of anesthesia according to its rate and depth of ventilation. For instance, as anesthetic depth increases the animal's ventilation decreases and less total gas is drawn through the vaporizer. Thus the animal inspires less anesthetic vapor and will begin to awaken as anesthesia lightens. Ventilation then increases, and more total gas is drawn through the vaporizer, vaporizing additional anesthetic drug. As a result the animal tends to inhale a higher concentration of the drug, and anesthesia is deepened.

DISADVANTAGES OF IN-CIRCUIT VAPORIZERS

- The glass jar is easily broken.
- They are unsafe for halothane, enflurane, or isoflurane anesthesia due to their high vaporization pressures.
- High total gas flows into the breathing circuit tend to cool the anesthetic liquid and decrease the vapor concentration available for inhalation, which can prolong anesthetic induction or result in a lighter level of anesthesia.
- Room temperature fluctuations can affect the degree of vaporization. Glass is a poor insulator against temperature changes. Cold room temperatures (below 18°C) decrease the amount of methoxyflurane vaporized. A warm room can raise the anesthetic liquid (combined with the animal's exhaled breath) to 25°C or higher, allowing methoxyflurane to vaporize at dangerously high concentrations.
- Dial settings are only relative numbers and do not provide accurate determination of inspired anesthetic concentrations.
- Positive pressure ventilation tends to create back pressure within the vaporization chamber and force more anesthetic vapor into the patient breathing circuit, which can lead to overdosage unless the vaporizer setting is reduced during positive pressure ventilation.

Anesthesia machines that incorporate two or more different types of vaporizers on the same machine are sometimes referred to as hybrid machines. (See Fig. 5-27). To prevent the accidental filling of one vaporizer with the wrong liquid anesthetic drug, a safety filler system is recommended (refer to Fig. 4-6).

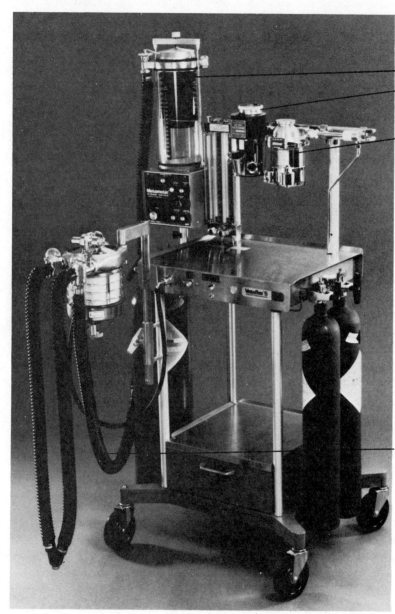

Ventilator

Halothane
vaporizer

Methoxyflurane
vaporizer

Ventilator hose
connected to
circle system

Fig. 5-27. Anesthesia machine equipped with two out-of-circuit anesthetic vaporizers and an automatic ventilator. (Courtesy Pitman-Moore, Inc.)

Mixing of compressed gas(es) with anesthetic vapor

Oxygen with or without nitrous oxide can either pass through the anesthetic vaporizer or be diverted into the vaporization chamber where it picks up anesthetic molecules and carries them into the patient breathing circuit. If the anesthesia machine contains an *oxygen flush* valve, oxygen can be routed directly into the patient breathing circuit without having to pass through the flowmeter or the out-of-circuit vaporizer. When the oxygen flush button is depressed, 100% oxygen flows into the breathing circuit at a rate of 30 to 50 L/minute (refer to Fig. 5-19, A). This feature, not present on all anesthesia machines, should be used only when a rapid flow of 100% oxygen is needed by the patient since any anesthetic in the breathing circuit and reservoir bag will be diluted. Filling the reservoir bag should not be a routine procedure during normal anesthetic induction or maintenance as it will tend to decrease the anesthetic concentration within the patient breathing circuit. At the end of the anesthetic period the oxygen flush may be used to dilute residual anesthetic drug being exhaled by the animal, although raising the oxygen flow rate on the flowmeter control will serve the same purpose and is not as wasteful. The oxygen flush must never be used to flush a semiopen breathing circuit as the high flow rate into the circuit can cause serious damage to the animal's lungs.

When nitrous oxide is used to supplement the volatile liquid anesthetic drug during induction and/or maintenance of anesthesia, it must be mixed with oxygen. Nitrous oxide cylinders contain 100% nitrous oxide, which, if inhaled for more than 30 to 60 seconds, would cause a serious or even fatal anoxia. Nitrous oxide (100%) and oxygen (100%) are piped from their cylinder regulators (or pipeline inlet) on the anesthesia machine to their respective *flowmeters*. Each gas enters its flowmeter at the bottom and, when turned on, flows upward and into a collecting manifold where the gases mix before entering the breathing circuit (see Fig. 5-19, A). The amount of each gas that reaches the manifold is determined by the flowmeter control. The flowmeter, then, controls the proportional mixture of nitrous oxide and oxygen that eventually reaches the animal. If, for instance, the nitrous oxide flowmeter control is set at the 2 L/minute position while the oxygen flowmeter is set at 1 L/minute, the resulting manifold mixture will be two parts nitrous oxide to one part oxygen, or a 2:1 ratio. When converted to a percentage figure, this ratio would represent approximately 66% nitrous oxide and 33% oxygen. Animals should never receive nitrous oxide in ratios greater than three parts nitrous oxide to one part oxygen (75% nitrous oxide, 25% oxygen).

Certain precautions should be observed to prevent damage to the flowmeter and assure its accurate function:

- Do not overtighten the control knob when turning flowmeter off.
- Do not turn on the compressed oxygen or nitrous oxygen cylinders (or connect machine to pipeline gases) with the flowmeter turned on. High pressure (50 psig) surging into a flowmeter may send the float to the top of the scale where it may lodge, making it impossible to turn off the flowmeter.

- Do not use a flowmeter that has a broken outer casing. Dirt within the flowmeter can alter the desired flow rate or cause the float to stick to the side of the tube. From the flowmeter manifold, oxygen and/or nitrous oxide is directed through one (or more) out-of-circuit vaporizers and then to a common inlet within the patient breathing circuit (see Fig. 5-19, A).
- Gases that enter the patient breathing circuit from the anesthesia machine are called "fresh" gas(es) since they have not yet mixed with any of the patient's exhaled gases.

The concentration of anesthetic vapor leaving an out-of-circuit vaporizer is regulated in one of two ways: variable bypass or measured oxygen flow.

The majority of modern direct reading vaporizers make use of the variable bypass method. The fresh gas flow from the flowmeter manifold is diverted into the vaporization chamber in variable amounts, according to the setting on the concentration dial. The diverted gas picks up anesthetic vapor before exiting from the vaporizer. In the "off" position all the fresh gas (oxygen or oxygen plus nitrous oxygen) is diverted by way of the bypass channel. When the dial is in the "full open" position, the maximal flow of fresh gas is diverted through the vaporization chamber. Dial settings in between allow for variable flows through both the vaporization chamber and bypass channel to produce a variety of anesthetic concentrations.

Measured oxygen flow vaporizers have a separate oxygen flowmeter to measure the amount of oxygen going into the vaporizer (see Figs. 5-19 and 5-23). The flowmeter for measuring this oxygen flow is not color coded green in order to bring attention to the fact that it is for vaporization of anesthetic liquid only. When anesthetic is not desired, this flowmeter must be turned off. The entire flow from the measured oxygen flowmeter enters the vaporizer and becomes saturated with anesthetic vapor before mixing with and becoming diluted by the fresh gas from the main flowmeter manifold. The measured oxygen flowmeter supplying the vaporizer is calibrated in cubic centimeters per minute rather than liters per minute since lesser oxygen flows are diverted through the vaporizer. Measured flow vaporizers require additional calculations to determine the concentration of anesthetic vapor actually arriving at the patient breathing circuit.

The concentration of anesthetic vapor exiting from a vaporizer can also be influenced by the following factors:

- Temperature of anesthetic liquid (increased temperature allows more anesthetic to vaporize)
- Fresh gas flow rate through the vaporization chamber (accuracy tends to decrease with very low or very high flow rates)
- Position of vaporizer inside or outside the patient breathing circuit, which is a consideration when a rebreathing circle system is used

• Back pressure (pumping effect). Positive pressure ventilation of the animal can force additional anesthetic vapor into the bypass channel, raising the delivered concentration above dial settings. The vaporizer dial setting should be reduced when using controlled ventilation unless it is back pressure compensated (see Chapter 6).

Examples of common anesthetic vaporizers. Modern out-of-circuit vaporizers have modifications to simplify and perfect the calibration of anesthetic liquids. Most of the newer vaporizers compensate in some way for the above four factors and are calibrated for a *single* anesthetic drug. Following is a brief summary of some commonly used anesthetic vaporizers by brand name. Each is discussed according to vapor regulation, position relative to the breathing circuit, temperature compensation, flow compensation, and pressure compensation:

Fluotec Mark III (manufactured by Fraser-Harlake, Inc.)

CLASSIFICATION. Variable bypass; out-of-circuit; temperature compensated by mechanical means; flow compensated; back pressure compensated; designed for halothane only

COMMENTS. Accurate over a wide range of fresh gas flows (500 ml/minute to 5 L/minute); automatic locking mechanism; safety filler system available; calibrated down to 0.5% halothane; concentration dial may stick or freeze with thymol preservative buildup; servicing at factory recommended on average of every 2 years; anesthetic liquid can enter control dial if vaporizer is tipped over. Older Mark II model is less accurate and is not back pressure compensated.

Pentec Mark II (manufactured by Fraser-Harlake, Inc.)

CLASSIFICATION. Same as Fluotec Mark III except designed for methoxyflurane only; out-of-circuit

COMMENTS. Similar to Fluotec Mark III except calibrated from 0.25% to 3% methoxyflurane (preservative within methoxyflurane can accumulate and affect the operation of the concentration dial)

Fluomatic (manufactured by Foregger Co.)

CLASSIFICATION. Variable bypass; out-of-circuit; temperature compensated by mechanical means; flow and back pressure compensated; designed for halothane

COMMENTS. Thymol preservative in halothane tends to build up, altering output concentration and causing the control dial to stick or freeze; calibrated in 0.5% increments to 5%; requires factory servicing periodically.

Pentomatic (manufactured by Foregger Co.)

CLASSIFICATION. Same as Fluomatic except designed for methoxyflurane; out-of-circuit

COMMENTS. Preservative buildup can cause dial to stick and alter output concentration; calibrated from 0.25% up to 3%

Vapor (manufactured by North American Drager Co.)

CLASSIFICATION. Variable bypass; out-of-circuit; back pressure compensated; temperature compensated by manual means; designed for halothane; manual locking shut-off control

COMMENTS. Vaporizers manufactured before the 1980 model require a manual adjustment for temperature changes within the anesthetic liquid. A thermometer at the top of the vaporizer registers the temperature of the liquid. The manual concentration dial is aligned to a temperature scale on the dial window in accordance with the anesthetic concentration desired. The manually controlled Vapor vaporizer is extremely accurate, has fewer internal moving parts, and requires servicing less often (an average of once every 5 years). The Vapor is quite heavy (about 16 kg) and can easily topple the machine if positioned above the center of gravity, especially when traversing uneven thresholds. In addition, the thermometer is vulnerable to breakage, rendering the vaporizer inaccurate until a replacement can be located.

Vernitrol (manufactured by Pitman-Moore, Inc.)

CLASSIFICATION. Measured oxygen flow; out-of-circuit; no wicks; temperature compensation by manual adjustments and copper casing; can be used for different anesthetic liquids (although most often used for vaporizing methoxyflurane)

COMMENTS. Versatile; requires compensation for variations in temperature, fresh gas flow rates, and specific anesthetic vapor pressure. Subject to anesthetist error when calculating the delivered concentration; requires a separate oxygen flowmeter; possible for anesthetic *liquid* to enter breathing circuit and animal's lungs if overfilled and/or the measured oxygen flowmeter is set at full open. All vaporizers mentioned thus far are composed of copper metal to conduct room heat into the anesthetic liquid in order to maintain a relatively constant temperature for vaporization. The copper metal adds considerably to the cost and weight of these vaporizers.

Ohio No. 8 (manufactured by Pitman-Moore, Inc.)

CLASSIFICATION. Variable bypass; glass jar drawover with string wick; in-circuit; no temperature compensation; no back pressure compensation; arbitrary concentration settings on control dial; most often used for vaporization of methoxyflurane; amount of anesthetic liquid vaporized influenced by animal's ventilation

COMMENTS. Self-regulating to a degree, depending on animal's rate and depth of breathing; should *never* be used to vaporize the more potent anesthetics with high vapor pressures (that is, halothane, enflurane, or isoflurane). Glass vaporization chamber breaks easily; old or corroded concentration dial will allow some vaporization even when in the "off" position.

Delivery of anesthetic vapor and fresh gas(es) to the patient

Up to this point the anesthesia machine has functioned to prepare a mixture of anesthetic vapor with fresh gas (oxygen or oxygen plus nitrous oxide). The anesthesia machine is but one of three integrated concerns when administering inhalation anesthesia. The other two are the *patient breathing circuit* and the *patient*. The anesthesia machine and the anesthetist must both work efficiently to ensure that the patient receives a safe concentration of anesthetic drug along with an oxygen flow sufficient for adequate ventilation and metabolic needs. The patient must never receive a hypoxic mixture of gases either through human negligence or machine failure. Such a risk is increased with the use of nitrous oxide. A minimum of 30% oxygen should be delivered to the patient at all times during the anesthesia period. Many newer anesthesia machines have built-in alarm systems designed to warn the anesthetist when oxygen cylinders fail and/or they automatically turn off the nitrous oxide flowmeter when oxygen pressure drops below 50 psig. These systems are referred to as "fail-safe" systems and vary somewhat according to manufacturers. It is important to become familiar with the system design when first learning to use a new anesthesia machine. One should never rely totally on a fail-safe system to warn of hypoxic gas mixtures, as such systems cannot be assumed foolproof.

The anesthesia machine delivers a mixture of fresh gas with (or without) anesthetic vapor to the patient for inhalation purposes. This gas mixture does not enter the patient's lungs directly but rather enters a breathing circuit of some kind before inhalation. The patient breathing circuit serves two major purposes:

1. It adapts and adjusts to the patient's changing ventilation pattern through the use of a reservoir bag, directional valves, and pressure relief valve. At the same time it maintains a constant input of fresh gas(es) and anesthetic vapor.

2. It prevents the patient from rebreathing exhaled carbon dioxide. Although patient breathing circuits vary, generally those used on animals weighing more than 8 to 10 kg employ a design that provides for the recirculation of exhaled gases after carbon dioxide has been removed from the breathing circuit. Animals weighing less than 8 to 10 kg can be placed on a breathing circuit that does not allow for rebreathing of any exhaled gases.

A major purpose in the design of any breathing circuit is to minimize resistance to gas flow. Resistance within a breathing circuit creates an additional stress on the anesthetized animal by increasing the energy expended in exhaling and inhaling through tubes. This is of particular concern with animals weighing less than 8 to 10 kg, especially if the animal has any degree of respiratory or cardiovascular depression. Resistance to gas flow within a breathing circuit is minimized by using wide diameter tubing of the shortest possible length and avoiding sharp bends or abrupt changes in the diameter of the breathing circuit. In general the major sources of airway resistance in a breathing circuit are:

- Movable valves
- Carbon dioxide absorbing canister
- Endotracheal tubes and their adapters
- Long, narrow diameter breathing tube(s)

Also of concern with the use of patient breathing circuits are:

- Absorption of anesthetic vapor by rubber tubing composing the circuit
- Mechanical dead space because of excessively long endotracheal tube, circuit design, or low rate of fresh gas flow into the circuit
- Alterations in the delivered concentration of anesthetic vapor and fresh gas before it is inhaled by the patient. Considerations include dilution of delivered concentration by use of oxygen flush valve, leaks in the circuit to room air, and absorption of anesthetic drug by rubber tubing. Anesthetic vapors that are highly soluble in rubber (for example, methoxyflurane) will be absorbed and released by the rubber tubing within the patient breathing circuit. The concentration of methoxyflurane that actually reaches the animal's lungs can be greater than the concentration being delivered from the anesthesia machine to the breathing circuit. However, during the induction period, the concentration of methoxyflurane inhaled by the animal would be less than the concentration delivered because rubber would absorb a considerable amount of the vapor. Rubber continues to absorb anesthetic vapor during anesthesia maintenance until it reaches a saturation point. When methoxyflurane concentration to the breathing circuit is decreased or discontinued toward the end of the anesthesia period, the animal will continue to inhale anesthetic vapor as it is released from the rubber tubing. When discontinuing methoxyflurane anesthesia, it is important to disconnect the animal from the breathing circuit as soon as possible to avoid unnecessary inhalation of this residual anesthetic drug. Absorption and release of anesthetic vapor from the breathing circuit is a concern primarily when administering methoxyflurane. Halothane, enflurane, and isoflurane are far less soluble in rubber (refer to Table 4-4).

SYSTEMS AND TECHNIQUES FOR DELIVERING INHALATION ANESTHESIA

Patients encountered in a small animal veterinary hospital vary tremendously in size and type. The choice of breathing circuits and techniques available for inhalation anesthesia also vary, both in design and in classification. No single technique is adaptable to all situations. It is important for the AHT to be aware of the available systems and to become familiar with the correct use of more than one technique for delivering inhalation anesthesia.

One of the major purposes of any anesthetic breathing circuit is to prevent the animal from rebreathing its exhaled carbon dioxide. If the breathing circuit fails to eliminate or remove carbon dioxide, the animal will be forced to reinhale it, becoming progressively hypercapnic. Normal arterial carbon dioxide tension ($PaCO_2$) is about 40 mm Hg (see Chapter 6). When carbon dioxide is reinhaled, the $PaCO_2$ rises rapidly, resulting in serious and potentially fatal physiologic alterations. Depending on the amount of carbon dioxide inhaled, it may take but a few minutes to raise the $PaCO_2$ from 40 mm Hg to over 100 mm Hg. Carbon dioxide tensions above 60 mm Hg can result in permanent or fatal damage to the CNS. High arterial levels of carbon dioxide (hypercapnia) can cause the following physiologic complications:

- Decreased capacity for hemoglobin to transport oxygen*
- Hypoxemia due to impaired alveolar ventilation*
- Respiratory acidosis
- Elevated blood pressure (hypertension)
- Elevated heart rate (tachycardia)
- Vasoconstriction of peripheral blood vessels
- Vasodilation of cerebral blood vessels (causes a rise of intracranial pressure that can result in damage to the CNS)
- Cardiac dysrrhythmias due to acidosis and hypoxemia

If hypercarpnia due to carbon dioxide rebreathing is left uncorrected and continues unabated, serious consequences will occur. The anesthetist must pay close attention to the patient under general anesthesia to prevent this complication. If hypercapnia occurs during inhalation anesthesia, there often is no clinical evidence of cyanosis. Clinical signs of hypercapnia include:

- Tachycardia
- Irregular respiratory pattern often associated with abdominal breathing; increased rate of ventilation
- Hypertension, followed by hypotension
- Flushed appearance to skin or, in some species, sweating
- Cardiac dysrhythmias (potentially fatal)

When signs of possible hypercapnia occur, immediate attention must be paid to supporting the animal's ventilation (see Chapter 6). At the same time the cause of the hypercapnia must be determined and corrected to prevent further rebreathing of carbon dioxide.

Carbon dioxide absorption

The potential for reinhaling carbon dioxide is greatest with systems that allow for recirculation of the patient's exhaled gases. In these systems a carbon dioxide absorber is incorporated into the breathing circuit to minimize the rebreathing of exhaled carbon dioxide (see Fig. 5-21). The material most commonly used in a

---

*Mucous membrane color may appear pink when the animal is receiving a high inspired oxygen concentration (for example, 30% to 100%), yet hypoxia may be present. The only sure means for detecting hypoxia and hypercapnia is by means of arterial blood gas analysis and hemoglobin determination.

canister for absorption of exhaled carbon dioxide is soda lime. For maximal efficiency the absorber canister should have an airspace volume one to two times the animal's tidal volume. The size of the granules used should be 4 to 8 mesh granules.

The carbon dioxide absorber is placed downstream from the exhalation valve and functions to remove carbon dioxide from the animal's exhaled gases before recirculating with fresh gas and anesthetic. (It is important to remember that, in addition to carbon dioxide, a patient under inhalation anesthesia will exhale oxygen and anesthetic vapor from its lungs and upper airway.) Commercially available carbon dioxide absorbent usually contains a pH-sensitive chemical that changes to a blue color, indicating that the absorbing granules are exhausted. When exhaled carbon dioxide comes in contact with active soda lime granules, a chemical reaction occurs that inactivates the carbon dioxide. This reaction also produces water along with considerable heat and carbonate precipitants:

$$H_2O + CO_2 \xrightarrow{\text{Soda lime}} H_2O + Heat + CaCO_3 + Na_2CO_3$$

Even in the most efficient absorbers some carbon dioxide will pass through the soda lime and return to the patient, the amount increasing as the soda lime becomes depleted. The heat produced can also be used as an indicator of the absorbing granules' ability to adequately remove carbon dioxide from the breathing circuit. If the carbon dioxide absorbing canister does not feel warm to the touch while in use, the absorbent should be replenished. One should not rely totally on the pH indicator, since the blue color will disappear after the canister sits unused for several hours or overnight. The following parameters should be used when evaluating absorbing granules for loss of activity:

- Lack of heat production during use
- Color indicator turning blue during use. It is common practice to replenish the absorbent when one third to one half of the granules undergo a color change.
- Hard and brittle granules. Fresh soda lime granules feel soft and crumble easily when rubbed between thumb and fingers.

When any or all of the above indicate that it is necessary to replenish exhausted carbon dioxide absorbent, the entire canister should be emptied and refilled with fresh absorbent. When filling the canister, care must be taken not to spill any granules into the patient breathing circuit. Further, granules must not be packed too tightly and a 1 to 2 cm air space should be present at the top of the canister. The animal's exhaled gases should pass through the absorbing granules evenly and with minimal resistance. Since water containing dissolved carbonate tends to collect in the bottom of the carbon dioxide canister, most carbon dioxide absorbers have a drain port located beneath the canister to allow removal of this caustic water (see Fig. 6-12). Proper maintenance includes removal of accumulated absorber water on a regular basis to prevent its backing up into the absorbing granules. Care should be taken when draining the canister not to spill the caustic water on skin or clothing. If accidental spillage does occur, it should be diluted immediately with tap water to prevent alkaline burning of mucous membranes, skin, or clothing.

Classification of breathing circuits

There are currently far too many systems for classifying different types of patient breathing circuits. As one investigates the English and American terminology, confusion begins to mount, as some systems are named after their originators while others attempt classification based on such terms as "open," "semiopen," "semiclosed," "closed," "nonrebreathing," "rebreathing," "circle," and "to and fro." In order to avoid some of the confusion, the student should concentrate on how each system accomplishes the two major purposes of breathing circuits previously discussed (p. 259). Breathing circuits should also be examined in terms of:

- Total fresh gas flow(s) required to provide the animal with adequate ventilation and oxygenation (Table 5-5)
- Type of equipment used to comprise the breathing circuit—for example, rubber tubing, valves, carbon dioxide absorbing canister, Y-piece, T-piece, reservoir bag, pop-off valve, and in-circuit vaporizer
- Means for removing the animal's exhaled carbon dioxide
- Relative positioning of fresh gas inlet to exhalation valve or port
- Mechanical dead space volume and resistance to gas flow
- Means for preventing waste anesthetic gases from entering room air

The system presented here classifies the various breathing circuits relative to the presence (or absence) of a reservoir bag and whether or not the patient rebreathes its exhaled gases. According to this classification there are four basic categories of breathing circuits:

- Open circuits
- Semiopen circuits
- Semiclosed circuits
- Closed circuits

Following is a brief discussion for each basic category. Within each category more than one system may exist for administering the inhalation anesthetic drug and fresh gas flow. Techniques of administration can also vary within each system according to the situation and personal preference. It is not the intent of this book to recommend one system over another. The dicussion, therefore, will be concerned with the basic concepts pertinent to each category. The techniques of administration mentioned are considered acceptable for routine anesthesia cases.

Open breathing circuits

Open circuits do not provide for rebreathing of exhaled gases. They have neither reservoir bag nor carbon dioxide absorber. The animal breathes only the

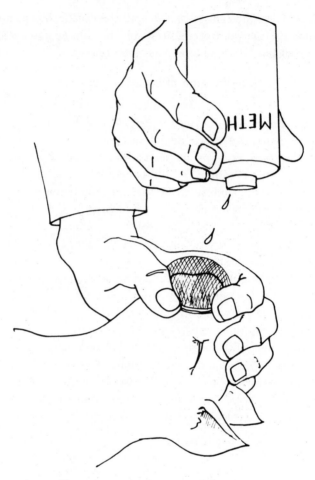

Fig. 5-28. Open drop technique for cat.

gas(es) and anesthetic vapor presented by the anesthesia machine or open drop mask. Open circuits are simply designed and minimally equipped. The systems and techniques used to deliver anesthesia via open drop technique represent the original methods employed to administer ether and chloroform anesthesia before the development of anesthesia machines. They are presently unpopular and considered unsafe compared to newer techniques. Open circuits are wasteful of anesthetic vapors, tend to dry the patient's respiratory tract, do not conserve patient body heat, and are highly polluting of the environment. Three types of open circuit systems are:

1. Open drop (see Fig. 5-28)
2. Insufflation
3. Anesthesia chamber (see Fig. 5-29)

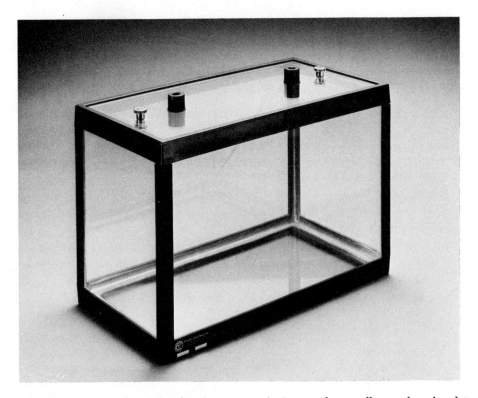

Fig. 5-29. Feline anesthesia chamber (open system). Cat or other small animal is placed in the chamber, and the lid is secured. A mixture of oxygen, nitrous oxide, and halothane is allowed to flow through one of the ports on the chamber lid while the other port serves as an exhalation valve. (Courtesy Fraser-Harlake, Inc.)

The open drop system is the oldest yet least popular of anesthetic techniques. Originally designed for administration of ether and chloroform to humans and animals, it is rarely used today. The technique is inherently wasteful, polluting, and inaccurate. Further, it affords very little control over anesthetic dosage and is considered a risky method of delivering general anesthesia.

Insufflation involves introduction of the anesthetic gas mixture into or near the patient's airway. For example, a wild animal can be sedated in its cage by dart gun and then induced by placing a small hose from the anesthesia machine into a nostril. Once the animal is unconscious, anesthesia is continued by face mask until the trachea can be intubated.

The anesthesia chamber is commonly used to induce inhalation anesthesia in cats and small animal patients weighing less than 6 to 7 kg. Induction chambers are commercially available and designed primarily for use on adult cats. The basic concept is to place the animal into a closed chamber into which a flow of fresh gas plus anesthetic drug is introduced (see Fig. 5-30). A mixture of nitrous oxide in oxygen with 3% to 5% halothane vapor is commonly used to rapidly induce unconsciousness. Fresh gas flows totaling 4 to 6 L/minute are used with a nitrous oxide–oxygen ratio of 2:1. It is advisable to have an exhalation port on the chamber to allow for escape of excessive gas pressure within the chamber. The exhalation port should be connected to a scavenger system to minimize pollution of room air with escaping anesthetic gases. Unconsciousness usually occurs within 3 to 5 minutes, whereupon the animal is removed from the chamber and the induction is continued by face mask and a semiopen breathing circuit system until intubation of the trachea can be accomplished (see Fig. 5-30, *B*).

The use of an anesthesia chamber is particularly helpful with healthy adult cats (or other species such as ferrets, rodents, rabbits, and snakes) that are difficult to restrain for intravenous induction. Animals with any form of upper airway obstruction or respiratory depression should *not* be induced by anesthesia chamber since such animals may become apneic in the chamber as a result of a compromised airway. In addition, animals with full stomachs should *not* be induced by chamber or mask as vomiting can easily occur before the trachea can be intubated.

Semiopen breathing circuits

Semiopen circuits do not provide for significant rebreathing of exhaled gases nor do they use a carbon dioxide absorber. Instead reservoir bags are used to accomplish the following objectives:

- Storage (and mixture) of anesthetic gases plus oxygen for inhalation. At the peak of inspiration the flow rate of gases into the lungs is greater than the fresh gas flow rate into the breathing circuit. The reservoir bag serves to supply the volume of gas needed during the peak of inspiration and should hold at least five times the animal's normal tidal volume.*
- Means for manually assisting or controlling the animal's ventilation

Semiopen breathing circuits are best suited for animals weighing less than 7 to 10 kg. When used on larger animals, the fresh gas flows needed make them less economical and more wasteful of anesthetic gases. Because they do not recirculate the animal's exhaled gases and water vapor, these systems can cause excessive drying of the upper respiratory tract with long-term use (100% oxygen and 100% nitrous oxide do not contain water and therefore tend to dry mucous membranes). Semiopen systems, like open systems, do not conserve the animal's exhaled body heat. In small patients this loss of body heat from the breathing circuit can contribute significantly to hypothermia during and following anesthesia. Warming blankets

---

*Since open breathing circuits employ no reservoir bag, room air is often taken into the lungs along with anesthetic gases during the peak of inspiration. This results in a dilution of anesthetic vapor and administration of an unknown concentration.

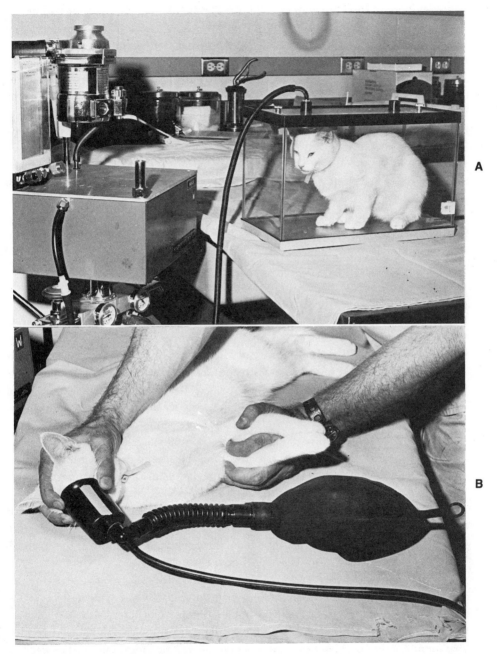

Fig. 5-30. A, Cat in chamber. **B,** Masking cat after it has been anesthetized in the chamber.

should be used on all animals under general anesthesia, especially animals on a semiopen type of breathing circuit. The smaller the patient, the greater will be the relative amount of body heat lost during anesthesia and surgery. Semiopen systems should be avoided in procedures lasting more than 1 to 2 hours unless adequate measures are taken to prevent hypothermia.

Semiopen circuits prevent rebreathing by utilizing either a pop-off valve or an open exhalation port on the reservoir bag to vent exhaled gases and carbon dioxide, thus providing a high fresh gas flowrate (see Table 5-5). Systems that use nonrebreathing valves increase the resistance against which the animal must breathe. These valves should be avoided with animals weighing less than 5 kg. In addition, moisture can accumulate on the valve disks, causing them to stick in the open or closed position, rendering the system inaccurate and subject to even greater air flow resistance.

Semiopen systems that do not use nonrebreathing valves are available by various names. The Mapleson system of classification categorizes five different systems based on the location of the fresh gas inlet relative to the exhalation port or pop-off valve (see Figs. 5-31 to 5-34).

Mapleson A (Magill system). This system employs a pop-off valve located at the patient end of the breathing tube. Fresh gases plus anesthetic drugs enter near the reservoir bag. The valve opens at the end of expiration, and exhaled gases are vented. This system is best suited for anesthetic procedures where the animal is breathing spontaneously. Total fresh gas flow into the system to prevent rebreathing need only be equal to the animal's respiratory minute volume, although higher flows are recommended (see Table 5-5). Due to the presence and location of the one-way valve, this system functions less efficiently for animals under 5 kg or when ventilation must be controlled.

Mapleson D system. This system employs a pop-off valve located at the reservoir bag end of the breathing tube. Fresh gases plus anesthetic drugs enter the patient end of the corrugated rubber tubing. The valve opens during the expiratory pause just before inspiration. Higher fresh gas flows are needed to flush the tubing of exhaled gases and carbon dioxide. A modification of the Mapleson D system (Bain circuit) has the fresh gas flow plus anesthetic drug passing through the corrugated tubing within a separate internal tube that allows for some warming of the fresh gas by surrounding exhaled gases (see Fig. 5-32).

The Mapleson D and Bain circuits are better suited for procedures where the animal's ventilation must be controlled. The volume of the corrugated breathing tube should accommodate at least one tidal volume. The total fresh gas flow into the breathing circuit must be two to three times greater than the animal's respiratory minute volume to prevent rebreathing. Therefore the Mapleson D system is more wasteful of anesthetic and fresh gases than the Mapleson A system. Recent studies with dogs suggest that a fresh gas flow rate of 70 to 100 ml/kg/minute is necessary to prevent rebreathing of exhaled carbon dioxide in this species.

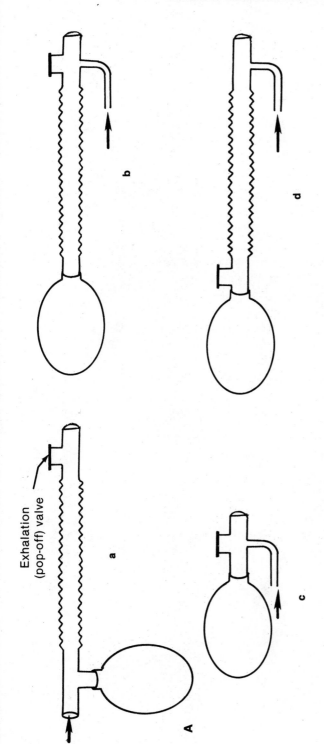

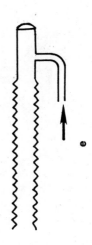

Fig. 5-31. A, Mapleson system for classification of semiopen patient breathing circuits. Systems *a*, *d* and *e* are in common use today. System *e* is the only circuit shown that does not use a pop-off valve.

Continued.

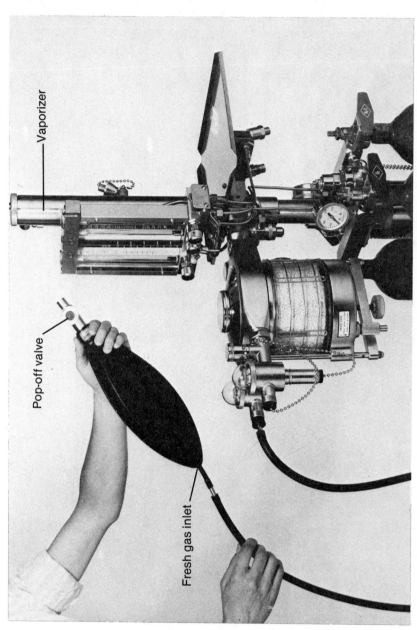

Fig. 5-31, cont'd. B, Inhalation anesthesia machine adapted for using a modified Mapleson A (Magill) breathing circuit. Note how the exhalation valve and reservoir bag port of the circle have been occluded with rubber stoppers. Fresh gas and anesthetic drug are supplied from the inhalation valve. (**B,** Courtesy Pitman-Moore, Inc.)

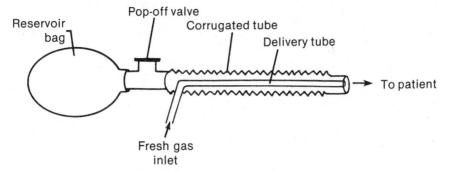

Fig. 5-32. Bain circuit. Fresh gas and anesthetic drug travels through the center of the corrugated tube to the patient. Exhaled patient gases travel around the delivery tube and exit from the one-way pop-off valve.

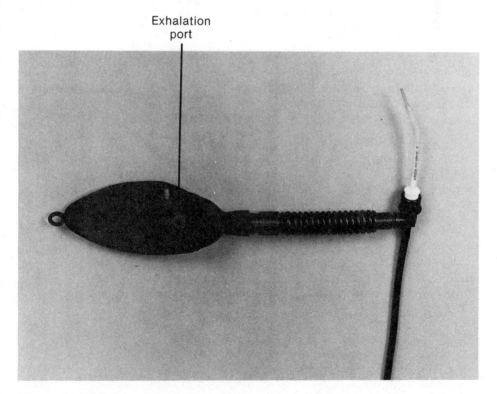

Fig. 5-33. Modified Mapleson E system (Kuhn circuit). Fresh gases enter near the patient end while exhaled gases exit through the hole in the reservoir bag.

TABLE 5-5
Recommended oxygen flow rates for various anesthetic breathing circuits

Breathing circuit	Recommended oxygen flow rate
Anesthesia chamber	5-6 L/minute*
Mask induction	<10 kg 3-5 L/minute ⎫ * >10 kg 5-12 L/minute ⎭
Semiopen circuits	2-4 L/minute* (or 2-3 times minute ventilation)†
Nonrebreathing valve in a semiopen circuit	1-2 L/minute*
Semiclosed circle	25-50 ml/kg/minute‡ (800 ml-1.5 L/minute)
Closed circle	10-15 ml/kg/minute§

*Indicates total gas flow rate to prevent rebreathing. If nitrous oxide is used, it is incorporated into the total flow rate as a 1:1 or 2:1 ratio with oxygen.
†Minute ventilation = Tidal volume (10 ml/kg) × Breathing rate (min^{-1}).
‡Indicates only the flow rate for 100% oxygen. If nitrous oxide is used, the total flow will increase two to three times, depending on its ratio with oxygen.
§Nitrous oxide not recommended for use in a closed circle system.

Mapleson E (modified Ayre's T-piece) (see Fig. 5-31, A). This is the only semi-open system that uses no valves. Its minimal dead space and low resistance to gas flow make it particularly useful with small dogs, cats, and neonates. Fresh gases plus anesthetic drugs enter the T-piece connector at the patient end of the breathing tube. Modifications of the original Ayre T-piece include the addition of a reservoir bag to the breathing tube. The reservoir bag is open at its end (Jackson-Rees system) or contains an exhalation port (Kuhn system) for elimination of exhaled gases (see Figs. 5-33 and 5-34).

The volume of the corrugated breathing tube should be equal to the animal's tidal volume (10 to 15 ml/kg). Fresh gas flow rates into the breathing circuit must be two to three times the animal's respiratory minute volume. Total gas flow rates of 3 L/minute are generally used for all animals weighing less than 8 to 10 kg. The Mapleson E system is suitable for either spontaneous or controlled ventilation. Vented gases can be collected by attaching a scavenger system to the opening in the reservoir bag. Special valves are available commercially for this purpose.

Disadvantages of semiopen breathing circuits. The major disadvantages of semi-open breathing circuits (relative to semiclosed and closed circuits) are that:
- They require high fresh gas flow rates to purge the system of the exhaled carbon dioxide and are therefore less economical and more wasteful of anesthetic drugs and compressed gases, especially in animals over 10 kg.
- They tend to be more polluting of the operating room environment unless adequate scavenging is available.
- They tend to dry the respiratory tract mucosa and increase the patients hypothermic state when used for procedures in excess of 90 minutes.

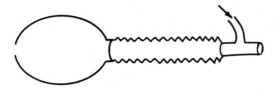

Fig. 5-34. Modified Mapleson E system. (Jackson-Rees circuit.) Double-ended bag is attached to the expiratory limb. Corrugated tubing is often used between the T-piece and bag. Bag allows assistance or control of breathing and monitoring of spontaneous breathing.

- They cannot be flushed by using the oxygen flush valve.
- The presence of the nonrebreathing valves between the animal and the fresh gas inflow tends to increase resistance and work of breathing.
- Nonrebreathing valves are subject to malfunction and can stick with moisture and/or preservative accumulation.
- Scavenger systems can add resistance to exhalation and/or become inadvertently occluded.

Semiclosed breathing circuits

Semiclosed circuits allow for partial rebreathing of exhaled gases. A carbon dioxide absorber is therefore an integral part of the system and is usually placed downstream from the pop-off valve to permit efficient removal of the animal's exhaled carbon dioxide (see Fig. 5-21). A reservoir bag is used for storage and mixing of fresh gas(es) plus anesthetic drug needed during peak inspiration. The reservoir bag is also a means for manually assisting or controlling the animal's ventilation. Semiclosed (and closed) breathing circuits require additional equipment and tend to be more expensive and complicated than semiopen circuits. The use of additional breathing tubes, carbon dioxide absorber, and one-way valves in the semiclosed and closed circuits increases the resistance to gas flow, mechanical dead space, and relative cost. Since carbon dioxide is being removed from the animal's exhaled breath by absorbing granules, a lower fresh gas flow can be used (see Table 5-3). The animal's exhaled anesthetic vapor and oxygen (with or without nitrous oxide) is mixed with the fresh gas plus anesthetic vapor before it is reinhaled. One-way (unidirectional) valves keep the gases within the breathing circuit moving in one direction to ensure that the patient's exhaled gases pass through the carbon dioxide absorber before reinhalation.

Animals weighing less than 10 kg must work harder to breathe when placed on a semiclosed or closed circuit, due to increased resistance of gas flow. If the animal is small and suffers from respiratory and/or cardiovascular depression, the energy it expends breathing through these systems could easily lead to exhaustion, apnea, or cardiopulmonary collapse. Semiclosed and closed breathing circuits, therefore, should be avoided when anesthetizing sick or debilitated animals weighing less than 10 to 15 kg.

Circle system. The most commonly used semiclosed breathing circuit is the circle system (see Fig. 5-35). A circle system can be used as either a semiclosed or closed breathing circuit—the difference between the two being a matter of how much rebreathing occurs. The circle system tends to conserve anesthetic drugs and fresh gases by allowing for lower flows and reuse of exhaled drugs. Since the patient's exhaled water vapor and heat are recirculated there is less drying of respiratory tract mucous membranes as well as a lesser degree of hypothermia during long procedures.

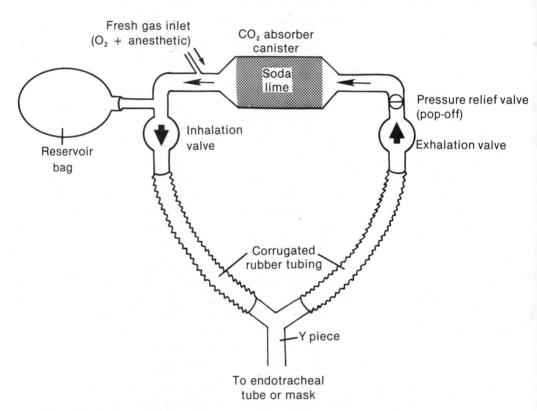

Fig. 5-35. Circle system breathing circuit components. System diagrammed shows fresh gas entering circle just downstream from the carbon dioxide absorber with the reservoir bag located on the inspiratory limb of the circuit. (The anesthetic vaporizer, positioned outside the circle, is not shown here.) (Redrawn with permission from Soma, L.R., and Klide, A.M.: Techniques and equipment for inhalation anesthesia in small animals, Journal of the American Veterinary Medical Association **152**:957, 1968.)

Following is a list of components that comprise the circle system, be it semi-closed or closed (see Fig. 5-35):

- Carbon dioxide absorber with either soda lime or barium hydroxide lime
- Unidirectional valves (inhalation and exhalation)
- Pop-off valve (also called a pressure relief or blow-off valve). When in the open position this valve acts to release excess pressure that may build up within the breathing circuit. When totally closed, this valve converts a semi-closed circle system to a closed circle system. Excessive pressure buildup within a circle system can result from obstructions to gas flow in the circle or within the animal's airway or endotracheal tube. Fresh gas flow rates in excess of the animal's needs will also cause a pressure buildup when the valve is in a closed position. The valve is usually located on the exhalation side of the circle.
- Reservoir bag (also called a rebreathing or breathing bag). The size of the bag should be three to five times greater than the animal's tidal volume. During use the bag should be about two-thirds filled with gas during the expiratory phase. An overdistended bag can add excess pressure to the breathing circuit and increase the effort expanded by the animal to exhale its lung gases. Excessively large bags make manual control of ventilation and monitoring of ventilation more difficult. The bag, which comes in 1, 2, 3, and 5 L sizes, can be positioned on the exhalation or inhalation side of the circle.
- Breathing tubes (composed of corrugated rubber to lessen the chance of kinking when placed in curved or bent positions). The corrugations on the inside diameter can collect exhaled water vapor and may act as a source of cross contamination (see Chapter 6).
- Y-piece adapter (allows for connection of the two breathing tubes with an endotracheal tube or face mask)
- Fresh gas inlet (introduces fresh oxygen with or without nitrous oxide and anesthetic vapor into the breathing circuit). The inlet position is most often placed between the carbon dioxide absorber and inhalation valve.

In addition to the above components, a circle system may also contain:

- An in-the-circuit anesthetic vaporizer such as the Ohio No. 8 for vaporization of methoxyflurane (see Figs. 5-21 and 5-25).
- A ventilation pressure gauge (also called a pressure manometer [see Fig. 5-19]). It allows for visual monitoring of pressures within the circle and hence the animal's lungs. This is of particular benefit when assisting or controlling the animal's ventilation (see Chapter 6). Pressures within the circle correlate closely with the pressure in the animal's airway and lungs. The ventilation pressure gauge is usually placed between the exhalation valve and carbon dioxide absorber in the vicinity of the pop-off valve. Routine patient monitoring should include periodic inspection of this gauge to ensure that pressures within the breathing circuit are not accumulating.

It should always be kept in mind that all breathing circuits, be they circle or semi-open systems, also include the entire animal as a major component!

Closed breathing circuits

The major difference between a closed and a semiclosed breathing circuit is the amount of rebreathing permitted. In a totally closed circuit all of the animal's exhaled oxygen and anesthetic drug mix with the fresh gas(es) and are reinhaled. Carbon dioxide is extracted when it passes through the carbon dioxide absorber. In the closed circle system the pop-off valve is closed, whereas it is open in the semi-closed circle system. With a totally closed system the fresh gas flow into the circuit is markedly reduced and need only be equal to the animal's ventilatory requirements. The oxygen flow rate can be lowered to the point where it will supply the animal's basic metabolic needs (see Table 5-5). At present, there are only two systems used for delivering anesthesia to the patient by means of a closed breathing circuit: the circle system and the to-and-fro system.

The closed circle system. Closed breathing circuits make use of the same components as does the semiclosed circle system. The closed circuit is the most economical system of all breathing circuits because of the low fresh gas flow and recirculation of anesthetic vapor. It conserves the animal's body heat and moisture more than any other system. In addition it is the least polluting of operating room environments since it does not allow release of gases from the pop-off valve. Closed circuits are safest when used on larger animals. Due to their inherent dead space and resistance to gas flow, they should not be used on animals weighing less than 15 to 20 kg. A major problem associated with their use is the potential for pressure buildup in the circuit when gas flows are greater than the animal's metabolic rate of oxygen consumption (10 to 15 ml/kg/minute). Nitrous oxide *should not be used* in a closed breathing circuit since it can decrease the amount of oxygen available to meet the animal's metabolic needs. Some older anesthetic vaporizers are not accurate when presented with a total gas flow rate of less than 500 ml/minute (see Fig. 5-36).

To-and-fro system. The to-and-fro circuit system is more simple in design than the circle system and has eliminated resistance from the unidirectional valves (see Fig. 5-37). Its major problem and the reason for its unpopularity are related to the carbon dioxide absorber being too close to the patient's lungs. As the patient breathes back and forth through the carbon dioxide canister the absorbing granules closest to the animal are exhausted first, which tends to increase the mechanical dead space of the system and may eventually result in hypercapnia. Another potential danger is the possiibility that the patient may inhale soda lime dust from the carbon dioxide absorber. In addition, the temperature generated by this system can be dangerous to the patient as temperatures of 40° to 42°C can develop after 30 minutes.

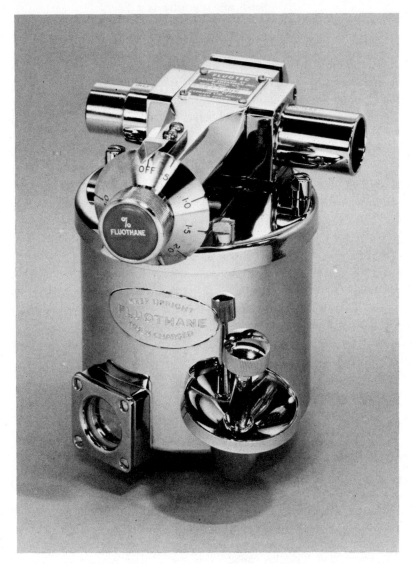

Fig. 5-36. Fluotec Mark II halothane vaporizer. When total fresh gas flowrate is less than 1 L/minute, the vaporizer will deliver a concentration greater than the dial setting. (Courtesy Fraser-Harlake, Inc.)

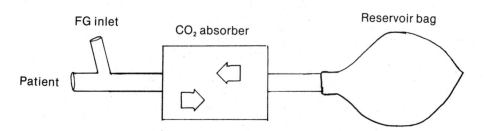

Fig. 5-37. Schematic drawing of to-and-fro closed rebreathing circuit. FG = Fresh gas.

Denitrogenation process (lung washout)

When an animal is first connected to the breathing circuit of an anesthesia machine, its lungs and air passages contain room air. During anesthetic induction this air, which contains approximately 80% nitrogen must be replaced as quickly as possible by the gas mixture from the anesthesia machine. High fresh gas flows into the breathing circuit are used for the first few minutes of induction to effect a rapid washout of air in the animal's lungs and breathing circuit. This process is known as "denitrogenation" and requires total fresh gas flows of 3 to 5 L/minute for the first 5 minutes of induction. After denitrogenation the fresh gas flow rates are reduced to the maintenance levels recommended for the particular breathing circuit being used (see Table 5-5).

Checklist for routine inhalation anesthesia

The practice of safe anesthesia requires a thorough check of the anesthesia machine and related equipment before beginning each case. The routine must be thorough and habitual if minor problems are to be caught before they become major complications during the anesthetic period.

Following is a summarized checklist presented for the AHT to observe when performing routine inhalation anesthesia on small animal patients. The checklist is divided into four periods:

I. Preanesthetic period
  A. Perform preanesthetic evaluation of animal: administer prescribed preanesthetic drugs
  B. Draw up required anesthetic drugs: prepare thiobarbiturate solution
  C. Check anesthesia machine for
    1. Presence of "E" cylinder wrench
    2. Sufficient supply of compressed oxygen and nitrous oxide (observe cylinder pressure gauges)
    3. Proper function of flowmeter controls
    4. Adequate anesthetic liquid in vaporizer
    5. Proper function of vaporizer dial
  D. Check anesthetic breathing circuit for
    1. Correct size and type for animal and situation
    2. Proper connection to anesthesia machine
    3. Presence of all necessary components (trace gas flow into and through the breathing circuit)
    4. Presence of functioning soda lime
    5. Leaks in the assembled circuit (see Chapter 6 for discussion of the procedure to leak-test anesthesia machine)
  E. Assemble necessary supplies
    1. Needles
    2. Syringes
    3. Adhesive tape (3 strips)
    4. Gauze
    5. Cuff syringe

6. Alcohol and cotton pads
7. Laryngoscope
8. Selected endotracheal tubes
9. Stylet for endotracheal tube
10. Sterile lubricating jelly
11. Lidocaine spray or paste
12. Esophageal stethoscope
13. Electric clipper
14. Indwelling catheter
15. Intravenous fluid assembly
16. Emergency drugs
17. Any other preferred supplies

F. Check laryngoscope blade bulb and endotracheal tube cuff to ensure their correct functioning

II. Induction period of anesthesia
A. Clip and prepare intravenous injection site (cephalic or lateral saphenous vein)
B. Assist with anesthetic induction
1. Intravenous thiobarbiturate (2%) to effect for dog or cat
2. Mask induction for cats or dogs with or without a slow thiobarbiturate injection
3. Anesthesia chamber for cats
C. Perform intubation of the trachea when animal is sufficiently unconscious
1. Use lubricated endotracheal tube of correct diameter and design
2. Be sure tube is correctly placed in the trachea (check by palpation and/or observe for exhaled breath); apply positive pressure and observe for bilateral chest expansion
3. Secure tube in place using a gauze tie around upper jaw or behind the ears
4. Connect endotracheal tube to breathing circuit; adjust fresh gas flow rate(s) and anesthetic concentration to effect denitrogenation and the desired level of stage III general anesthesia*
5. Check endotracheal tube cuff for evidence of leaks, and correct, if necessary, by inflating the cuff while applying positive pressure to the lungs and listening for air leakage around tube
6. Check tube and breathing hoses for kinking or constriction; support animal's head and breathing tubes to prevent drag on the endotracheal tube
7. Premeasure and insert esophageal stethoscope and/or other monitoring devices
8. Instill bland ophthalmic ointment in both eyes
D. Adjust intravenous fluid drip rate and ensure patency of intravenous line
1. Maintenance flow rate for healthy dog or cat = 10 ml/kg/hour
2. Administer up to 70 ml/kg/hour for severe blood loss or shock
E. Protect animal's airway and ensure its safety during the entire process, including surgical preparation, diagnostic procedures, and positional changes; avoid entanglement of various monitoring lines with intravenous fluid line and anesthetic circuit

III. Maintenance period of anesthesia
A. Use thermal padding or circulating warm water pad to prevent hypothermia (monitor body temperature [esophageal] in long procedures, and/or in small animals)

*Vital signs and reflexes are monitored throughout the anesthesia period, while steps 1 through 4 should be accomplished in 1 minute or less.

B. Monitor depth of anesthesia and check equipment for proper functioning
1. Monitor vital signs at least once every 5 minutes
2. Maintain anesthetic record
3. Check compressed gas and anesthetic liquid levels periodically
C. Adjust fresh gas flow rates for adequate ventilation
D. Adjust anesthetic vaporizer to minimal concentration setting necessary to maintain desired anesthetic depth: 1.5% halothane, 0.5% methoxyflurane, 2% enflurane, or 1.5% isoflurane

IV. Recovery period
A. Gradually decrease concentration of inhalation anesthetic toward the end of the procedure; allow time for postsurgical procedures such as radiographs or splinting of a fracture
B. To prevent diffusion hypoxia, discontinue nitrous oxide at least 5 minutes before allowing animal to breathe room air
C. Increase oxygen flow rate to aid in the elimination of anesthetic vapor from the animal's lungs and breathing circuit; remove reservoir bag and evacuate its contents into scavenging system to hasten anesthetic elimination when indicated
D. Extubate trachea when the animal swallows or attempts to chew on the tube; deflate cuff before extubation
E. Provide animal with a warm, quiet, and softly lit recovery cage; remove food or water dishes from the recovery cage
1. Provide padding and insulation between the animal and the cage floor
2. Provide warmth by circulating warm water blanket or indirect heat lamp if animal is hypothermic (below 36°C)
F. Administer 100% oxygen, when necessary, to avoid hypoxemia
G. Maintain an unobstructed airway
1. Keep head extended
2. Pull tongue anteriorly
3. Free mouth and/or pharynx of any accumulated blood or secretions
H. Continue intravenous fluids if indicated; assure adequate flow rate
I. Monitor body temperature
J. Rotate animal (unless contraindicated) once every 10 to 15 minutes, especially after long procedures
K. Monitor mucous membrane color and other vital signs closely until the animal regains full consciousness and is sternal (brachycephalic breeds require close monitoring until they are able to stand and breathe normally)

ADDITIONAL READINGS

Dorsch, J.A., and Dorsch, S.E.: Understanding anesthesia equipment: construction, care and complications, Baltimore, 1975, The Williams & Wilkins Co.

Eger, E. I., II: Anesthetic uptake and action, Baltimore, 1981, The Williams & Wilkins Co.

Hubbell, J., et al.: An outline of veterinary anesthesia, Columbus, Ohio State University Press, 1981.

Lichtiger, M., and Moya, F.: Introduction to the practice of anesthesia, ed. 2, New York, 1978, Harper & Row, Publishers, Inc.

Lumb W.V., and Jones, E.W.: Veterinary anesthesia, Philadelphia, 1973, Lea & Febiger.

Pinniger, R.S., editor: Jones' animal nursing, Oxford, 1972, Pergamon Press, Inc.

Quimby, C.W., Jr.: Anesthesiology—a manual of concept and management, New York, 1972, Appleton-Century-Crofts.

Sawyer, D.C., Evans, A.T., and DeJoung, D.J.: Anesthetic principles and techniques, East Lansing, Michigan State University Press, 1977.

Short, C.E.: Clinical veterinary anesthesia, a guide for the practitioner, St. Louis, 1974, The C.V. Mosby Co.

Soma, L.R.: Textbook of veterinary anesthesia, Baltimore, 1971, The Williams & Wilkins Co.

6

Controlled ventilation, care of equipment, and anesthetic pollution

PERFORMANCE OBJECTIVES

After completion of this chapter, the student will:

- List the primary and secondary functions of the respiratory system

- Differentiate among the terms "anatomic," "physiologic," and "mechanical" dead space

- List the indications and disadvantages of positive pressure ventilation for small animal patients during general anesthesia

- Prepare a step-by-step procedure for the routine cleaning and disinfecting of anesthetic rubber and plastic goods

- List four disinfectant preparations advocated for use on anesthetic equipment and mention a disadvantage for each method

- List the sources of potential health hazards associated with an operating room environment

- Describe a method to check for leaks in the high pressure gas lines of an anesthesia machine

- Discuss the common sources for gas leaks occurring in the low pressure circuitry of an anesthesia machine and a method for detection and assessment of such leaks

- List and discuss the various practices by which the levels of waste anesthetic gases can be reduced in a small animal surgical hospital

FUNDAMENTALS OF PULMONARY FUNCTION

The ability to safely administer inhalation anesthesia requires a basic under-standing of pulmonary physiology.* The two most important functions of the lungs are *ventilation* and *gas diffusion*. Secondarily, the lungs serve as immunologic de-fense mechanism, a buffering system for the blood, and a means for eliminating body heat. The upper respiratory tract also serves to warm and humidify inhaled air and remove inhaled particles through the action of cilia that line the passage-ways from the nostrils to the bronchi.

Ventilation

As defined here, ventilation involves the mechanisms that provide for the up-take of oxygen (O_2) from the lungs into the pulmonary circulation as well as the elimination of carbon dioxide (CO_2) from the pulmonary circulation into the lungs and its subsequent exhalation. In the normal, spontaneously breathing animal, ven-tilation has an active phase (inhalation) and a passive phase (exhalation). The term "respiration" is more encompassing than ventilation since it is concerned with the entire complex of physiologic events involved with oxygen delivery to tissues, me-tabolism of oxygen by tissues, and transport of carbon dioxide back to the lungs. Ventilation refers only to the physical movement of air (or anesthetic gases) into and out of the lungs and upper respiratory passageways. Ventilation as measured by tidal volume is only one part of overall respiration.

Under normal conditions the act of ventilation (or breathing) is controlled by the respiratory center in the brain, which is stimulated primarily by the tension of carbon dioxide in the arterial blood. The term "tension" is synonymous with "level," or "partial pressure." When referring to the tension of a gas such as carbon dioxide in arterial blood the symbol $PaCO_2$ is used (P = the symbol for partial pressure; a = the symbol for arterial blood).

As the $PaCO_2$ of blood supplying the brain rises above a threshold level, the respiratory center is stimulated to initiate the active inspiratory phase of ventila-tion. The muscles of respiration (intercostals and diaphragm) are stimulated to pro-duce an effort resulting in expansion of the thorax. As the thoracic cavity expands, the lungs also expand to a greater volume (similar to a bellows). As the lungs are expanded, a negative pressure is created within the intrapleural space and alveoli relative to the atmosphere (see Fig. 6-1). Air then moves from an area of relative positive pressure (the atmosphere) to an area of relative negative pressure (the lungs). Normal inhalation involves the movement of air from the animal's nostrils into the alveoli of the lungs by negative attraction. When the lungs are stretched

*Since this subject (as well as controlled ventilation, especially as it relates to anesthetic management and the use of mechanical ventilators), is not specifically discussed in great detail in this chapter, the student is urged toward further reading in these areas in order to appreciate their importance to suc-cessful anesthesia.

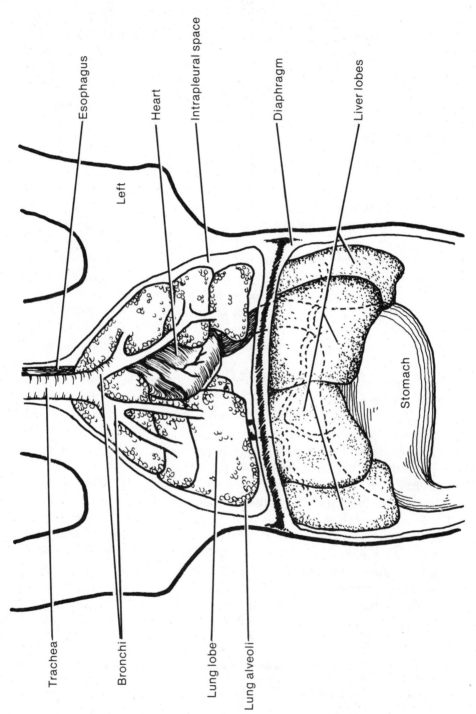

Fig. 6-1. Cutaway view of thoracic cavity.

to a certain volume, nerve impulses are sent back to the respiratory center to stop any further work on the part of the muscles of respiration. At this point the active inhalation phase is complete. The intercostal and diaphragmatic muscles relax, causing the thorax (and lungs) to passively collapse. Like a balloon that is allowed to deflate, air and carbon dioxide contained within the lungs are forced out due to the elastic recoil of lung tissue. This exhalation phase usually requires twice the time to expel air from the lungs as it did to expand them during inhalation. In normal, resting animals, the time relationship between inspiration (I) and expiration (E) is expressed as a ratio: I/E = 1/2 (I requires about 1 second and E requires 2 seconds or longer).

Following exhalation the $PaCO_2$ level begins to rise again until it stimulates the respiratory center to initiate another active inspiratory effort. During this phase the lungs are in a state of rest. The exhalation phase of ventilation normally requires no work on the part of the animal so long as the lungs are able to recoil passively. Obstructions to an animal's airway or diseases of the lung that interfere with their ability to collapse and expel air from alveoli will increase the work of ventilation. The term used in reference to the lungs' capacity for collapsing is "elasticity" while "compliance" (the reciprocal of elasticity) is a measurement of the lungs' capacity for expanding. When compliance is increased, the lungs are said to be more distensible. Compliance decreases with conditions that tend to make the lung more rigid. It is computed as the ratio of a change in lung volume produced by a specified increase in airway pressure (see Fig. 6-2). When compliance decreases the effort expended on the part of the animal to breathe becomes excessive, often leading to collapse and/or respiratory arrest due to physical exertion. Tranquilizers, narcotics, and general anesthetic drugs depress ventilation in two ways. (1) they decrease the responsiveness of the respiratory center to $PaCO_2$, thereby allowing a buildup of carbon dioxide in arterial blood (hypercapnia) and (2) they cause varying degrees of muscle relaxation and may even paralyze the muscles of respiration with overdosage.

The functional unit of the lungs is the alveolus, where all gas diffusion into or out of the bloodstream occurs. The respiratory tract consists of conducting passageways (mouth, nose, pharynx, larynx, trachea, bronchi, and bronchioles) and the various lobes of the lung. There are between 200 and 600 million alveoli in a normal adult human lung, and the total surface area encompassed within the lung's divisions is approximately equal in area to the surface of a tennis court—that is, approximately 100 square meters. The purpose of such a large surface area is to allow for adequate gas exchange between the lung and pulmonary circulation.

The amount of air that passes into or out of the lungs in a single breath is called the *tidal volume* (V_T). The tidal volume is expressed in cubic centimeters (or milliliters) and is a measure of the "depth" of breathing (see Fig. 6-3). The number of tidal volumes occurring in 1 minute determines the *respiratory rate* or breaths per minute. A more meaningful value when assessing an animal's adequacy of ventila-

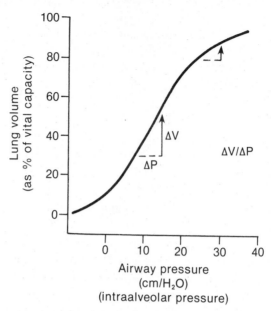

Fig. 6-2. Compliance of the lung is the ratio of an increase in volume to the increase in pressure used to produce that volume change. As intraalveolar pressure increases, lung volume increases, as represented by the curved line. Compliance is greatest in the region where the line is approximately linear and decreases at the lower and upper extreme of lung volume. The lung therefore is more difficult to inflate when it is either overly distended (for example, in emphysema) or collapsed (for example, with atelectasis and pneumothorax). Normal lung compliance in the dog is approximately 3.65 ml/cm H_2O/kg of body weight. Adequate inflation of the lungs of a dog or cat with positive pressure requires about 20 cm/H_2O pressure applied to the upper airway.

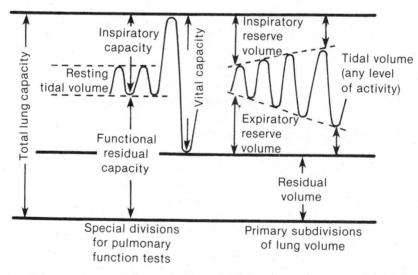

Fig. 6-3. Lung volumes and capacities. See Appendix D for abbreviations.

TABLE 6-1

Expected arterial blood gas values in the dog—awake and during anesthesia

	Normal awake values	Values during general anesthesia
Pa_{O_2} (mm Hg)	90-98	250-500 (on 100% O_2)
		125-250 (on 50% O_2)
Pa_{CO_2} (mm Hg)	38-45	50-70
Base excess (mEq/L)	0 ± 1	-2 to -10
pH	$7.38 - 7.42$	$7.20 - 7.30$

tion is the *respiratory minute volume,* or *minute volume* ($\dot{V}_E$). An animal's minute volume is simply its tidal volume multiplied by the respiratory rate: $\dot{V}_T \times$ Respiratory rate $= \dot{V}_E$. For example, if a 20 kg dog has a tidal volume of 200 ml and a respiratory rate of 18 breaths per minute, its minute volume is 200×18, or 3.6 L/minute.

An estimate of an animal's awake, at-rest tidal volume can be made by multiplying its kilogram weight by 10 to 15 ml/kg. General anesthetic drugs decrease an animal's tidal volume by 30% to 50%. In addition they decrease the rate of respiration so that minute volume is reduced proportionally. Under anesthesia an animal's tidal volume may be reduced to 6 to 8 ml/kg. Using the 20 kg dog as an example and assuming it has a tidal volume of 140 ml and a respiratory rate of 12 breaths per minute under pentobarbital anesthesia, it is easy to see how ventilation is depressed:

$$\dot{V}_E = 140 \text{ ml} \times 12 = 1.68 \text{ L/minute}$$

In this example the dog's tidal volume under anesthesia was reduced by 30% yet its minute volume was reduced even more (55%). The result is a decrease in alveolar ventilation with a consequential reduction in oxygen uptake by the blood and carbon dioxide elimination. When ventilation is depressed to this degree, carbon dioxide tends to accumulate in arterial blood. Because anesthetic drugs also depress the respiratory center's response to Pa_{CO_2} levels, there is no immediate increase in ventilation to stimulate carbon dioxide elimination by the lungs. As carbon dioxide accumulates in the blood, it acts as a weak acid and lowers the pH of circulating blood, eventually leading to acidosis—more specifically, respiratory acidosis—a condition caused by respiratory depression, pulmonary disease, airway obstruction, or anything that impairs normal ventilation. In addition to a diminished elimination of carbon dioxide, depressed ventilation can also cause a decrease in the uptake of oxygen from the lungs. This leads to a lowered arterial oxygen tension (Pa_{O_2}) and, eventually, hypoxemia. Table 6-1 gives the values for Pa_{O_2}, Pa_{CO_2}, and pH of arterial blood in both awake and anesthetized dogs.

During prolonged anesthesia it is recommended that the animal's ventilation be intermittently assisted or controlled to compensate for a decreased minute ventilation. In normal, awake animals the respiratory center periodically initiates a greater than normal inspiratory inhalation effort known as a *"sigh."* It is generally believed that this greater than normal tidal volume is designed to reexpand partially collapsed lung alveoli and remove residual carbon dioxide gas trapped in nonfunctioning alveoli. Normal sigh responses are, for the most part, involuntary and occur unconsciously while awake or asleep. Sedentary life-styles and lack of physical exercise tend to produce an increased frequency of sigh reflexes. Normal sigh reflexes are approximately three to four times the resting tidal volume or about 60% to 70% of the lung's inspiratory capacity. General anesthetic drugs, in addition to decreasing minute volume, also eliminate the animal's ability to perform periodic sighs. Thus an animal's ventilation is intermittently assisted during anesthesia to prevent long-term collapse of lung alveoli (atelectasis) and to overcome any ventilation to perfusion irregularities that result from nonfunctioning alveoli. Periodic sighs should be administered once every 5 to 10 minutes at approximately three times the animal's normal tidal volume, especially when the animal is under anesthesia for longer than 20 to 30 minutes. An animal's tidal volume under anesthesia is estimated by observing bilateral chest expansions and movement of the reservoir bag. However, sighing may be contraindicated in animals with lung disease and/or cardiac instability. When the lungs recoil after inhalation, they never completely collapse. Even if one were to forcefully exhale as much air from the lungs as physically possible, some air will remain. This is referred to as the lungs' *residual volume* (see Fig. 6-3), which prevents total atelectasis of alveoli.

Because of the anatomy of the respiratory tract a significant amount of the air (or anesthetic gases) inhaled with each tidal volume never reaches the alveoli. Gas exchange occurs only in the terminal alveolar sacs. Since air contained in the mouth, nose, pharynx, larynx, trachea, bronchi, and bronchioles does not take part in gas exchange, it is referred to as "dead space" air and the passageways containing this air are termed "anatomic dead space." In addition, there are always some alveoli in the lungs that receive no blood supply due to perfusion shunts, and the air within these nonfunctioning alveoli is termed "physiologic dead space." With conditions of pulmonary and/or cardiovascular disease, physiologic dead space can increase anatomic dead space.

Anatomic dead space air contains a mixture of both inspired and expired gases. At the end of exhalation, anatomic dead space gas is high in expired carbon dioxide, which means it will be taken back into the lungs with the next inhalation. Some rebreathing of expired lung gases will always occur because of the anatomy of the respiratory tract. When an animal inhales, some fresh air has to displace this dead space air before it reaches the alveoli. In humans anatomic dead space has been calculated at 30% of a normal resting tidal volume. Anatomic dead space remains fairly constant* no matter what happens to tidal volume or minute ventilation. Since both decrease under general anesthesia, dead space gas becomes a major concern when assessing the adequacy of ventilation. Anatomic dead space can be decreased by use of a proper size endotracheal tube since it bypasses a large volume of dead space air normally contained in the mouth, nose, and pharynx. Excessively long or narrow endotracheal tubes, however, can add another form of dead space, referred to as "mechanical dead space." Thus endotracheal tubes should not extend more than 1 to 2 cm beyond the animal's incisor teeth. Inhalation anesthetic machines also increase mechanical dead space, (depending on the form and type of breathing circuit used) and the use of atropine can add to anatomic dead space by dilating the bronchi. The animal cannot afford to have its dead space increased while under anesthesia since alveolar ventilation will be inadequate for proper gas exchange.

Gas diffusion

Gas exchange occurs by simple diffusion across the alveolar membrane and pulmonary capillary membrane into the pulmonary capillary blood (see Fig. 6-4). The greater the number of gas molecules in the alveolus relative to blood, the faster will be the rate of diffusion of the gas into the pulmonary capillary blood. The partial pressure of a gas within the blood is determined by its partial pressure in the alveolus (see Fig. 6-4, *B*). If the partial pressure of the gas is high in the alveolus, it will also be high in the blood. The rate of speed with which a gas is removed from the alveolus into the blood vessels supplying the alveolus is governed by the solubility of the particular gas in blood. A gas that is highly soluble in blood (for example, methoxyflurane and ether) will be removed from the alveolus quite rapidly, thereby reducing its partial pressure within the alveolus. When alveolar partial pressure is low, the partial pressure in blood is also low. Blood acts to dissolve the more soluble gases, thus decreasing their partial pressure in blood as well as in the alveoli. On the other hand, gases that are relatively insoluble in blood (such as halothane, enflurane, and isoflurane) are removed from the alveolus into the blood at a slower rate than are soluble gases, which results in the partial pressure of the gas within the alveolus remaining high. This tends to maintain a high partial pressure in blood as well because insoluble gases are not readily dissolved in the blood (see Table 4-2). Since rapid induction of anesthesia with an inhalation anesthetic gas depends, in part, on maintenance of a high alveolar partial pressure, the insoluble anesthetic drugs tend to produce a more rapid induction and recovery. The lower the blood/gas solubility coefficient (λ) for an inhalation anesthetic drug, the more rapidly will that drug tend to induce general anesthesia.

Following is a list of the common inhalation anesthetic drugs in decreasing order of their induction speed in the dog, each with its blood/gas solubility coefficient:

*Normal anatomic and physiologic dead space is estimated to be 2 to 3 ml/kg of body weight.

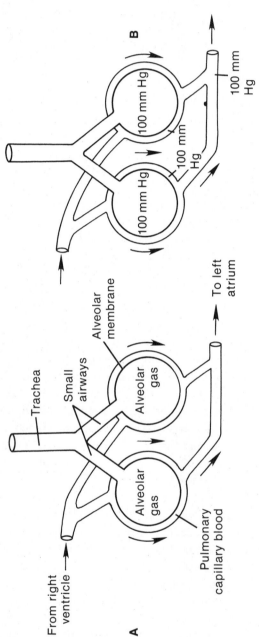

Fig. 6-4. Normal alveolus–pulmonary capillary relationship. **A,** Blood entering the alveolus is low in oxygen tension relative to the alveolar oxygen tension, causing oxygen to diffuse from alveolus to blood. The reverse is true for carbon dioxide since entering blood has a higher CO_2 tension in terms of the alveolus (see Table 6-2). **B,** Theoretical situation showing how pulmonary capillary blood equilibrates with alveolar gas tensions, provided there are no barriers to gas diffusion or pulmonary shunts. In this case, both alveoli contain a gas whose partial pressure is 100 mm Hg. As blood circulates around these alveoli, diffusion occurs rapidly so that, at the end of the pulmonary capillary, equilibration has taken place and the blood now contains the gas at a similar partial pressure. In this example, it is assumed the blood entering the alveoli contains none of the gas that is present in the alveoli.

Speed of induction	Anesthetic	λ
Fast	Nitrous oxide	0.45
	Enflurane	1.9
	Halothane	2.3
	Ether	12.0
Slow	Methoxyflurane	13.0

In addition to the partial pressure of the gas being inhaled, the alveolus will contain water vapor at a partial pressure of about 48 mm Hg, which will reduce the partial pressure of inhaled gases proportionately as they enter the alveoli (see Table 6-2).

TABLE 6-2

Partial pressures of major respiratory gases in inspired and alveolar air and in blood (mm Hg)

Gas	Inspired atmospheric air	Alveolar air	Arterial blood	Venous blood
Oxygen	160	102	100	40
Carbon dioxide	0.2	40	40	45
Nitrogen	595	570	572	572
Water vapor	4.8	48	48	48
TOTAL	760	760	760	705

When the partial pressure of a gas becomes greater in the venous blood than in the alveolus, diffusion takes place in reverse; that is, gas will leave the pulmonary capillary blood for the alveolus and be expelled from the lungs on exhalation. This is what occurs during normal carbon dioxide elimination since its partial pressure within the pulmonary capillary blood is always greater than in the alveoli.

Oxygen

Table 6-3 gives the approximate percentages of atmospheric gases found in room air, alveolar air, and expired air. The partial pressure (tension) for any gas is found by multiplying its percentage times the atmospheric pressure. The partial pressure for oxygen in room air is 160 mm Hg (0.21×760 mm Hg). When room air reaches the alveoli of the lungs, the oxygen tension is diluted with water vapor and residual carbon dioxide so that its partial pressure drops from 158 to about 103 mm Hg. The partial pressure in arterial blood is 95 to 100 mm Hg, and in venous blood returning to the lungs, it is approximately 40 mm Hg as body tissues extract oxygen along the way for metabolism. When an animal receives 100% oxygen during inhalation anesthesia, its arterial partial pressure (Pa_{CO_2}) is elevated (see Table 6-1). Any condition that interferes with normal ventilation or perfusion of the lungs will decrease Pa_{O_2}, which can cause hypoxemia ($Pa_{O_2} < 70$ mm Hg). Vital tissues like the brain and

TABLE 6-3

Approximate values of major respiratory gases (in humans) at standard temperature and pressure as they are found in room air, alveolar air, and exhaled air

Gas	Inspired air(%)	Alveolar air(%)*	Exhaled air(%)
Oxygen	20	15	16
Carbon dioxide	0.04	5	4
Nitrogen	79	80	79.9

*Alveolar air at 37° C is fully saturated with water vapor, which contributes approximately 48 mm Hg pressure to the alveolar gas.

heart require arterial oxygen tensions of at least 60 to 70 mm Hg. Cellular anoxia occurs when arterial oxygen tension drops below 50 to 60 mm Hg. If this condition exists for a prolonged period, the myocardium may develop dysrhythmias and/or arrest may occur. Furthermore, prolonged cellular anoxia to brain tissue can result in permanent cell death, leading to nervous disorders, coma, or death due to respiratory paralysis. Administration of a high inspired oxygen concentration (30% to 100%) is recommended during anesthesia as a safeguard against pulmonary shunting, atelectasis, hemorrhage, hypotension, decreased cardiac output, and depressed ventilation—any of which can lead to a lowering of arterial oxygen tension and hypoxia.

Carbon dioxide

Carbon dioxide tensions in the blood are regulated by the respiratory center's control over ventilation. Since carbon dioxide is produced as an end product of cellular metabolism, it is a continuous process. In the normal awake animal the respiratory center adjusts ventilation to maintain arterial carbon dioxide levels at between 38 to 40 mm Hg. Since the P_{CO_2} of venous blood is higher than the P_{CO_2} within the alveoli (see Table 6-2), the diffusion gradient is reversed from oxygen. Carbon dioxide normally diffuses from the pulmonary capillaries into the alveoli and is expelled during the exhalation phase of ventilation. If an animal becomes apneic or ventilation is in anyway impaired, the Pa_{CO_2} will increase rapidly since the cells of the body continue to produce carbon dioxide in spite of respiratory arrest. Thus respiratory acidosis can develop within minutes unless corrective measures are begun immediately. A blood pH of 7.25 or less can be life threatening unless corrected and stabilized to a more normal value of 7.43. Respiratory acidosis is best treated by controlling the animal's ventilation manually or mechanically. Large, heavily muscled dogs or overweight animals tend toward higher Pa_{CO_2} levels under anesthesia since weakened respiratory efforts, combined with the additional weight compressing the chest wall, add a further depression to ventilation.

The $PaCO_2$ level in spontaneously breathing dogs or cats under general anesthesia can be as high as 55 to 65 mm/Hg or more if ventilation is in any way impaired. When blood gas analysis is available, it is desirable to maintain a $PaCO_2$ of 35 to 45 mm Hg during the anesthetic period.

CONTROLLED (ARTIFICIAL) VENTILATION

The respiratory center in the brain responds primarily to increased carbon dioxide levels in the arterial blood. Control of ventilation in the conscious animal is also influenced peripherally by aortic and carotid chemoreceptor bodies. These specialized receptors are stimulated to increase ventilation when blood pH or PaO_2 are low. General anesthesia depresses all of these chemoreceptor responses. Consequently, a slight degree of hypoxia during anesthesia may not stimulate increased ventilation. However, some anesthetic drugs (for example, halothane) tend to produce a rapid rate of ventilation (tachypnea). At deep planes of anesthesia all general anesthetic drugs depress the ability of intercostal muscles to contract and fully expand the thorax. Even though the animal's diaphragm may have sufficient strength to continue spontaneous breathing efforts, it does so with a significant decrease in tidal volume. This decreased tidal volume results in decreased alveolar ventilation, which results in both lowered PaO_2 (hypoxemia) and elevated $PaCO_2$ (hypercapnia). Increasing the animal's inspired oxygen concentration by administering an anesthetic drug mixed with 100% oxygen (or 33% oxygen plus 66% nitrous oxide) is usually sufficient to correct for the hypoxemia; however, $PaCO_2$ remains unchecked and when elevated can quickly lead to respiratory acidosis. The severity of acidosis during anesthesia depends to a large extent on the particular drug(s) used, the animal's physical status, the depth and length of anesthesia, and the degree of hypothermia. Narcotic drugs such as morphine depress the sensitivity of the respiratory center and its ability to respond to rising $PaCO_2$ tensions (see Fig. 6-5).

Positive pressure ventilation (PPV)

In the absence of a practical "iron lung" machine to deliver negative pressure to an animal's body, artificial ventilation traditionally involves the forceful introduction of air into the lungs. Thus expansion of lung alveoli occurs by a positive rather than negative inspiratory force. Because PPV is not a normal physiologic procedure, it is associated with certain disadvantages and is not without its potential hazards. Therefore it should be performed only by those thoroughly trained in its principles and applications.

During PPV the normal alveolar pressure gradient during inspiration is reversed by creating a positive pressure on the upper airway and pushing gas into the lungs rather than having them drawn in as a result of negative intrathoracic pressure. PPV may be provided *manually* or *mechanically*. In either case it requires an airtight endotracheal tube seal and a reservoir bag or bellows that squeezes the gas

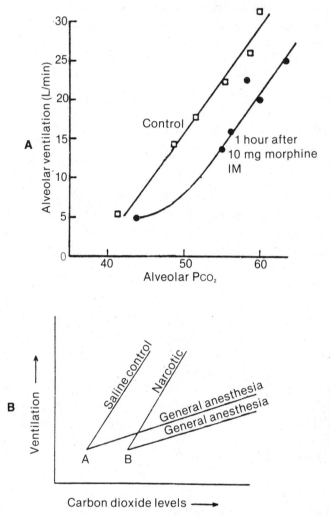

Fig. 6-5. Carbon dioxide response curves demonstrating how narcotics and general anesthetic drugs depress an animal's alveolar ventilation as a result of their suppression of the respiratory center's ability to respond to elevated arterial P_{CO_2} levels. **A,** Alveolar P_{CO_2} is taken to be the same as arterial P_{CO_2}. **B,** Saline control represents the normal CO_2 response. As CO_2 tension in arterial blood increases, the respiratory center responds by increasing alveolar ventilation. Narcotics shift the curve to the right while general anesthesia changes the slope of the line. (**A,** Redrawn from Belleville, J.W., and Seed, J.C.: The effect of drugs on the respiratory response to carbon dioxide, Anesthesiology **21:**727, 1960. **B,** Redrawn from Soma, L.R.: Textbook of veterinary anesthesia, Baltimore, 1971, The Williams & Wilkins Co.)

into the patient's lungs. Exhalation is accomplished passively by removing the positive inspiratory pressure and allowing the lungs to empty by natural recoil action. A brief explanation of the different techniques used to administer positive pressure ventilation to anesthetized animals follows.*

Manual control of ventilation

Movement of gases into or out of an animal's lungs while it is under anesthesia often requires assisting or totally controlling the ventilation cycle. Positive pressure is accomplished by closure of the exhalation (pop-off) valve and compression of the reservoir bag until the lungs are bilaterally inflated (see Fig. 6-6). Exhalation is accomplished by releasing the reservoir bag and allowing the lungs to deflate by elastic recoil. Manual PPV may also be accomplished during emergency stituations by use of a portable Ambu bag until the animal can be connected to an anesthesia machine or a mechanical respirator. The anesthesia machine can serve as a source of 100% oxygen and a means for ventilating animals in need of immediate resuscitation (it takes about 20 cm H_2O pressure to adequately inflate the lungs of most dogs and cats [see Fig. 6-8]).

When positive pressure is used to assist or control an animal's breathing efforts during the inspiratory phase, it is termed *inspiratory positive pressure ventilation* (or breathing)— *IPPV* or *IPPB*. Most healthy dogs and cats will breath spontaneously during anesthesia even though their tidal volume is decreased and the respiratory center of the brain is less sensitive to rises in $PaCO_2$. For the most part these patients may need nothing more than a periodic hyperinflation (sigh) once every 5 to 10 minutes to lessen the likelihood of atelectasis. If the procedure requiring anesthesia is short (20 to 30 minutes) and the animal is healthy, there may be no need for PPV. IPPV is most often used to assist ventilation in older, overweight, heavily muscled, or hypoventilating animals or during prolonged operative procedures. Usually positive pressure assistance is given every third or fourth breath to augment the animal's spontaneous breathing effort and ensure adequate alveolar ventilation. When positive pressure is used to totally replace an animal's spontaneous breathing effort, it is referred to as controlled ventilation (CV).

Animals that have suffered traumatic injuries to the lungs or rib cage and animals with certain forms of pulmonary disease (for example, pneumothorax, emphysema, or lung cyst) may require little or no PPV under anesthesia. Care must be taken in such cases not to hyperinflate the lungs and risk lung laceration from a fractured rib, overexpansion of emphysematous alveoli, or rupture of a lung cyst. When positive pressure is contraindicated, as in the above situations, the animal must be closely observed to ensure that its spontaneous ventilation is adequate to prevent hypercapnia, hypoxemia, and atelectasis. In addition, analysis of arterial blood gases may be necessary to properly assess the animal's ventilation status.

*Appendix D gives symbols commonly used when referring to gases, lung volumes, and blood.

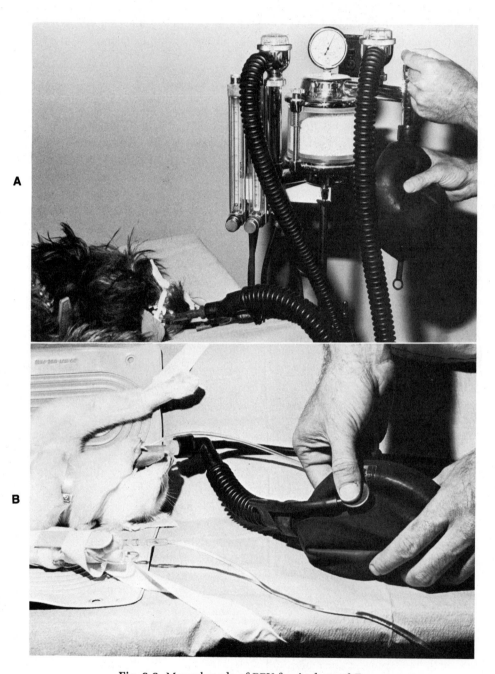

Fig. 6-6. Manual mode of PPV for **A,** dog and **B,** cat.

When positive pressure is applied to the airway during both the inspiratory and the expiratory phases of ventilation, it is termed *continuous positive pressure ventilation* (or breathing)—CPPV or CPPB. The term "constant positive airway pressure" (CPAP) is used interchangeably by some respiratory therapists. The terminology referring to the various uses of positive end-expiratory pressure (PEEP) relates to whether the patient is breathing spontaneously or is being ventilated mechanically.

When positive pressure ventilation is indicated it is often necessary to begin manual control of the animal's ventilations immediately following anesthetic induction and endotracheal intubation. Animals with respiratory disease, diaphragmatic hernia, or space-occupying lesions in the chest require rapid control of ventilation in order to promote the gaseous exchange of oxygen and anesthetic gas(es) between alveoli and blood. Preoxygenation of such cases with 100% oxygen by face mask for several minutes before induction may improve oxygenation and help to speed denitrogenation of the lungs. Rapid induction of anesthesia and tracheal intubation are essential for controlling ventilation and lessening the chance of aspiration pneumonitis. The use of a functioning inflatable cuff and correct endotracheal tube placement are paramount to successful ventilation control, which, if delayed, can quickly lead to serious disturbances in cardiopulmonary physiology and/or cardiac arrest.

When manually controlling an animal's ventilation, it is necessary initially to increase the rate and tidal volume in order to prevent spontaneous breathing efforts. Superimposing positive pressure on the animal's spontaneous breathing efforts at a rate of 12 to 16 ventilations per minute and an inspiratory pressure of 15 to 20 cm H_2O will usually effect control within 3 to 5 minutes. Although the use of muscle-paralyzing drugs to remove the animal's ability to ventilate spontaneously is sometimes indicated, it is often unnecessary for controlling ventilation. Endobronchial intubation must be avoided, and proper endotracheal tube position should be checked as soon after intubation as possible. Observance of bilateral chest expansion and auscultation of bilateral breath sounds should be part of a routine checklist when controlling an animal's ventilation. Once the animal's spontaneous breathing efforts have been abolished, control can be maintained by administering adequate tidal volumes at a rate of 8 to 12 ventilations/minute.

The use of a ventilation pressure gauge (pressure manometer) (see Fig. 6-7) is often helpful during positive pressure ventilation to determine proper inspiratory pressures. The ventilation pressure gauge may also be used to monitor pressures within the animal's airway and/or within the breathing circuit of the anesthesia machine. Most gauges read in centimeters of water (cm H_2O) pressure and have both a positive and negative scale. Inspiratory pressure should be sufficient to provide an adequate tidal volume with bilateral chest wall expansion. Inspiratory pressure under most circumstances will be 15 to 20 cm H_2O for both dogs and cats. When the thorax is opened to atmospheric pressure, additional inspiratory pressure

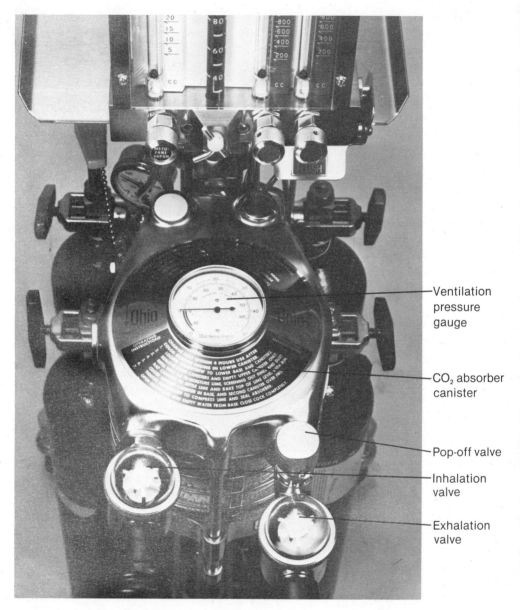

Ventilation pressure gauge

CO_2 absorber canister

Pop-off valve

Inhalation valve

Exhalation valve

Fig. 6-7. Ventilation pressure gauge (pressure manometer). Dial is calibrated in centimeters of water pressure (inner scale) and millimeters of mercury pressure (outer scale). The dark scale below zero indicates negative airway pressure while the scale above zero reflects positive airway pressure. (Courtesy Pitman-Moore, Inc.)

Controlled ventilation, care of equipment, and anesthetic pollution

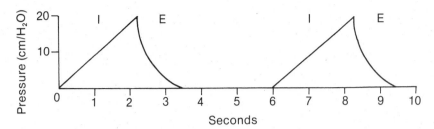

Fig. 6-8. Diagram illustrates the mean airway pressure as reflected in the ventilation pressure gauge during IPPV. The inspiratory/expiratory ratio is approximately 1:2. The concept of mean airway pressure involves looking at the area under each positive inspiratory curve and averaging the total pressure over the time for the ventilation cycle. When positive pressure is excessive or incorrectly applied, the mean airway pressure can cause serious cardiovascular depression and/or barotrauma.

is needed to adequately expand all lung lobes (20 to 30 cm H_2O). Inspiratory time should last 1 to 2 seconds. Expiratory time should be about twice as long as inspiratory time, (2 to 4 seconds), so that a rate of about 8 to 12 ventilations/minute is achieved. During the expiratory phase of each ventilation, airway pressure should quickly return to zero (see Fig. 6-8).

It is good practice to completely remove one's grip on the reservoir bag except when applying positive inspiratory pressure. Should the ventilation pressure gauge read more than +2 to 3 cm H_2O during the expiratory phase, either the fresh gas flow rate(s) into the breathing circle are set too high or an obstruction to flow exists somewhere within the patient's airway or breathing circuit. It is important to correct the situation since excessive positive pressure can overinflate alveoli, resulting in collapse of pulmonary capillaries and decreased venous return to the heart. To avoid uneven ventilation of lung alveoli, sufficient time should be allowed for passive exhalation while also maintaining a smooth and reasonable inspiratory flow rate. The force exerted on the reservoir bag should allow the peak of respiration to occur within 1 to $1^1/_2$ seconds, followed immediately by passive exhalation. The inspiratory flow rate determines the speed with which each tidal volume is delivered to the lungs. In general, slower inspiratory rates (1 to 2 seconds) allow for a more even distribution of gases within the lungs. Overly rapid inspiratory flow rates (less than 1 second) tend to create turbulence to air flow and an uneven inflation of lung aveoli. Although tidal volume cannot be measured accurately without the use of a spirometer, experience with manual ventilation allows use of bilateral chest wall expansion and resistance to forced inspiration as a guide for delivering adequate tidal volume. When controlling or assisting an animal's ventilation, somewhat higher than normal tidal volumes are generally used to prevent atelectasis and provide adequate ventilation. Tidal volumes of about 15 ml/kg are generally used unless contraindicated due to pulmonary and/or cardiovascular instability.

Semiopen breathing circuits generally do not incorporate a ventilation pressure gauge. When administering positive pressure ventilation to animals on any of these circuits, one must rely primarily on sight and touch to determine adequate tidal volume and minute ventilation. When manually controlling ventilation with semi-open circuits, it is generally necessary to use high total fresh gas flow rates of 2 to 3 times the animal's minute volume (or approximately 300 to 500 ml/min/kg) to prevent rebreathing of expired alveolar gases.

Weaning from controlled ventilation

At the end of an anesthetic period where controlled ventilation was used, weaning from positive pressure ventilation should be done gradually. With thoracic surgery, weaning should not be attempted until the thorax is completely sealed and any air trapped within the chest is removed. Successful weaning can only occur when the animal has the ability to maintain an adequate rate and tidal volume through spontaneous breathing efforts. Muscle-paralyzing drugs administered during the procedure must be *completely* reversed or metabolized before discontinuing controlled ventilation. Although weaning from controlled ventilation to spontaneous breathing can usually be accomplished within minutes, hours (or days) may be required, depending on many factors. Generally, the longer the period of controlled ventilation, the older or more debilitated the animal, and the greater the concomitant use of muscle-paralyzing drugs, the longer will be the weaning time from PPV to spontaneous ventilation.

Weaning from manually controlled IPPV is accomplished by gradually decreasing the rate and tidal volume until the animal shows evidence of spontaneous breathing efforts. Initially the animal will tend to breathe with a shallow tidal volume, and assisted IPPV may be indicated for a short period. Until it is ventilating normally and showing signs of recovery, the animal should be allowed to breath 100% oxygen from the anesthesia machine. However, the endotracheal tube is left in place until the animal demonstrates the ability to move adequate volumes of air into and out of its lungs and is able to maintain proper respiratory function while breathing room air. Blood gas analysis may be necessary to assess proper respiratory function before extubation. In any case, the endotracheal tube must remain in place as long as possible to ensure that the animal has recovered sufficiently from the anesthetic drug as well as from the controlled ventilation.

Mechanical ventilation

Machines that could both automatically ventilate and administer anesthesia to humans were introduced in the mid-1950s. Once controlled ventilation was recognized as a necessity for successful thoracic surgery, manual techniques were replaced by mechanical ventilators in order to free the hands of the anesthesiologist and allow for more precise control of the patient's ventilation parameters. In human anesthesia, manual ventilation is seldom used for long-term control of ventilation. Since the introduction of the first anesthesia ventilators, newer and more complex machines have been developed, along with changing concepts of how to manage and care for patients requiring ventilatory support. Mechanical anesthesia ventilators used for veterinary patients are essentially machines for human use that may or may not have special adaptations for animals. Essentially, mechanical ventilators function by automatically compressing a bellows-type reservoir bag. Hence they serve as an extra pair of hands. Anesthesia ventilators use the principle of positive pressure inspiration to deliver oxygen mixed with anesthetic gas(es) to the patient. A variety of ventilators are commercially available ranging in complexity (and price) from a simple volume-cycled ventilator that can be incorporated into the breathing circle of an anesthesia machine (see Fig. 6-9) to a complete anesthesia-ventilator unit capable of performing various modes of controlled ventilation while also delivering anesthetic gases. The bellows of the anesthesia ventilator is usually driven by compressed oxygen.

The majority of small animal veterinary hospitals do not use mechanical anesthesia ventilators routinely. Failure of machines is not uncommon; however, failure is often the fault of improperly trained personnel. It is essential that the person responsible for the use of a mechanical ventilator be thoroughly trained in its particular mode(s) of action as well as its proper care and management since no two ventilators are exactly alike. It is also essential that an alternative means of manual ventilation be available in the event of a mechanical failure. In anesthesia of small animals there is no good substitute for the anesthetist properly trained in the control of ventilation by manual technique!

Classification of anesthesia ventilators

Mechanical anesthesia ventilators used most often for small animal patients can be classified according to how they regulate and deliver inspiratory gases:

1. Through pressure cycle (pressure preset = pressure limited)
2. Through volume cycle (volume preset = volume limited)
3. Through time cycle (time + volume limited)

Most ventilators allow for either assisted or controlled ventilation. Some incorporate both volume and pressure settings in the same machine to allow for situations where one mode may be preferred over another. For example, an older animal may have decreased lung compliance and require a preset tidal volume rather than a preset inspiratory pressure to provide more constant alveolar ventilation and $PaCO_2$. Volume-cycled ventilators usually incorporate a high pressure override control to vent excessively high pressures that may develop in the patient's airway due to obstructions to air flow or attempts on the part of the patient to cough or exhale during a positive pressure inspiration. Most ventilators also have an adjustment to control the rate of ventilation by either increasing or decreasing the time allowed

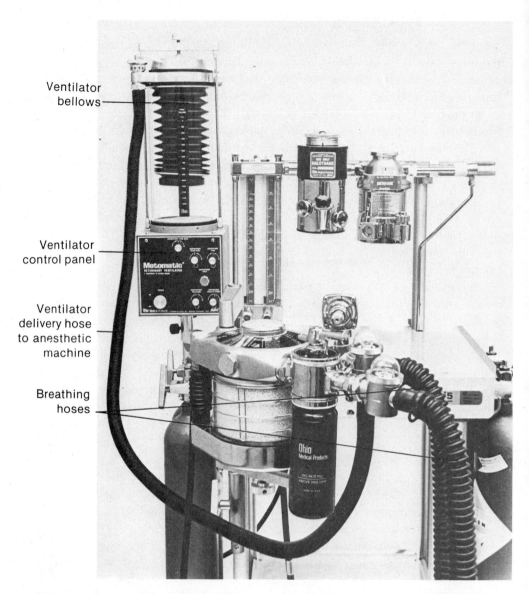

Ventilator bellows—

Ventilator control panel—

Ventilator delivery hose to anesthetic machine—

Breathing hoses—

Fig. 6-9. Volume-cycled anesthesia ventilator replaces the reservoir bag of the circle breathing circuit. Note that the anesthesia machine has two out-of-circuit and one in-circuit anesthetic vaporizers, making it a hybrid. (Courtesy Pitman-Moore, Inc.)

for the expiratory phase of the ventilation cycle (see Fig. 6-10). For instance, if one wished to double the rate of ventilation from 6 to 12 breaths/minute, the control knob would be adjusted to decrease expiratory time by 50%, thereby allowing twice as many inspiratory phases per minute. The inspiratory time is usually maintained at 1 to 1½ seconds by adjusting the inspiratory flow control knob.

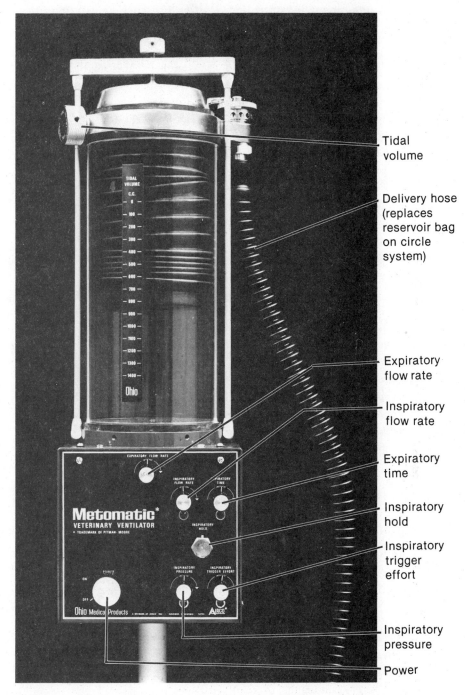

Fig. 6-10. Ventilator controls for volume-cycled anesthesia ventilator shown in Fig. 6-9. (Courtesy Pitman-Moore, Inc.)

Indications for using controlled positive pressure ventilation

The decision to use controlled PPV must be made by the veterinarian. In many small animal hospital practices the actual administration of intermittent or continuous PPV is a duty of the trained technician. Any animal that is unable to maintain adequate ventilation under anesthesia by spontaneous breathing may be considered a candidate for artificial ventilation. Whether or not PPV is assisted or controlled depends on the severity of the respiratory inadequacy and the particular procedure involved. For example, the use of controlled IPPV during and sometimes after the anesthesia period is a necessity with the use of muscle-paralyzing drugs and/or for a thoracotomy procedure.

Following is a general listing of causes of acute or chronic ventilatory inadequacy that should be considered possible indicators for controlling an animal's ventilation while under anesthesia.

A. Central respiratory depression
   1. Drug induced: for example, narcotics, tranquilizers, general anesthetic drugs
   2. Physiologically induced: metabolic or respiratory acidosis, hypothermia, ventilation-perfusion mismatching, metabolic coma states (for example, uremia and hypoglycemia)
   3. Physically induced: head trauma, cerebral edema
B. Inadequate lung expansion/contraction
   1. Chronic obstructive lung disease: for example, bronchitis, collapsing trachea, pleuritis
   2. Pneumonia, pneumonitis
   3. Atelectasis
   4. Emphysema
   5. Tension pneumothorax
   6. Diaphragmatic hernia
   7. Pulmonary edema
   8. Space-occupying thoracic tumor
   9. Phrenic or intercostal nerve disease or trauma
   10. Thoracic surgery
   11. Hyperventilation
   12. Apnea
C. Inadequate chest wall expansion
   1. Muscle-paralyzing drugs such as curare, succinylcholine, pancuronium, certain antibiotics (for example, neomycin and kanamycin)
   2. Obesity
   3. Rib fractures (unless contraindicated)
   4. Restrictive bandaging
   5. Pain (for example, because of chest trauma)

6. Abdominal distention: gastric torsion or impairment of diaphragmatic excursion due to excessive abdominal pressure
7. Restrictive positioning: use of sandbags or padding on surgical or x-ray table (head down position and/or dorsal recumbency cause weight of abdominal viscera to impair diaphragmatic excursion)
D. Acute cardiopulmonary depression
1. Respiratory and/or cardiac arrest
2. Cardiac dysrythmias such as atrial or ventricular tachycardia, heart block, hypovolemic shock, sudden hypotension
3. Congestive heart failure
E. Other indications
1. Prolonged anesthesia
2. Certain orthopedic or abdominal procedures

Disadvantages of positive pressure ventilation

A. *Cost considerations.* Mechanical ventilation requires expensive and often intricate equipment such as
1. Mechanical ventilator
2. Inhalation anesthesia machine
3. Ventilation pressure gauge (optional)
4. Back pressure–compensated out-of-circuit vaporizer
5. Abundant compressed oxygen source to drive ventilator
6. Blood gas analyzer (optional)
7. Trained personnel
B. *Physiologic considerations*
1. *Cardiovascular system.** During inspiration the positive pressure created in the airway and lung is transmitted into the thoracic cavity, causing a reversal of the normal subatmospheric intrathoracic pressure, the consequences of which include
   a. Loss of thoracic "pump" mechanism that draws venous blood and lymph toward the heart
   b. Decreased cardiac output due to compression of thoracic veins, resulting in decreased venous return to the heart. May precipitate circulatory collapse or shock
   c. Decreased arterial blood pressure
   d. Decreased pulmonary blood flow that can lead to poor perfusion of alveoli

---

*The anesthetic vaporizer setting should be reduced during initiation of PPV to prevent unnecessary depression of the cardiovascular system. In the case of halothane anesthesia in 100% oxygen, the vaporizer setting can be reduced by 0.25% to 0.5% when beginning either manual or mechanical controlled ventilation.

      e. Increased vagal tone resulting in bradycardia and/or cardiac stand-still

      f. Reduced urine output

  2. *Pulmonary system.* PPV results in several undesirable effects on the lungs and airway (many of which tend to be of greater significance when either the positive pressure applied is excessive [that is, greater than 30 to 40 cm H_2O] or the period of controlled ventilation is prolonged [that is, more than 90 to 120 minutes])

      a. Uneven inflation of lungs resulting in a relative hypoventilation of peripheral lung tissue

      b. Pulmonary edema due to water retention

      c. Progressive reduction in lung compliance, possibly leading to a decline in overall lung volume so that delivered tidal volumes also decline, resulting in atelectasis, hypoxemia, and possibly hypercapnia*

C. *Barotrauma.* Overzealous and prolonged administration of excessive positive pressure ventilation (>40 to 60 cm H_2O pressure) can produce additional complications, especially in very small animals or animals with lung disease—for example

      a. Pneumothorax (leakage of air into the thorax from ruptured alveoli)

      b. Subcutaneous emphysema (leakage of air from ruptured alveoli, with dissection along the mediastinum and expansion beneath the skin along the dorsum of the body)

      c. Air embolism (forceful entry of air into the pulmonary capillaries with dissemination into the general circulation. Although rare, this condition can occur with inspiratory pressures exceeding 60 cm H_2O and may lead to cardiac arrest or serious postanesthetic complications, depending on where the air bubbles may lodge [such as the CNS, or a coronary artery]).

In summary, PPV, whether by hand or by hardware, is an unnatural and potentially harmful technique. It may be totally contraindicated in those animals with diseased or decompensated conditions relating to the cardiovascular and/or respiratory systems. Knowing the potential dangers associated with PPV, many veterinarians prefer the sole use of manual PPV for those cases where it is indicated, since they believe that a trained individual is more likely to detect and correct a change in the animal's ventilatory and cardiovascular status than is a machine.

The degree of cardiovascular depression that results from PPV depends on the animal's age, size, and cardiovascular status. Mature, healthy animals are able to

---

*Volume-cycled mechanical ventilators protect against this effect more than do pressure-cycled ventilators. As lung compliance decreases, pressure-cycled ventilators must be readjusted to deliver a higher inspiratory pressure to compensate for stiffer lungs.

compensate for the adverse effects on the circulatory and pulmonary systems while the animal that is hypovolemic from any cause or unable to compensate for the decreased arterial blood pressure through vasoconstriction may become seriously hypotensive. The degree of hypotension is related to the amount of positive pressure applied to the airway and to the length of time it is administered throughout the ventilatory cycle. High airway pressures applied for longer than $1^1/_2$ to 2 seconds with short expiratory times are more likely to produce hypotension, since such practice tends to increase the mean (average) airway pressure (see Fig. 6-8). The lower the mean airway pressure during the ventilation cycle, the less reduction in cardiac output and the less will be the degree of hypotension. The pressures observed on the ventilation pressure gauge of the anesthesia machine or mechanical ventilator reflect the pressures at the mouth or upper trachea, but they do not indicate the actual pressures of the alveoli or intrathoracic cavity. During PPV the pressures at mouth level are considerably higher than at the intrathoracic level; however, they are directly proportional in most cases. When $+20$ cm H_2O pressure is used to inflate the lungs during PPV, the intraalveolar and intrathoracic pressures will also become positive, but they will not approach the $+20$ cm H_2O pressure registered by the ventilation pressure gauge.

Mechanical ventilators, with their intricate control dials and constancy of operation, are still unable to differentiate among changing physiologic conditions in the patient. *Volume-cycled ventilators*, because they deliver a constant tidal volume, are capable of creating excessive airway pressure when lung compliance decreases and/or resistance is placed in the airway. These ventilators automatically raise airway pressure to deliver a constant tidal volume, yet they are unable to compensate for an air leak within the breathing circuit. Indeed, such ventilators will continue to cycle normally even when they have become disconnected from the patient and/ or there is a major leak around the endotracheal tube cuff or pop-off valve. *Pressure-cycled ventilators*, on the other hand, are able to compensate for small leaks within the circuit but will not cycle correctly if the leak is large—as in an open pop-off valve or if the machine is disconnected. Pressure-cycled ventilators cannot deliver a constant tidal volume with changes in pulmonary compliance or airway resistance. The volume of gas delivered to the patient will decrease as compliance decreases and/or airway resistance increases (for example, with bronchoconstriction, partial airway obstruction, atelectasis, kinked endotracheal tube, or breathing hose). As a result, the preset inspiratory pressure is rapidly attained and delivered tidal volumes are reduced. Thus the proper duration of inspiration is never obtained, and the rapid, short inspiratory cycles lead to ineffective alveolar ventilation. Such ventilators require frequent adjustments of inspiratory pressure and inspiratory flow rate to ensure that adequate alveolar ventilation is maintained throughout the procedure.

If they are allowed to, mechanical ventilators can lend a feeling of false security to the anesthesia period. Often their rhythmic cycling sound is used as an inappropriate monitor of the patient's ventilatory status. Due to their shortcomings and the fact that they will ventilate the room as well as the patient (whether alive or dead), ventilators must never be relied on as substitutes for complete patient monitoring. Mechanical ventilators are acceptable replacements only for the hands but not for the brain of the anesthetist.

Summary of advantages of controlled ventilation

- Ensures adequate oxygen supply to alveoli
- Spares body oxygen requirements by decreasing the energy expended during spontaneous breathing
- Prevents hypoxia and hypoventilation
- Provides for a more ideal surgical field by preventing hyperventilation movements
- Ensures a more adequate elimination of carbon dioxide and prevents hypercapnia
- Provides a more constant delivery of inspired anesthetic gas

Summary of disadvantages of controlled ventilation

- Has potential for cardiovascular depression or collapse
- Has potential for pulmonary complications such as barotrauma and pulmonary edema
- Denies information on anesthetic depth by interfering with cardiopulmonary mechanics
- May necessitate use of muscle-paralyzing drug
- Lowers lung compliance and surfactant activity with loss of elasticity
- Has potential for respiratory alkalosis due to overventilation
- Includes possibility for mechanical ventilator malfunction

• • •

Some of the more recent techniques employed during controlled ventilation of patients with various degrees of respiratory failure are:
- Positive end-expiratory pressure (PEEP)
- Constant positive airway pressure (CPAP)
- Intermittent mandatory ventilation (IMV)
- Negative end-expiratory pressure (NEEP)
- High frequency ventilation (HFV)

CARE AND MAINTENANCE OF ANESTHETIC EQUIPMENT

The majority of anesthetic equipment requires minimal daily care. In most cases the manufacturer of a particular apparatus supplies instructions for its regular care and cleaning, and these should be adhered to whenever possible. Defects or malfunctions in such components as the anesthetic vaporizer, flowmeter control, and compressed gas regulator require repair by qualified service representatives. The information presented here is a guide for the routine cleaning and sterilization of anesthetic equipment that may act as a nosocomial infecting agent.

Evidence for cross-infection among human patients has been substantially documented, yet the means for effecting safe and effective sterilization of anesthetic equipment has been both difficult and time-consuming. The greatest danger of cross-contamination among patients comes from those parts of an anesthesia setup that are close to or in contact with the animal, such as the endotracheal tube, esophageal stethoscope, breathing tubes, Y-piece, reservoir bag, IV administration tubing, and laryngoscope blade. Even within the human hospital environment there is a great deal of debate over how much and how often sterilization of such items should be performed. Within the veterinary field less emphasis is placed on cross-contamination and sterilization protocols for anesthetic equipment. This is due, in part, to the rare occurrence of cross-contamination and the additional cost involved in sterilization equipment, personnel, storage, and inventory facilities.

Sterilization of bulky items and rubber goods is difficult and not without certain dangers to personnel and patients. However, equipment should always be sterilized after it is used on an animal with a known or highly suspected case of respiratory infection (such as rhinotracheitis or canine distemper) or on an animal known or suspected of harboring a highly virulent organism (such as canine parvovirus, rabies, feline panleukopenia, or feline leukemia). Routine cleaning and disinfection of anesthesia equipment will reduce the population of contaminating organisms and lessen the chance of transmitting an infective dose to subsequent animals. It is especially important that clean equipment and sterilized breathing circuits be used on animals with lowered resistance to infections. Use of the newer disposable polyethylene breathing circuits and endotracheal tubes are indicated for those cases where cross-infection is a real risk. Many human hospitals are using disposable plastic endotracheal tubes, breathing tubes, reservoir bags, and absorbers for each patient. Since this solution is not economically practical for the small animal practitioner, the practice of cleaning and disinfecting those items nearest the animal (endotracheal tube, face mask, laryngoscope blade, and breathing tubes) greatly reduces the contamination of those parts of the anesthesia machine further from the animal. Bacterial filters, which can be incorporated into the inspiratory or expiratory limb, may also prove beneficial in protecting the anesthesia machine and ventilator from contamination.

The anesthesia machine and ventilator should be monitored regularly for bacteria, as should other anesthetic equipment such as laryngoscope blades, endotracheal tubes, and esophageal and rectal probes. Anesthesia machines and ventilators are difficult to clean and disinfect because of the many dust and water traps inherent in their design. Routine disinfection of the rubber breathing tubes, ventilator bellows, reservoir bag, one-way valves, and soda lime absorber should be part of an established care and maintenance program. Periodically it may be necessary to dismantle and sterilize individual components of the anesthesia machine and ventilator. Such practice, unfortunately, requires that the machine or ventilator be out of service for as long as 1 to 2 days, especially if ethylene oxide gas is used to sterilize the rubber and plastic components.

Sterilization of plastic and rubber goods is difficult, time-consuming, and not without potential harm to the animal. Rubber deteriorates rapidly when sterilized by heat or certain chemicals while chemicals used for cold "sterilization" can be absorbed into the rubber or plastic and cause chemical burns when subsequently placed on the animal's skin or within its airway. Ethylene oxide is particularly harmful to mucous membranes, and several incidents of tracheal inflammation and necrosis have been reported following its use as a sterilizer of endotracheal tubes.[1,2] Further, ethylene oxide, once absorbed into rubber or plastic, requires a particularly long aeration period before the equipment can be considered safe for use in, on, or near the patient: between 5 to 7 days. This period can be reduced only by the use of an aerator that is designed to function as a sterile, heated (50° to 60° C) chamber. Under these conditions the aeration time for most items can be reduced to 8 to 12 hours. Polyvinylchloride (PVC) items absorb ethylene oxide readily yet require a considerably longer aeration period than rubber. In addition, some PVC endotracheal tubes are presterilized by the manufacturer with gamma irradiation and are therefore designed for single use. They must never be resterilized with ethylene oxide since a toxic substance, ethylene chlorohydrin, is formed, which can be extremely harmful to skin and mucous membranes.

A multitude of disinfectants have been advocated for control of cross-contamination. Their number and variety emphasize the fact that each has its own set of attributes and deficiences. No single disinfectant can be considered totally safe to the patient and personnel or can serve as the sole means for disinfecting all types of anesthetic equipment. Some of the disinfectants advocated for use on anesthesic apparatus include:

- Buffered solutions of gluteraldehyde for rubber and plastic items (solution or vapor can be irritating to skin or mucous membranes)
- Autoclaving of masks, endotracheal tubes, and connectors (shortens the life of rubber and plastic)
- 1% bichloride of mercury for immersing corrugated breathing tubes and reservoir bags (time-consuming—requires 5 hours)
- Soaking in chlorhexidine, followed by 2 minutes of boiling (impractical and damaging to plastic and rubber goods)

Cold "sterilization" of anesthetic equipment is rarely 100% effective at destroying all forms of viruses, bacteria, and spores. Many gram negative bacteria are resistant to chemical solutions like chlorhexidine. Alcohol, hexachlorophene, and quaternary ammonium compounds are not effective against bacterial spores or the tubercle bacilli (tuberculosis). Some cold sterilizing agents can be inactivated by material contained in the solution. For instance, quaternary ammonium compounds

TABLE 6-4

Properties of chemical sterilizing compounds

| Classification | General usefulness as | | Effectiveness against | | Miscellaneous properties |
	Disinfectants	Antiseptics	Tubercle bacilli	Spores	
Mercurial compounds	None	Poor	None	None	Bacteriostatic only Inactivated by organic matter Bland
Phenolic derivatives	Good	Poor	Good	Poor	Bad odor Irritating Not inactivated by organic matter or soap
Chlorine (inorganic)	Good (a)	Fair	Fair (a)	Fair (a)	Inactivated by organic matter Corrosive
Alcohol (ethyl and isopropyl)	Good (b)	Good (b)	Very good (b)	None	Volatile Strong concentration required Rapidly bacteriocidal Not inactivated by soap
Formalin (aqueous)	Fair	None	Good (c)	Fair	Toxic Irritating fumes
Cationic detergents (Quats)	Good	Good	None	None	Neutralized by soap Relatively nontoxic Odorless Absorbed by gauze and fabrics
Glutaraldehyde (activated)	Good	None	Good	Good	Low protein coagulability Useful for lensed instruments and rubber articles Irritating
Combinations: Formaldehyde-alcohol	Good (c)	None	Very good (c)	Good (c)	Toxic Irritating fumes Volatile

Continued.

TABLE 6-4—cont'd

Properties of chemical sterilizing compounds

| Classification | General usefulness as | | Effectiveness against | | Miscellaneous properties |
	Disinfectants	Antiseptics	Tubercle bacilli	Spores	
Iodine-alcohol	Fair	Very good	Very good	None	Stains fabrics
Iodine-detergents (iodophors)	Good	Good	Good (d)	Poor (d)	Stains temporarily
					Relatively nontoxic
					Corrosive
Chlorine-phenolic (hexachlorophene)	Fair	Good	None	None	Slow acting
					Not neutralized by soaps
					Water insoluble
					Inactivated by organic matter

(a) 4 to 5 percent concentrate
(b) 70 to 90 percent concentrate
(c) 5 to 8 percent formaldehyde (12 to 20 percent formalin)
(d) 450 + ppm [parts per million] available iodine

From Holland, B.F., and Anderson, R.W.: Selecting hospital disinfectant agents. Reprinted from Hospital Formulary © 1967 by Harcourt Brace Jovanovich, Inc.

are inactivated by soap; mercurials by protein, and halogens (for example, chlorine) by organic debris (see Table 6-4).

The chemical glutaraldehyde (Cidex) is one of the most effective sterilizing solutions presently in use. It is both bactericidal and sporicidal. Its main disadvantage is that equipment must be thoroughly rinsed and dried before use, thereby permitting the chance for recontamination. In addition, glutaraldehyde fumes and solutions are extremely irritating to the skin and mucous membranes so that rubber gloves should be worn to protect the skin against repeated exposure. The container of glutaraldehyde should be covered at all times and kept in an area where accidental spillage cannot expose hospitalized animals to its irritating fumes. Further, glutaraldehyde should not be used to wash cages or floors. At a concentration of 2%, vegetative bacteria are killed instantly, viruses are destroyed after 10 to 15 minutes, and spores are killed in 10 hours. Once glutaraldehyde has been made up into a 2% solution, it can be used for 2 to 4 weeks before it requires replacing with a fresh solution. Unlike many other chemical agents, glutaraldehyde is not inactivated by blood, protein, or other organic material. Details concerning the use and precautions for this or any other disinfectant sterilizing agent should be obtained from the manufacturer. An automatic washing machine (Cidematic) is available that accommodates large loads of anesthetic equipment without exposing the operator to glutaraldehyde. Although the Cidematic provides a fully automated sterilization-soaking-drying time of 90 minutes, its cost and size make it impractical except for large volume surgical practices.

Cleaning and sterilizing of rubber and plastic items*

Following is a recommended guideline for the routine cleaning and sterilization of rubber or plastic anesthetic equipment. Depending on the volume and nature of the anesthetic case load, the following procedures should be performed on a daily basis.

1. Place endotracheal tube, breathing tubes, and reservoir bag into a *soaking* barrel of soapy water *immediately* after use.
   a. Remove metal connectors and Y-piece before soaking.
   b. Do not use harsh detergents or soaps; use a low-sudsing soap that is noncorrosive and will not harm rubber or plastic.
2. *Clean* equipment to remove surface contamination. *Rinse* in fresh water.
   a. Surgical scrub brushes can be used for most equipment; bottle brushes and test-tube brushes should be used for cleaning the inner surface of breathing tubes and endotracheal tubes.

*The importance of proper cleaning and drying cannot be disregarded, especially when dealing with potentially contaminated equipment. Since surface contamination prevents adequate contact between equipment and the sterilizing agent, the item must be actively cleaned for effective sterilization. The collapsible rubber bellows of the anesthetic ventilator should be similarly processed after any prolonged use or whenever known contamination has occurred.

    b. Replace or sterilize brushes once or twice weekly.

    c. Use protective rubber gloves.

3. Allow equipment to *dry* for 8 to 12 hours.

    a. Do not place wet items into chemical sterilizer or disinfectant as this will dilute the chemical and decrease its potency.

    b. Do not place wet items into ethylene oxide as a toxic precipitate (ethylene glycol) can form within water droplets.

4. Place dried equipment into a large container of 2% glutaraldehyde for chemical sterilization.

    a. Allow 10 to 12 hours for soaking.

    b. Use protective rubber gloves; avoid contact with solution or inhalation of fumes.

5. *Rinse* equipment under running water, then allow additional soaking in fresh water for an hour or longer.

    a. Use protective gloves when handling equipment from glutaraldehyde container.

    b. When rinsing corrugated tubing, additional effort should be made to thoroughly rinse and drain the inherent water traps, especially on the inner ridged surface. Proper drying may be difficult unless the ridges are expanded, thereby allowing for adequate drainage (see Fig. 6-11). Reservoir bags must also be thoroughly rinsed and drained.

    c. Rerinse equipment that has any residual odor of glutaraldehyde.

Cleaning and sterilization of other anesthetic equipment*

Following is an abbreviated guide for the routine cleaning and decontamination of anesthetic equipment that cannot be handled according to those guidelines already presented. It is based on the approach that items difficult to sterilize are cleaned after each use and periodically sterilized or disinfected, the exception being mandatory sterilization after known cases of contamination.

Compressed gas cylinders

1. Remove wrapper, if present.

2. Clean cylinder with water; wipe with cloth soaked in germicide before attaching to machine or bringing into sterile OR.

Anesthesia machine (and/or ventilator)

1. Daily

    a. Remove blood or other collected debris promptly.

*Always consult manufacturer's recommendations regarding the proper dismantling, cleaning, and disinfecting of apparatus.

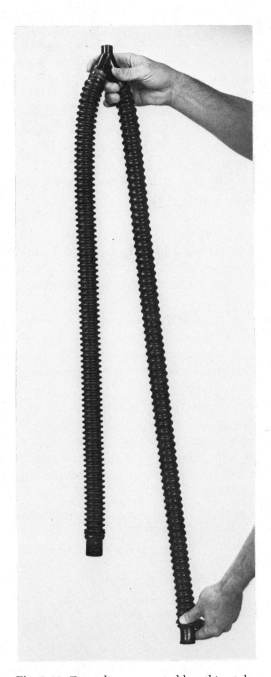

Fig. 6-11. Expanding corrugated breathing tubes.

    b. Wipe top, front, sides, and wheels with a germicidal detergent if machine is taken out of sterile OR.

    c. Do not use grease or oil on *any* part of the machine or breathing circuit; use only an approved noncombustible lubricant on moving parts.

2. Weekly (or more often)

    a. Clean unidirectional valves and inside of valve dome cover by wiping with 70% alcohol or approved detergent.

    b. Clean pop-off valve by wiping with approved detergent or disinfectant.

    c. Drain absorber canister of collected water; avoid skin contact with alkaline water (see Fig. 6-12).

    d. Drain anesthetic liquid from vaporizer; discard if discolored. Allow vaporizer to air overnight or longer.

3. After known contamination

    a. Wear protective gown, gloves, cap, and mask.

    b. Sterilize entire absorber, pop-off valve, and unidirectional valves, using glutaraldehyde or ethylene oxide.

    c. Sterilize breathing tubes, Y-piece, absorber bag, and endotracheal tubes (as previously discussed).

    d. Spray machine surfaces with a bactericidal for hospital use, then clean as during routine daily care.

    e. Discard such items as contaminated sponges, cloths, rubber gloves, gowns, and syringes into a plastic bag for proper disposal.

4. Quarterly

    a. Perform bacterial surveillance of all components contacting the patient either directly or indirectly. This involves aseptic technique when sampling such components as the endotracheal tube (both surfaces), mask, laryngoscope blade, Y-piece, inspiratory valve, breathing tubes, reservoir bag, pop-off valve, carbon dioxide absorber, and fresh gas inlet area. After routine daily use, machines should be cultured only after being unused for 12 to 24 hours.

    b. Dismantle and sterilize all components of the circle system with ethylene oxide. Care must be taken to allow for adequate aeration time. Before it is used on an animal, 100% oxygen should be allowed to flow through the system for several minutes to remove any residual gas. (Glutaraldehyde may also be used for sterilization of dismantled components provided it is not contraindicated by the manufacturer.)

Y-piece

Reusable Y-pieces are composed of a hard neoprene plastic or stainless steel and are relatively expensive items. Disposable Y-pieces are commercially available but often come as an integral part of a disposable breathing tube assembly. Because of their proximity to the animal's exhaled lung gases, the possibility of contamina-

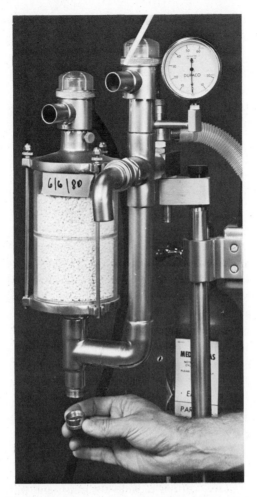

Fig. 6-12. Drainage port on CO_2 absorbing canister.

tion is high. Generally, the Y-piece is easy to sterilize by a variety of methods and should undergo daily cleaning and sterilization along with quarterly culturing:

1. Remove Y-piece from breathing hoses; rinse, clean, dry, and sterilize as individual item.
2. Sterilize by one or more of the following methods: boiling, autoclaving, or using gluteraldehyde or ethylene oxide gas. Boiling and autoclaving can also be used for corrugated tubing; however, these methods will tend to make the rubber brittle and subject to premature aging.

Face masks

Face masks are among the most heavily contaminated items since they are exposed to a variety of potential pathogens, including skin, mouth, nose, pharynx, ocular discharge, saliva, mucus, and vomitus. Disposable masks are available for use on known infectious cases. Masks, like endotracheal tubes, should be handled in as near an aseptic manner as possible:

1. Clean daily after each case (as previously discussed).
2. Sterilize by any of the previously mentioned methods. Autoclaving or boiling will shorten the life of rubber while some plastics will melt with autoclaving.
3. Seventy percent alcohol can also be used as a 10 minute soak, followed by a liberal rinse in tap water.

Endotracheal tubes

The use of a sterile endotracheal tube for every anesthetized patient is not a widespread practice in veterinary medicine. Although the distal trachea is a relatively sterile structure, insertion of a totally aseptic tube is, in most cases, impractical since the tube must be passed through a nonsterile oral cavity. Tracheostomy tubes, on the other hand, must be handled and inserted into the tracheotomy site as sterile objects. Thoroughly cleaned and disinfected endotracheal tubes should be used routinely. They should be stored in a clean and dust-free area or packaged individually until ready for use. The patient end of the tube should not be touched or placed on a contaminated surface. When passing the tube, every effort should be made to avoid touching structures within the mouth or pharynx. Following extubation, the endotracheal tube should be rinsed, cleaned, and sterilized as previously discussed.

1. Seal the pilot tube before immersing the endotracheal tube in water or other liquid in order to prevent water from entering the inflatable cuff. A three-way stopcock may be used for this purpose.
2. Remove items such as adapter, gauze tie, and adhesive tape before soaking them.
3. Brush inner and outer surfaces; use care not to damage the cuff, and rinse thoroughly.
4. Allow sufficient time for drying; arrange so that tube drains from cuff end toward adapter.
5. Reinsert adapter when tube is dry.

Sterilization may be accomplished by any of several methods. With gas sterilizing, the pilot tube is left open, and the tube must be totally free from water. Tubes previously sterilized by gamma irradiation must never be exposed to ethylene oxide. If tubes are autoclaved, the adapter is removed, and the pilot tube is left open. Many of the plastic tubes, as well as coiled tubes, will be damaged by the high autoclave temperature. Repeated autoclaving of any endotracheal tube will lead to premature deterioration, especially the rubber or latex components. Bubble formation with separation of the inner latex lining of coiled tubes may result from the autoclave or gas sterilization process. When liquid chemicals are used for disinfecting or sterilizing endotracheal tubes, the pilot tube should be sealed and the tubes held submerged during the sterilization period. Thorough rinsing in water is imperative to prevent chemically induced tracheitis. Care must be taken not to contaminate the tube when drying and storing, and the tube should always be handled by the adapter end.

Semiopen breathing circuits

Breathing systems such as the T-piece and Mapleson circuit systems (see Fig. 5-31) are subject to contamination by the animal's exhaled breath. After use, the circuit should be disassembled and the components processed as for cleaning and sterilizing of rubber and plastic items. The fresh gas inlet hose and scavenger hose should also be included as part of this routine cleaning, especially after known cases of contamination.

Gas sterilization

Sterilization of rubber or plastic items can also be accomplished using gas (ethylene oxide) sterilization. The student should become thoroughly familiar with gas sterilization techniques before attempting this method (see *Small Animal Surgical Nursing*).

POLLUTION IN THE OPERATING ROOM

Based on numerous epidemiologic and animal studies conducted in eight different countries, there now appears to be sufficient evidence to *suggest* an increase in the rate of certain diseases among personnel working in the OR environment. Exposure of OR personnel to waste anesthetic gases has been incriminated as the most likely cause for this increased disease risk, especially in women. The National Institute for Occupational Safety and Health (NIOSH) estimates that 214,000 workers (including anesthesiologists, nurse-anesthetists, OR nurses, OR technicians, oral surgeons, dentists, dental assistants, and veterinarians and their assistants) in the United States are potentially exposed to waste anesthetic gases. The American Veterinary Medical Association (AVMA) estimates the number of veterinarians, veterinary technicians, and veterinary students potentially exposed to waste anesthetic gases to be approximately 50,000.

Waste anesthetic gases, by definition, are those inhalation anesthetic gases and vapors released in work areas associated with, or adjacent to, the administration of a gas or volatile liquid used for anesthetic purposes. At the present time the six most commonly used anesthetic gases and vapors are nitrous oxide, halothane, methoxyflurane, enflurane, diethyl ether, and cyclopropane.

The major epidemiologic studies that have led to the present concern over the effects of waste anesthetic gases on exposed personnel were conducted between 1967 and 1975 in Russia, Denmark, the United Kingdom, and the United States.

The most comprehensive study in the United States was a joint effort by NIOSH and the Ad Hoc Committee of the American Society of Anesthesiologists (ASA) to study the effects of trace levels of anesthetics on the health of OR personnel.[3] Results from this and other epidemiologic studies suggest that women working in ORs had (1) an increased risk of spontaneous abortion and (2) an increased incidence of congenital abnormalities in their live-born children. In addition, some of the studies indicated an increased incidence of liver and kidney disorders in exposed females and an increased incidence of congenital abnormalitites among the children of males who worked in the OR environment. A recent study of dentists has suggested an increased risk to women involving adverse reproductive effects from trace levels of nitrous oxide.[4] Although these and animal studies indicate the likelihood that chronic exposure to trace (that is, subclinical) levels of anesthetic gases may be a major contributing factor to these health risks, it must be pointed out that a cause and effect relationship remains to be proved. At present there is still a great deal of controversy as to the real cause or causes for such epidemiologic findings. The mechanism by which these disease risks occurs remains a subject of great debate and considerable research.

Exposure to trace levels of anesthetic gases is but one of many potential hazards affecting the health of personnel working in an OR environment. Other health hazards that may also be contributing to adverse effects on reproduction among OR personnel are:

1. Exposure to x-radiation
2. Exposure to ultraviolet radiation
3. Exposure to electromagnetic radiation in environments such as electrocautery and defibrillator units
4. Exposure to fluorinated hydrocarbon propellants such as Freon (used in many aerosol spray cans)
5. Exposure to methyl methacrylate (used as a surgical cement)
6. Exposure to stress, both physical and mental, associated with a job involving long hours and a high degree of responsibility

As a result of the data from the ASA As Hoc Committee and other reports NIOSH was concerned enough in 1977 to submit a "Criteria Document" to the Department of Labor's Occupational Safety and Health Administration (OSHA), recommending standards for controlling exposure to waste anesthetics.[5] Although NIOSH concluded that a safe level of exposure to waste anesthetic gases could not be defined at that time, it recommended maximal *permissible* levels as a means for controlling employee exposure to anesthetic gases:

- 25 parts per million (ppm)* for nitrous oxide (N_2O)

---

*"Parts per million" is a means for measuring small concentrations of a substance within a mixed solution, for instance, anesthetic gases mixed with room air. As an example, if nitrous oxide were present in room air at a concentration of 70%, it would be equal to 700,000 ppm! In other words, 1% of a gas in air equals 10,000 ppm concentration.

- 2 ppm for halogenated anesthetics (including halothane, enflurane, methoxy-flurane and isoflurane)

When halogenated anesthetics are used in combination with nitrous oxide, the level should be reduced to 0.5 ppm or less.

The "Criteria Document" proposed by NIOSH recommends a scavenging program in combination with good room ventilation as the primary means for reducing employee exposure. Most anesthetic machines and breathing circuits can be adapted with workable scavenging systems that are simple in design and relatively inexpensive. Measures to reduce inadvertent dumping of anesthetic gases into room air, along with daily leak tests of the anesthetic machine, are also important practices to help reduce the level of waste anesthetic gases in the work area. In anticipation of a NIOSH standard eventually becoming law, many veterinary hospitals and most human hospitals have implemented measures to control and monitor the level of waste anesthetic gases in the operating room environment.

Methods for reducing exposure to waste anesthetic gases

Investigations into levels of anesthetic gases in human operating rooms that use no measures to control anesthetic pollution show concentrations of room air samples for:

- Nitrous oxide at 500 ppm
- Halothane at 10 to 20 ppm

Concentrations in veterinary hospitals have only recently attracted attention and seem to show a range similar to that found in unscavenged human operating rooms. Levels for both nitrous oxide and halothane can be expected to be even higher when using high flow rates with semiopen breathing circuits and/or an open anesthesia chamber. (Most people are unable to detect halothane odor at levels below 35 to 50 ppm.) Significant reductions in the levels of waste anesthetic gases can be accomplished by:

- Proper room ventilation
- Effective scavenger system(s)
- Practice of nonpolluting techniques
- Periodic leak testing of anesthetic machines and nitrous oxide pipelines

Room ventilation

Operating rooms and areas where anesthetic gases are used on a regular basis should make use of nonrecirculating ventilation systems. Present recommendations are that the system provide at least 10 total air exchanges per hour to reduce the accumulation of anesthetic gases. Ideally, each room should have an accessible low resistance exhaust grill to accommodate the scavenger hose from the anesthesia machine.

Effective scavenger system(s)

A variety of scavenger systems are now commercially available, ranging in design from simple to complex. Fig. 6-13 shows two systems applicable to small animal anesthesia. In order for any scavenger system to be effective and safe it must:

1. Attach to the exhalation valve of the anesthesia machine or anesthetic ventilator (the "pop-off" valve with circle systems and the exhalation port or nonrebreathing valve with semiopen systems)
2. Adapt to a wide variety of exhalation valves, depending on the particular machine in use and the type of breathing circuit
3. Direct the collected gases to a vacuum interface or exhaust duct for transport out of the work area
4. Protect the patient from the extremes of both positive and negative pressure that could accidentally be applied to the scavenger valve or hosing. Occlusion of the collecting valve or scavenger hose will cause excessive positive pressure to be transferred back into the patient breathing circuit with serious results. Systems using wall suction to evacuate collected gases can create excessive negative pressure within the patient's breathing circuit with equally undesirable results. A scavenger system should make use of a vacuum interface to prevent the likelihood of excessive negative pressure affecting the breathing circuit.

Not all scavenger systems meet these requirements. Safe and effective scavenging of anesthesia chambers, semiopen breathing systems, and anesthetic ventilators may require different scavenger systems according to the particular system in use. One disadvantage of the charcoal filter system (see Fig. 6-13, *B*) is that it absorbs only halogenated hydrocarbons, allowing nitrous oxide to pass through and back into room air. In addition, the filter requires periodic replenishing.

Still to be developed is a single, safe scavenging system adaptable to all situations within a veterinary practice. Although scavenging systems are available that are efficient and inexpensive, none of the present systems is 100% effective in reducing to zero the level of trace anesthetic gases under all circumstances.

Practice of nonpolluting techniques

Significant concentrations of anesthetic gases can accumulate rapidly within a room when high flow rates are used for open, semiopen, or semiclosed techniques, especially if the room is inadequately ventilated. The use of high gas flow rates is a common practice during the induction and emergence phases of anesthesia. Some anesthesiologists are now advocating the use of a low-flow closed circle technique for maintenance of inhalation anesthesia to decrease the amount of gases "popped off." When such techniques are used, there is less control over the inspired concentrations of oxygen and anesthetic gas. Consequently, the use of an oxygen monitor is recommended to ensure that the patient receives adequate concentrations of

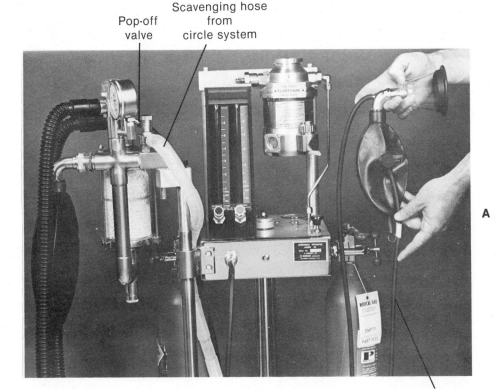

Fig. 6-13. Scavenger system for **A,** semiopen circuit and **B,** activated charcoal filter designed for collection and absorption of hydrocarbon anesthetic waste gases. The system in **A** employs the use of suction to collect waste gases from the reservoir bag in both breathing circuits. *Continued.*

inspired oxygen. When an anesthesia chamber is used for induction of cats, some means for scavenging the exhalation port should be considered part of a routine for reducing room air pollution.

Other practices that help to prevent unnecessary pollution of the room air with anesthetic gases include[6,7]:

- Using tight-fitting face masks during induction of anesthesia and performing endotracheal intubation with an inflatable cuff tube for maintenance
- Avoiding the use of nitrous oxide or anesthetic vaporizer until the patient is connected to the breathing circuit. All flowmeters and vaporizer should be turned off when machine is not directly attached to patient or when it is not in use, and the scavenger should be connected before anesthetic gases are turned on.

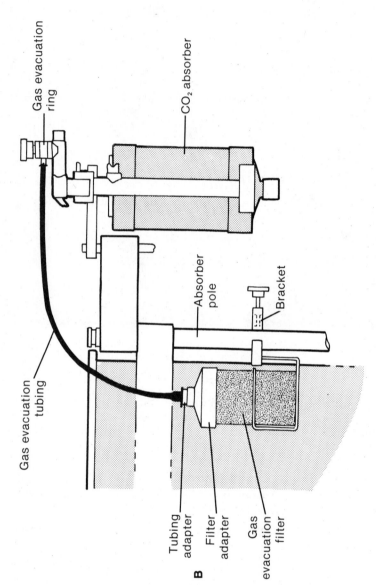

Gas evacuation ring

CO₂ absorber

Absorber pole

Bracket

Gas evacuation tubing

Tubing adapter

Filter adapter

Gas evacuation filter

B

Fig. 6-13, cont'd. B. For legend see p. 323.

- Using only leak-proof breathing tubes and reservoir bag
- Avoiding disconnection of the patient from the machine during a procedure and then only when the flowmeter is off or the Y-piece occluded
- Turning off anesthetic vaporizer and nitrous oxide flow before disconnecting the animal from the machine at the end of a procedure. (The animal should remain attached to the breathing circuit [using only oxygen flow] as long as possible.) The reservoir bag gases should be dumped into the scavenger system rather than into the room air, and a high oxygen flow rate (that is, 3 to 5 L/minute) should be used to wash residual anesthetic gases from the breathing circuit and animal.

Leak testing of anesthetic machine

A major contribution to pollution of room air with anesthetic gases can be attributed to inaudible leaks within the gas circuitry of the anesthesia machine or the patient breathing circuit. Even with adequate room ventilation, efficient scavenging, and good technique, significant levels of pollution can occur when leaks are present in the anesthesia machine or its breathing circuit. Older anesthesia machines are especially prone to leaks within the high pressure gas circuit due to loose connections, dried and cracked rubber hoses, improperly functioning flowmeter valve, or leaks within the breathing circuit. A slight leak, for instance, around the "O" ring seal on a nitrous oxide yoke can add considerable amounts of the gas to the room air. The major source of leaks within any breathing circuit are from an *unscavenged* "pop-off" valve.

Small leaks may be present in the reservoir bag or breathing tube(s) of any breathing circuit, especially as the rubber ages with use. In addition, anesthetic gases delivered to the patient may leak around the outside diameter of the endotracheal tube if the tube is uncuffed or too small in diameter, or if it has a leak within the cuff.

High pressure leaks. In terms of anesthetic pollution of room air, nitrous oxide is of primary concern. The high pressure portion of the anesthesia machine includes the nitrous oxide compressed gas cylinder, pressure gauge, pressure regulator, and flowmeter plus all seals and connectors between the nitrous oxide cylinder and nitrous oxide flowmeter. Although leakage of oxygen into room air is not a source of anesthetic pollution, it should be eliminated because it may be expensive and dangerous should a fire ever occur in the OR area. Nitrous oxide pipeline systems may leak anywhere from their source to the point of connection on the anesthesia machine. Common points for leaks to occur are where the large nitrous oxide cylinder attaches to the main pressure manifold, the pressure regulator connection, or the switch-over connection within the main manifold and the connection to the nitrous oxide outlet line within the hospital. A high pressure leak of 1 L/minute is practically impossible to hear, yet it may leak 24 hours a day if undetected. Such a leak would contribute about 1500 L of nitrous oxide to the room air on a daily basis. If the leak went uncorrected for a year, it would cost about $2,000 (based on a cost of $50 per "G" cylinder of nitrous oxide). Major leak sources of nitrous oxide, when used as "E" size cylinders on the anesthesia machine, are from faulty cylinder valves or an improper seal between the "O" ring on the machine yoke and the outlet port of the compressed gas cylinder. The "O" ring washer should be checked for wear and replaced on the average of every second or third cylinder change.

Gas leaks in the high pressure lines of a pipeline system can be detected by covering the suspected leak site with a dilute soap and water solution (for example, 10% mild dish detergent in water) and observing for bubble formation. To check for leaks in the high pressure lines of the anesthesia machine with attached "E" cylinder(s), the following procedure is recommended:

1. Close flowmeter control.
2. Turn on "E" cylinder for nitrous oxide (if machine uses two nitrous oxide yokes, check each separately).
3. Note the cylinder gauge pressure for nitrous oxide.
4. Close "E" cylinder valve and set machine aside for 1 hour.
5. Recheck cylinder gauge after 1 hour.

If the pressure gauge remains constant, the system is considered leak-free to the point of the flowmeter control. If the pressure is at or near zero, there is a leak somewhere between the cylinder yoke, up to and including the flowmeter control valve. If the leak cannot be detected at the connection of the cylinder with the machine yoke, the leak is probably somewhere within the internal gas circuitry or pressure-reducing valve and should be corrected by a qualified service representative of the manufacturer. This test should be performed once a week or every time a new "E" cylinder of nitrous oxide is attached to the machine.

Low pressure leaks. The low pressure gas circuitry portion of an anesthesia machine system extends from the flowmeter control up to and including the patient. Common sources of leaks that can occur include:

- Poor connections to the inlet or outlet portion of the anesthetic vaporizer(s)
- Cracks within the carbon dioxide absorbing canister
- Worn, cracked, or absent seals around the absorbing canister
- Improper positioning or tightening of the absorbing canister on its mount
- Inadvertent disconnections of a breathing hose, reservoir bag, endotracheal tube, or fresh gas connection
- Small holes in the rubber hoses or reservoir bag
- Loose or defective directional valve dome covers or an open drainage port on the absorbing canister

In addition, anesthetic gases delivered to the patient can leak around the outside diameter of the endotracheal tube and exit through the animal's mouth or nostrils into the room air. Use of correct sized endotracheal tubes with a functional cuff helps reduce this source of pollution.

Gas leaks within the low pressure circuitry of a circle system can be detected according to the following procedure:

1. Close pop-off valve.
2. Occlude the end of the Y-piece.
3. Flow oxygen into the circle by use of the oxygen flush valve until the pressure within the circuit reaches about 40 cm H_2O. A ventilation pressure gauge is required to perform this leak test properly. Alternatively one can pressurize the circle until the reservoir bag is fully distended and observe for rapid collapsing of the bag; however, this is a crude measure at best.
4. Observe the ventilation pressure gauge for a decline in pressure, indicating a leak somewhere between the flowmeter up to and including the breathing circle. If the pressure gauge holds at 40 cm H_2O pressure, the system is considered free from polluting leaks. Nitrous oxide should not be used for low pressure leak testing since it is both unnecessary and undesirable in that it would pollute the air during the testing sequence.
5. The extent of any leak can be determined by repressuring the circle to 40 cm H_2O and flowing oxygen at a rate necessary to keep the pressure gauge from falling below 40 cm H_2O pressure. The flow rate required to maintain pressure in the circle in the presence of a leak is considered equivalent to the leak in the system. Any flow rate in excess of 100 to 200 ml/minute is excessive, and measures should be taken to detect and correct the source of the leak (or leaks).

Ideally a low pressure leak test should be done at the beginning of each day, especially in a high volume surgical practice. At the very least is should be performed twice weekly and/or with each change of soda lime. The NIOSH "Criteria Document" proposes daily low pressure leak tests of the anesthesia machine and seeks a requirement that written accounts of both low and high pressure leak tests be maintained on a quarterly basis.[5]

Monitoring of waste anesthetic gases

The "Criteria Document" also recommends quarterly air monitoring of the anesthetic gas or gases most often used in those areas where workers face potential exposure.[5] In spite of periodic leak testing, practice of nonpolluting techniques, preventive machine maintenance, and scavenging of pop-off gases, leakage of anesthetic gases into room air is still possible. The recommended level of exposure to anesthetic drug such as halothane is usually far less than can be detected by the sense of smell. The only assurance that waste gases are below recommended concentrations is through the use of periodic air sampling of the work area. Waste gas monitoring is best if based on a weighted sample taken over a specific period of time, preferably in the breathing zone of the anesthetist or surgeon. The sample is then analyzed for nitrous oxide and/or halothane, preferably nitrous oxide since it serves as an indicator of its own pollution as well as that of the volatile anesthetic drug being administered in combination with it. The analysis may be performed immediately with an infrared nitrous oxide analyzer, or it may be sent to a commercial laboratory for analysis of nitrous oxide (and volatile anesthetic if indicated). Some companies will perform quarterly "in house" waste gas monitoring for a modest fee. In certain areas of the country contracts are available that provide all the services and consultation necessary to ensure that minimal exposure levels are maintained in accordance with federal guidelines.

REFERENCES

1. The physician and the law, Anesthesia and Analgesia **49**:889, 1970.
2. Marx, G.F., et al.: Hazards associated with ethylene oxide sterilization, New York State Journal of Medicine **69**:1319-1320, 1969.
3. Cohen, E.N., et al.: Occupational disease among operating room personnel: a national study, Anesthesiology **41**:321-340, 1974.
4. Cohen, E.N., et al.: Occupational disease in dentistry and chronic exposure to trace anesthetic gases, Journal of the American Dental Association **101**:21-31, 1980.
5. Criteria for a recommended standard . . . occupational exposure to waste anesthetic gases and vapors, DHEW (NIOSH) Pub. No. 77-140, Washington, D.C., March 1977, Department of Health, Education and Welfare.
6. Manley, S.V., and McDonnell, W.N.: Recommendations for reduction of anesthetic pollution, Journal of the American Veterinary Medical Association **176**:519-524, 1980.
7. Whitcher, C., et al.: Development and evaluation of methods for the elimination of waste anesthetic gases and vapors in hospitals, DHEW (NIOSH) Pub. No. 75-137, Cincinnati, 1975, USDHEW, Public Health Service, Center for Disease Control, National Institute for Occupational Safety and Health.

ADDITIONAL READINGS

Cohen, E.N.: Anesthetic exposure in the workplace, Littleton, Mass., 1980, John Wright • PSG, Inc.
Dorsch, J.A., and Dorsch, S.E.: Understanding anesthesia equipment, Baltimore, 1981, The Williams & Wilkins Co.
Egan, D.F.: Fundamentals of respiratory therapy, ed. 3, St. Louis, 1977, The C.V. Mosby Co., Chapters 1, 3, 4, 5, and 9.
Ganong, W.F.: Review of medical physiology, Los Altos, Calif., 1981, Lange Medical Publications, Chapters 28-37.
Murray, J.F.: The normal lung, Philadelphia, 1976, W.B. Saunders Co.
Soma, L.R.: Textbook of veterinary anesthesia, Baltimore, 1971, The Williams & Wilkins Co., Chapters 14, 22, 35, 36, and 38.
West, J.B.: Respiratory physiology—the essentials, Baltimore, 1979, The Williams & Wilkins Co.

A

Normal values for clinical chemistry and CBC in the dog and cat

TABLE A-1
Normal clinical chemistry values

	Units	Dog	Cat
CO_2 combining	mEq/L	19-27	14-22
Calcium	mg/dl	9.6-11.1	6.8-10.8
Phosphorus	mg/dl	3.6-6.0	2.1-6.9
Glucose	mg/dl	55-96	52-110
Creatinine	mg/dl	0.4-1.0	0.9-1.3
Bilirubin (total)	mg/dl	0-0.8	0.1-1.0
Bilirubin (direct)	mg/dl	0-0.2	0-0.2
Albumin	gm/dl	2.3-3.2	2.1-3.3
Protein	gm/dl	5.4-7.1	5.4-7.8
BSP		<5% R	5% R
BUN	mg/dl	9-29	22-40
Cholesterol	mg/dl	125-250	98-130
Alkaline phosphatase	IU/L	0-67	1-37
Amylase	IU/L	300-1000	800-2000

TABLE A-2
Normal CBC values

	Dog	Cat
Plasma protein (gm/dl)	5.4-7.1	5.4-7.8
PCV (%)	37-55	30-45
Hb (gm/dl)	12-18	10-15
Total leukocytes (1000 cells/ml)	5-12	5-15
Neutrophil—segmented (1000 cells/ml)	4-8	4-9
Neutrophil—band (cells/ml)	0-500	0-500
Lymphocyte (1000 cells/ml)	1-4	1-5
Monocytes (cells/ml)	0-500	0-400
Eosinophil (cells/ml)	0-600	0-1000
Basophil (cells/ml)	Rare	Rare

B

Standard values and equivalents

STANDARD VALUES
Metric weights

1 gram (1 gm)	= Weight of 1 cc water at 4° C
1,000 gm	= 1 kilogram (kg)
0.1 gm	= 1 decigram (dg)
0.01 gm	= 1 centigram (cg)
0.001 gm	= 1 milligram (mg)
0.001 mg	= 1 microgram (μg)

Metric volumes

1 liter (L)	= 1,000 milliliters (ml) or 1,000 cubic centimeters (cc)
0.001 L	= 1 ml
1 deciliter (dl)	= 100 ml

Solution equivalents

1 part in 10	=	10.00% (1 ml contains 100 mg)
1 part in 50	=	2.00% (ml contains 20 mg)
1 part in 100	=	1.00% (1 ml contains 10 mg)
1 part in 200	=	0.50% (1 ml contains 5 mg)
1 part in 500	=	0.20% (1 ml contains 2 mg)
1 part in 1,000	=	0.10% (1 ml contains 1 mg) = 1,000 μg per ml
1 part in 1,500	=	0.066% (1 ml contains 0.66 mg)
1 part in 2,600	=	0.038% (1 ml contains 0.38 mg)
1 part in 5,000	=	0.02% (1 ml contains 0.20 mg)
1 part in 50,000	=	0.002% (1 ml contains 0.02 mg)
1 part in 200,000	=	0.0005% (1 ml contains 5 micrograms)

The number of milligrams in 1 ml of any solution of known percentage strength is obtained by moving the decimal one place to the right. For example, a 1% solution contains 10 mg/ml. By definition, a percent solution contains the specified weight (in grams) of the solute in 100 ml of total solution. For example, a 5% dextrose and water solution contains 5 gm of dextrose dissolved in each 100 ml of water.

Apothecaries' or troy weight (used in prescriptions)

1 pound (lb)	= 12 ounces = 5,760 grains
1 ounce (ʒ)	= 8 drams = 480 grains
1 dram (ʒ)	= 60 grains

Apothecaries' volume

1 pint (O)	= 16 fluid ounces
1 fluid ounce (f ʒ)	= 8 fluid dram = 480 minims (min)
1 fluid dram (f ʒ)	= 60 min

Avoirdupois or imperial weight (used in commerce in the United States and in the British pharmacopoeia)

Grain	= 64 mg
Ounce (oz)	= 437½ grains
Pound (lb)	= 16 oz = 454 gm = 7,000 grains
Ton	= 2,000 lb = 909 kg

Approximate equivalents
Weights

1 kg	= 2.2 avoirdupois or imperial pounds
1 kg	= 2.6 apothecary or troy pounds
1 gm	= 15 (15.4) grains
1 mg	= 1/60 (1/64) grain
1 oz	= 30 gm
(Avoirdupois or imperial	= 28.350 gm)
(Apothecary or troy	= 31.1035 gm)
1 dram	= 4 gm
1 grain	= 60 mg

Volumes

1 L	= 1 quart (qt)
1 ml or cc	= 15 min
1 pt	= 500 cc
1 f ʒ	= 30 cc
1 f ʒ	= 4 cc

Length

1 mile	= 5,280 feet (ft) = 1.61 kilometers (km)
1 km	= 0.62 mile
1 meter	= 39.37 inches (in)
1 in	= 1/12 ft = 2.54 centimeters (cm)

Pressure

1 lb per sq in (psi)	= 0.070 kg/sq cm
	= 51.7 mm of mercury (Hg)
	= 70.3 cm of water (H_2O)
1 mm Hg	= 1.36 cm H_2O
1 cm H_2O	= 0.73 mm Hg

Pressure—cont'd

1 atmosphere
= 760 mm Hg
= 14.7 lb/sq in
= 29.9 in Hg
= 1.03 kg/sq cm
= 33.9 ft H_2O
= 760 torr
= 1013.25 millibars
= 100 kilopascals (kPa)

Household measures

1 drop = $1/_{20}$ ml
1 teaspoon = 5 ml
1 tablespoon = 15 ml
1 glass = 250 ml

EQUIVALENTS OF CENTIGRADE AND FAHRENHEIT THERMOMETRIC SCALES

Fahrenheit to centigrade: $°C = °F - 32 × 5/_9$
Centigrade to fahrenheit: $°F = °C × 9/_5 + 32$

Centigrade degree	Fahrenheit degree	Centigrade degree	Fahrenheit degree	Centigrade degree	Fahrenheit degree
−17	+ 1.4	5	41.0	27	80.6
−16	3.2	6	42.8	28	82.4
−15	5.0	7	44.6	29	84.2
−14	6.8	8	46.4	30	86.0
−13	8.6	9	48.2	31	87.8
−12	10.4	10	50.0	32	89.6
−11	12.2	11	51.8	33	91.4
−10	14.0	12	53.6	34	93.2
− 9	15.8	13	55.4	**35**	**95.0**
− 8	17.6	14	57.2	**36**	**96.8**
− 7	19.4	15	59.0	**37**	**98.6**
− 6	21.2	16	60.8	**38**	**100.4**
− 5	23.0	17	62.6	**39**	**102.2**
− 4	24.8	18	64.4	**40**	**104.0**
− 3	26.6	19	66.2	41	105.8
− 2	28.4	**20**	**68.0**	42	107.6
− 1	30.2	**21**	**69.8**	43	109.4
0	**32.0**	22	71.6	44	111.2
+ 1	33.8	23	73.4	45	113.0
2	35.6	24	75.2	⋮	
3	37.4	25	77.0		
4	39.2	26	78.8	100	212.0

C

Catheter comparison scale

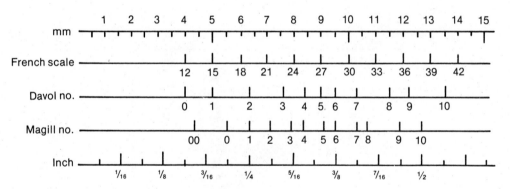

Modified from Lumb, W.V., and Jones, E.W.: Veterinary anesthesia, Philadelphia, 1973, Lea & Febiger.

D

Special symbols

—Dash above any symbol indicates a *mean* value.
.Dot above any symbol indicates a *time derivative*.

For gases

Primary symbols
(large capital letters)

Examples

V	= gas volume	Va	= volume of alveolar gas
$\dot{V}$	= gas volume/unit time	$\dot{V}O_2$	= O_2 consumption/min
P	= gas pressure	PAO_2	= alveolar O_2 pressure
$\overline{P}$	= mean gas pressure	$\overline{P}O_2C$	= mean capillary O_2 pressure
F	= fractional concentration in dry gas phase	FIO_2	= fractional concentration of O_2 in inspired gas
f	= respiratory frequency (breaths/unit time)	DO_2	= diffusing capacity for O_2 (ml O_2/min/ mm/Hg)
D	= diffusing capacity	R	= $\dot{V}CO_2/\dot{V}O_2$
R	= respiratory exchange ration		

Secondary symbols
(small capital letters)

Examples

I	= inspired gas	$FICO_2$	= fractional concentration of CO_2 in inspired gas
E	= expired gas	VE	= volume of expired gas
A	= alveolar gas	$\dot{V}A$	= alveolar ventilation/min
T	= tidal gas	VT	= tidal volume
D	= dead space gas	VD	= volume of dead space gas
B	= barometric	PB	= barometric pressure
STPD	= 0° C., 760 mm Hg, dry		
BTPS	= body temperature and pressure saturated with water vapor		
ATPS	= ambient temperature and pressure saturated with water vapor		

Continued.

For blood

Primary symbols *(large capital letters)*		*Example*	
Q	= volume of blood	Qc	= volume of blood in pulmonary capillaries
$\dot{Q}$	= volume flow of blood/unit time	$\dot{Q}c$	= blood flow through pulmonary capillaries/min.
C	= concentration of gas in blood	Cao_2	= ml. O_2 in 100 ml. arterial blood
S	= % saturation of Hb with O_2 or CO	$S\bar{v}o_2$	= saturation of Hb with O_2 in mixed venous blood

Secondary symbols *(small letters)*		*Examples*	
a	= arterial blood	$Paco_2$	= partial pressure of CO_2 in arterial blood
v	= venous blood	$P\bar{v}o_2$	= partial pressure of O_2 in mixed venous blood
c	= capillary blood	$Pcco$	= partial pressure of CO in pulmonary capillary blood

For lung volumes

VC	= vital capacity	= maximal volume that can be expired after maximal inspiration
IC	= inspiratory capacity	= maximal volume that can be inspired from resting expiratory level
IRV	= inspiratory reserve volume	= maximal volume that can be inspired from end-tidal inspiration
ERV	= expiratory reserve volume	= maximal volume that can be expired from resting expiratory level
FRC	= functional residual capacity	= volume of gas in lungs at resting expiratory level
RV	= residual volume	= volume of gas in lungs at end of maximal expiration
TLC	= total lung capacity	= volume of gas in lungs at end of maximal inspiration
V_T	= tidal volume	= volume of air inhaled or exhaled in one breath
$\dot{V}_E$	= respiratory minute volume	= volume of gas exhaled in one minute

APPENDIX

E

Drugs and equipment (described in text)*

DRUGS

Generic name	Trade name	Manufacturer†
Acetaminophen	Tylenol	48
Acetylpromazine maleate	Acepromazine	7
Adrenocorticosteroids		
Prednisolone Na succinate	Solu-Cortef, Delta-Cortef	71
Dexamethasone	Azium	64
Apomorphine hydrochloride		44
Atropine sulfate		31, 50
Calcium chloride solution		71
Carbon dioxide		45, 51, 60
Chloroform		49
Chloroprocaine hydrochloride	Nesacaine	73
Chlorpromazine hydrochloride	Thorazine	59
Cyclopropane		51, 53, 60
Dextran	Expandex	18
	Macrodex	58
	Rheomacrodex	58
Diazepam	Valium	63
	Tranimul	63
Dibucaine hydrochloride	Nupercaine	17
Dimethyl tubocurarine	Metubine	44
	Mecostrin	68 *Continued.*

Derived in part from Lumb, W.V., and Jones, E.W.: Veterinary anesthesia, Philadelphia, 1973, Lea & Febiger, pp. 647-654; and Physicians' Desk Reference (PDR), ed. 36, Oradell, N.J., 1982, Medical Economics Books.

*Inclusion of a drug or item of equipment does not imply an endorsement of the product and is for informational purposes only.

†The numbers in this column are keys to the names and addresses of manufacturers appearing in Appendix F.

DRUGS—cont'd

Generic name	Trade name	Manufacturer†
Diprenorphine hydrochloride	M50-50	61
Dobutamine hydrochloride	Dobutrex	44
Dopamine hydrochloride	Intropin	5
Doxapram hydrochloride	Dopram	62
Enflurane	Ethrane	53
Epinephrine hydrochloride	Adrenalin	57
Ether		68
Ethyl chloride		34
Etorphine hydrochloride	M-99	61
Fentanyl citrate	Sublimaze	54
Fentanyl citrate + droperidol	Innovar-Vet	59
Gallamine triethiodide	Flaxedil	3
Glycopyrrolate	Robinul-V	62
Halothane	Fluothane	7
Heparin sodium		71
Hexobarbital sodium	Evipal	75
Isoflurane	Forane	53
Isoproterenol hydrochloride	Isuprel	75
Ketamine hydrochloride	Vetalar	57
	Ketaset	15
Lactated Ringer's solution		1, 20, 47, 70
Levallorphan tartrate	Lorfan	39
Levarterenol bitartrate	Levophed	75
Lidocaine hydrochloride	Xylocaine	6, 41
Meperidine hydrochloride	Demerol	75
Meprobamate	Equanil	76
Methohexital sodium	Brevital	26
Methoxyflurane	Metofane	59
	Penthrane	1
Methylatropine nitrate	Brophen	36
	Metropine	69
Morphine sulfate		44
Nalorphine hydrochloride	Nalline	49
Naloxone hydrochloride	Narcan	28
Neostigmine methylsulfate	Prostigmin	39
Nitrous oxide		45, 51, 53, 60
Oxymorphone hydrochloride	Numorphan	28
Pancuronium bromide	Pavulon	54
Pentazocine lactate	Talwin	75
Pentobarbital sodium	Nembutal	1
	Bulk powder (for euthana-sia solution)	33
Pentobarbital sodium, chloral hydrate, and magnesium sulfate	Equithesin	43
	Sedax (for birds)	22

DRUGS—cont'd

Generic name	Trade name	Manufacturer†
Pentobarbital sodium and thiopental sodium	Combuthal	23
	Pento-Short	37
Phenobarbital sodium		50
Phenylephrine hydrochloride	Neo-Synephrine	75
Potassium chloride solution		70
Procaine hydrochloride	Novocain	75
Promaxine hydrochloride	Sparine	76
Propiopromazine hydrochloride	Tranvet	23
d-Propoxyphene hydrochloride	Darvon	44
Propranolol hydrochloride	Inderal	7
Scopolamine hydrobromide		35
Secobarbital sodium	Seconal	44
	Somosal	26
Sodium bicarbonate		1, 20, 41, 47, 70
Succinylcholine chloride	Anectine	16
	Sucostrin	68
Tetracaine hydrochloride	Pontocaine	75
	Cetacaine (spray)	37
Thiamylal sodium	Surital	57
	Biotal	12
Thiopental sodium	Pentothal	1
Tiletamine hydrochloride	CI-634	57
Trichloroethylene	Trimar	53
Triflupromazine hydrochloride	Vetame	68
Xylazine hydrochloride	Rompun	9

EQUIPMENT*

Description or trade name	Manufacturer†
Ambu Resuscitator	29
Anesthesia machines, breathing circuits, and related equipment	13, 25, 30, 32, 52, 53, 59, 66
Baralyme	51
Bird respirator	13
Blood gas analyzers	19, 40, 46
Blood pressure recorder	10, 38
Cap-Chur Gun	55
Cardiac monitors	14, 27, 38
Endotracheal catheters	24, 25, 30, 32, 52, 53, 59, 66
Intravenous catheters	8, 21, 42, 65, 67
Oximeter	74
Oxygen regulators	45, 51, 53, 60
Scavenging systems	13, 25, 30, 32, 52, 53, 59, 66, 72
Soda lime	53
Thermometer (thermistor)	77
Transfusion equipment (pressurized)	5, 47
Ultrasonic Doppler	56
Vaporizers:	
Copper Kettle	30
Enflurane	53
Fluomatic	30
Fluotec	32
Goldman	32
Isoflurane	53
Ohio No. 8	53
Pentec	32
Pentomatic	30
Vapor	52
Vernitrol	53, 59
Ventilators	2, 11, 13, 32, 52, 59

*Inclusion of a drug or item of equipment does not imply an endorsement of the product and is for informational purposes only.

†The numbers in this column are keys to the names and addresses of manufacturers appearing in Appendix F.

F

Alphabetical listing of manufacturers

Manufacturers

1. Abbott Laboratories
   North Chicago, IL 60064
2. Air Shields, Inc.
   Hatboro, PA 19040
3. American Cyanamid Co.
   P.O. Box 400
   Princeton, NJ 08540
4. Amsco Division
   American Sterilizer Co.
   Erie, PA 16512
5. Arnar-Stone, Inc.
   Aguadilla, PR 00604
   Distributed by:
   American Critical Care
   Division of American Hospital Supply Corp.
   McGaw Park, IL 60085
6. Astra Pharmaceutical Products
   Worcester, MA 01600
7. Ayerst Laboratories
   685 3rd Ave.
   New York, NY 10017
8. Bard-Parker
   Division of Becton, Dickinson and Co.
   Rutherford, NJ 07070
9. Bayvet
   Division of Cutter Laboratories
   Shawnee, KS 66201
10. Beckman Instruments Co.
    Palo Alto, CA 94300

11. Bennett Respiration Products
    1639 Eleventh St.
    Santa Monica, CA 90406
12. Bio-Ceutic Laboratories, Inc.
    P.O. Box 999
    St. Joseph, MO 64502
13. Bird Corp.
    Richmond, CA 94804
14. Birtcher Corp. (The)
    4371 Valley Blvd.
    Los Angeles, CA 90032
15. Bristol Laboratories
    Division of Bristol-Myers Co.
    Syracuse, NY 13201
16. Burroughs Wellcome and Co., Inc.
    Tuckahoe, NY 10707
17. Ciba Pharmaceutical Co.
    Summit, NJ 07901
18. Commercial Solvents Corp.
    245 Park Ave.
    New York, NY 10017
19. Corning Scientific Instruments
    Medfield, MA 02052
20. Cutter Laboratories
    Fourth & Parker Sts.
    Berkeley, CA 94710
21. Deseret Pharmaceutical Co., Inc.
    Sandy, UT 84070
22. Detroit Veterinary Supply
    Detroit, MI 48200   *Continued.*

Derived in part from Lumb, W.V., and Jones, E.W.: Veterinary anesthesia, Philadelphia, 1973, Lea & Febiger, pp. 647-654; and Physicians' Desk Reference (PDR), ed. 36, Oradell, N.J., 1982, Medical Economics Books.

23. Diamond Laboratories, Inc.
    2538 Southeast 43rd St.
    Des Moines, IA 50304
24. Dow Corning Corp.
    Midland, MI 48640
25. Dupaco
    205 North Second Ave.
    Arcadia, CA 91006
26. Elanco Products Co.
    Division of Eli Lilly and Co.
    Indianapolis, IN 46206
27. Electrodyne Co., Inc.
    Norwood, MA 02062
28. Endo Laboratories, Inc.
    Garden City, NY 11530
29. Ethical Veterinary Supply Co.
    34 31st St.
    Long Island, NY 11102
30. Foregger Co., Inc. (The)
    2 Lambert St.
    Roslyn Heights, NY 11577
31. Fort Dodge Laboratories
    Fort Dodge, IA 50501
32. Fraser-Harlake, Inc.
    145 Midcounty Dr.
    Orchard Park, NY 14127
33. Ganes Chemical Works
    535 5th Ave.
    New York, NY 10017
34. Gebauer Chemical Co.
    Cleveland, OH 44100
35. Gotham Pharmaceutical Co., Inc.
    Brooklyn, NY 11200
36. Hall Veterinary Drug Co.
    P.O. Box 467
    Garden Grove, CA 92642
37. Haver-Lockhart Laboratories
    Kansas City, MO 64100
38. Hewlett-Packard
    Medical Electronics Division
    175 Wyman St.
    Waltham, MA 02154
39. Hoffmann-LaRoche Inc.
    Nutley, NJ 07110
40. Instrumentation Laboratory Inc.
    113 Hartwell Ave.
    Lexington, MA 02173
41. Invenex Pharmaceuticals
    Division of the Mogul Corp.
    337 Genessee St.
    P.O. Box 708
    Buffalo, NY 44102
42. Jelco Laboratories
    Raritan, NJ 08869

43. Jensen-Salsbery Laboratories, Inc.
    520 West 21st St.
    Kansas City, MO 64141
44. Lilly, Eli and Co.
    Indianapolis, IN 46200
45. Liquid Air Corp.
    Industrial Gases Division
    One Embarcadero Center
    San Francisco, CA 94111
46. London Co. (The)
    811 Sharon Dr.
    Cleveland, OH 41145
47. McGaw Laboratories
    Division of American Hospital Supply Corp.
    Irvine, CA 92714
48. McNeil Laboratories
    Camphill Rd.
    Fort Washington, PA 19304
49. Merck & Co.
    Rahway, NJ 07065
50. Moore Kirk Laboratories, Inc.
    Worcester, MA 01600
51. National Cylinder Gas Division
    Chemetron Corp.
    840 North Michigan Ave.
    Chicago, IL 60611
52. North American Dräger
    Box 121
    Telford, PA 18969
53. Ohio Medical Products
    P.O. Box 1319
    3030 Airco Dr.
    Madison, WI 53701
54. Organon, Inc.
    West Orange, NJ 07052
55. Palmer Chemical and Equipment Co., Inc.
    Atlanta, GA 30300
56. Park Electronics Laboratory
    Box BB
    Beaverton, OR 97005
57. Parke, Davis & Co.
    Joseph Campau Ave. at the River
    Detroit, MI 48232
58. Pharmacia Laboratories, Inc.
    800 Centennial Ave.
    Piscataway, NJ 08854
59. Pitman-Moore Co.
    P.O. Box 344
    Washington Crossing, NJ 08560
60. Puritan Compressed Gas Corp.
    13th and Oak Sts.
    Kansas City, MO 64106

61. Reckitt & Colman
    Damsom Lane
    HU8 7DS
    Hull, England

62. Robins, A.H.
    1407 Cummings Dr.
    Richmond, VA 23220

63. Roche Laboratories
    Division of Hoffmann-La Roche Inc.
    Nutley, NJ 07110

64. Schering Corporation
    Bloomfield, NJ 07003

65. Sherwood Medical
    Brunswick Co.
    St. Louis, MO 63103

66. Snyder Laboratories
    New Philadelphia, OH 44663

67. Sorensen Research Co.
    4387 Atherton Dr.
    Salt Lake City, UT 84107

68. Squibb, E.R., & Sons
    745 5th Ave.
    New York, NY 10022

69. Strasenburgh Laboratories
    755 Jefferson Rd.
    P.O. Box 1710
    Rochester, NY 14600

70. Travenol Laboratories, Inc.
    Morton Grove, IL 60053

71. Upjohn Company (The)
    301 Henrietta St.
    Kalamazoo, MI 49006

72. Vital Signs, Inc.
    1 Madison St.
    East Rutherford, NJ 07073

73. Wallace Laboratories
    Half Acre Rd.
    Cranbury, NJ 08512

74. Waters Corp. (The)
    Rochester, MN 55904

75. Winthrop Laboratories
    1450 Broadway
    New York, NY 10012

76. Wyeth Laboratories
    Box 8299
    Philadelphia, PA 19101

77. Yellow Springs Instrument Co., Inc.
    Yellow Springs, OH 45387

G

Equipment and drugs for use during cardiopulmonary arrest and/or shock

1. Equipment and supplies
   a. Endotracheal tubes (cuffed and of various sizes)
   b. Laryngoscope (with several blade sizes)
   c. Adhesive tape (1 inch)
   d. Gauze roll (2 inch)
   e. Sterile gauze pads (3 × 3 inch)
   f. IV fluid administration set
   g. Blood administration set
   h. Intravenous catheters (18, 20, and 22 gauge sizes)
   i. Hypodermic needles (18, 20, 22, and 25 gauge); at least one $1^{1}/_{2}$ inch and one $2^{1}/_{2}$ inch 20 gauge needle for cardiac injection
   j. Syringes (3, 5, 12, and 30 ml sizes)
   k. Alcohol dispenser
   l. Tongue depressors
   m. Flashlight
   n. Sterile surgery pack (to include scalpel handle and blades, hemostats (3), thumb forcep, Metzenbaum scissors (1), needle holder, Mayo scissors (1), suture material with swedged-on needle, ten 4″ × 4″ gauze pads)
   o. Sterile water or saline for injection (50 ml vial)
   p. Sterile saline or 5% dextrose in water (500 ml container)
   q. Sterile lactated Ringer's or equivalent fluid (1000 ml)
   r. Ambu resuscitation bag

2. Drugs (injectable)
    Epinephrine (1:1000)
    Isoproterenol
    Ephedrine
    Dopamine
    Dobutamine
    Sodium bicarbonate
    Atropine sulfate
    10% calcium chloride
    2% lidocaine (without epinephrine)
    Doxapram
    Dexamethasone
    Prednisolone sodium succinate
    Mannitol (20%)
    Diazepam
    Diphenhydramine (Benadryl)
    Naloxone
    Neostigmine

3. A source of compressed oxygen and flowmeter plus two or three sizes of face masks should be available in the area(s) where they will most likely be needed—for instance, the recovery room and radiology.

Index